# Evolving Industrial Biotechnology in Developing Countries

### *About the Centre*

The Centre for Science and Technology of the Non-Aligned and Other Developing Countries (NAM S&T Centre) is an inter-governmental organisation with a membership of 47 countries spread over Asia, Africa, Middle East and Latin America. Besides this, 11 S&T agencies and academic/research institutions of Bolivia, Brazil, India, Nigeria and Turkey are the members of the S&T-Industry Network of the Centre. The Centre was set up in 1989 to promote South-South cooperation through mutually beneficial partnerships among scientists and technologists and scientific organisations in developing countries. It implements a variety of programmes including international workshops, meetings, roundtables, training courses and collaborative projects and brings out scientific publications, including a quarterly Newsletter. It is also implementing 7 Fellowship schemes, namely, Research Training Fellowship for Developing Country Scientists (RTF-DCS), Joint NAM S&T Centre – ZMT Bremen Fellowship, Joint NAM S&T Centre – ICCBS Fellowship, Joint CSIR/CFTRI (Diamond Jubilee) – NAM S&T Centre Fellowship, Joint NAM S&T Centre – DST (South Africa) Training Fellowship on Minerals Processing and Beneficiation, NAM S&T Centre Research Fellowship, NAM S&T Centre – U2ACN2 Research Associateship in Nanosciences and Nanotechnology in Indian institutions. These activities provide, among others, the opportunity for scientist-to-scientist contact and interaction, training and expert assistance, familiarising the scientific community on the latest developments and techniques in the subject areas, and identification of technologies for transfer between member countries. The Centre has so far brought out 79 publications and has organised 108 international workshops and training programmes.

For further details, please visit www.namstct.org or write to the Director General, NAM S&T Centre, Core 6A, 2nd Floor, India Habitat Centre, Lodhi Road, New Delhi-110003, India (Phone: +91-11-24645134/24644974; Fax: +91-11-24644973; E-mail: namstcentre@gmail.com; namstct@bol.net.in).

# Evolving Industrial Biotechnology in Developing Countries

— *Editors* —

**Prof. Lucy Ogbadu**

**Prof. Godwin Ogbadu**

**Prof. Courtie Mahamadi**

CENTRE FOR SCIENCE & TECHNOLOGY OF THE NON-ALIGNED AND OTHER DEVELOPING COUNTRIES (NAM S&T CENTRE)

2019

DAYA PUBLISHING HOUSE®

*A Division of*

ASTRAL INTERNATIONAL PVT. LTD.

New Delhi – 110 002

ISBN: 9789389569087 (Int. Edition)



*Published by* : **Daya Publishing House®**
*A Division of*
**Astral International Pvt. Ltd.**
– ISO 9001:2015 Certified Company –
4736/23, Ansari Road, Darya Ganj
New Delhi-110 002
Ph. 011-43549197, 23278134
E-mail: info@astralint.com
Website: www.astralint.com

*Digitally Printed at* : **Replika Press Pvt. Ltd.**

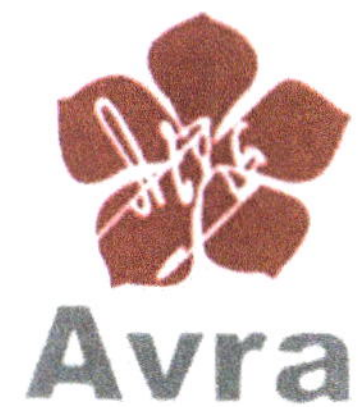


**Dr. A.V. Rama Rao** Ph.D.(Tech) D.Sc.F.N.A.
*(Former Director. Indian Institute of Chemical Technology)*
*Chairman/Managing Director*

# Foreword

Industrial Biotechnology is the application of new biotechnology-based tools to traditional industrial processes ('bio-processing') and manufacturing of bio-based products such as fuels, chemicals and plastics from renewable feedstock, in which microbes, microorganisms, enzymes and their genetic engineering form the basis of technologies and processes. The process works by transforming biomass, *e.g.* agricultural (by) products, organic waste and algae, into bio-fuels and bio-based chemicals in the same way as crude oil is used as a feedstock in the production of chemicals and fuels. Thus industrial biotechnology saves energy in production processes and also leads to significant reductions in greenhouse gas emissions, helping to fight global warming. This is also reflected in improved performance and sustainability for industrial and higher value products. Industrial biotechnology is one of the most promising new approaches to pollution prevention, resource conservation and cost reduction and is considered as a potential tool for societal and economical development.

Industrial biotechnology is often referred to as the third wave in new biotechnology, next to healthcare and agricultural biotechnology. It deals not only in transforming how we manufacture products but also in its application in new products development. It can also lead to improved performance and sustainability for industry and higher value products. There are several bio-based products already on the market include biopolymer fibres used in both construction and household applications, biodegradable plastics, bio-fuels. lubricants and industrial enzymes such as those used in detergents or in paper and food processing. Biotechnological processes also constitute a key element in the manufacturing of antibiotics, vitamins, amino acids and other tine chemicals.

The present book is a follow up of the 2 Training Workshop on 'Industrial Biotechnology: Driving Value Addition and Beneficiation' that was organised by the Centre for Science and Technology of the Non-Aligned and Other Developing Countries (NAM S&T Centre) in Harare, Zimbabwe in August 2017 in partnership with the Ministry of Higher and Tertiary Education, Science and Technology Development and the National Biotechnology Authority (NBA) of Zimbabwe.

I am very happy with the initiative of the NAM S&T Centre in bringing out this important publication comprising 21 papers from the contributors of 14 developing countries which reflects on their technological endeavours, status of developments and strategies for future growth in the area of industrial biotechnology for maximising the benefits for the mankind.

14th Aug. 2018.

*Dr. A.V. Rama Rao*

**Avra Laboratories Pvt. Ltd**

*Plot No 9/15 (2&3), Road No. 6, IDA Nacharam, Hyderabad - 500 076*
*Tel: +91 40 2717 8566/6567/8568 Fax: +91 40 2717 9149*
*Email : corporate@avralab.com, info@avralab.com*

# Preface

This book is a compilation of notable biosciences research efforts in developing countries that are members of the non-aligned movement. It presents in the main part the status of research advances by the various nations that participated in the workshop. Given the importance of Industrial biotechnology in national development, the workshop-participants have in their quest to impact on the economies of their countries through science, submitted relevant reports on topics where they stand strong.

By classification, the book contains either overview reports touching on national strategic road maps for the major sectors of biosciences, or reports on specific research efforts relating to industrial biotechnology. In both categories, the book provides readers with reading materials towards a better understanding of how these holistic strategic plans or specific research efforts have assisted these countries in the progress they have recorded as a nation.

The book is recommended for government officials in national planning, science policy makers, technocrats and regulatory officers involved in biotechnology practice.

## Strategic Development Programs

The papers under this section include Master Plans covering policies, regulatory frameworks and systematic action agendas developed and followed by the respective governments, as well as using mathematical modelling as a predictive tool for biological systems. Programs developed and implemented following these plans and models with precision are and would be result oriented. Of equal importance is the level of budgetary commitment as well as funding which these papers document. That scientific language, processes and products are global, is demonstrable through their international interaction, participation and patronage recorded. This part of the book as provided in particular by Cuba and India elucidates the keys to unlock doors of the secret to leapfrogging as envisaged by developing countries. There are great lessons contained in this section for all member countries to tap from.

## Specific Biotechnology Efforts

The section on specific biotechnology efforts contains a collection of papers on advances in specific processes of biotechnology application in agriculture, environment and industrial fields. Recent advances in the field of biosciences and techniques have featured and have been largely deployed in the experimentations.

Those in agriculture range from *in vitro* deployment of tissue culture techniques and biofertilizer development in enhancing commodity plantation output for national economic benefit, as well as biological control to molecular techniques in identification of microbial agents of infection in agriculture.

Various processes exploring metabolic pathways and techniques for production of useful metabolic compounds including bioleaching and my core mediation techniques among others are presented.

***Prof. Lucy Ogbadu***

***Prof. Godwin Ogbadu***

***Prof. Courtie Mahamadi***

# Introduction

Industrial Biotechnology is the application of biotechnology to industrial processes leading to synthesizing and creating innovative products in a sustainable manner. It is one of the most promising new approaches to pollution prevention, resource conservation, cost reduction and creation of new markets while protecting the environment. Most of the countries, including those with emerging economies, acknowledge the role being played by this upcoming area in the conversion of natural resources into value added products of benefit to humans. For example, Industrial Biotechnology can be a game changer in the mineral extraction, metals recovery and entire process chain by providing environmentally friendly higher productivity and yields. Novel biotechnologies for adding economic value to under-utilized biological resources in developing countries are capable of meeting specific developmental and biodiversity conservation goals. Industrial Biotechnology is among the most efficient and growing sectors today with enormous scope for innovation, research and development, and by innovative advancements in this area a country can achieve new heights in the fields of agriculture, medicine, renewable energy, climate sustainability and many more.

In order to gather collective wisdom for use by all the stake holders to accelerate the pace of industrial development and intensely deliberate on the issues concerning potential of industrial biotechnology and the strategies for its exploitation and application across a variety of areas in the developing countries, the NAM S&T Centre in partnership with the Ministry of Higher and Tertiary Education, Science and Technology Development, Zimbabwe and the National Biotechnology Authority (NBA) of Zimbabwe organised the 2nd Training Workshop on 'Industrial Biotechnology: Driving Value Addition and Beneficiation' during 22-24 August, 2017 in Harare which brought various stake holders, *viz.* scientists, experts and professionals engaged in R&D, policy making and implementation to a common platform for improving their skills and sharing views and experiences in various aspects of Industrial Biotechnology. The overall programme of the Training

Workshop comprised Technical Sessions, Training Lecture Sessions, Hands-On Training Sessions and also tours to biotechnology industries with the purpose of industry familiarization.

The Harare Training Workshop was attended by 68 scientists, experts and professionals from 17 developing countries, including Cuba, Egypt, The Gambia, India, Indonesia, Kenya, Malaysia, Mauritius, Myanmar, Nepal, Nigeria, South Africa, Sri Lanka, Sudan, Tanzania, Togo and Zimbabwe.

As a follow up of the above workshop, the present book – 'Evolving Industrial Biotechnology in Developing countries' has been brought out by the NAM S&T Centre, which has been edited by Prof. Lucy Ogbadu, Prof. Godwin Ogbadu and Prof. Courtie Mahamadi.

There are 21 scientific and technical papers contributed by the experts from 14 countries, reflecting on their status of technological developments and applications in this area of industrial biotechnology with the efforts to derive the maximum economic and environmental gains from the promising technology.

The publication of the book has been possible due to the commitment and valuable efforts of the entire team of the NAM S&T Centre, especially of Dr. Kavita Mehra, Mr. M. Bandyopadhyay, Ms. Keerti Mishra and Ms. Jasmeet Kaur at all the stages of the publication process. The contribution of Mr. Pankaj Buttan in designing of the cover page, formatting and liaising with the printers is worthy of mention.

I sincerely trust that this book will be useful to the policy experts and technology service providers, business, civil societies and multi-lateral agencies amongst developing countries with the objective of harnessing the benefits of promising Industrial Biotechnology.

***Prof. Dr. Arun P. Kulshreshtha***

*Former Director-General,*

*NAM S&T Centre*

# Contents

# Strategic Development Programs

# Chapter 1

# Advances of Biotechnology in Cuba

*Marisol Romeu Hernández*

*Head,*
*Biotechnology Unit in the Ministry of Science, Technology and Environment,*
*Havana City, CUBA*
*E-mail: marisol@delegcha.cu; jbiocitma@ceniai.inf.cu*

## ABSTRACT

This presentation on the development of biotechnology in Cuba is focussing on the period starting with the creation of the professional base and infrastructure necessary for its development since the 1980s. The major achievements are recorded in different areas, such as; the production of medicines; the creation of new therapies for the treatment of diverse diseases such as cancer Hepatitis B, meningitis and HIV; as well as in the agro food and allied, energy, chemical and even computer industries. Development of biotechnology in Cuba has greatly impacted on the quality of life of the population as well as on those in other collaborating countries with limited economic resources through technology transfer.

The Cuban health system has more than 400 biotechnology products which are all derived from the development of the concept of closed cycle, from the take-off of productive forces in a cycle of research, production and marketing. Significant social impacts have been achieved, mainly based on national programs for the development of prophylactic vaccines for disease prevention; early diagnosis and treatment of pathologies of different types of cancer; treatment of diabetes and its complications, such as diabetic foot ulcers; diagnosis of non-infectious diseases with novel medical equipment and the program for the discovery of malformation and hereditary metabolic diseases.

The country's economic model includes foreign investment, with the commercial proposal of 43 biomedical products and 10 agro-biotechnological products, providing the experience in the design of industrial facilities, a highly qualified staff and the portfolio of generic and innovative products.

***Keywords:*** *Biotechnology, Health, Research, Development, Innovation, Foreign investment.*

# INTRODUCTION

When we speak of biotechnology today, we often refer to processes that involve genetic engineering techniques. However, Biotechnology includes age long bio-activities that have been associated with man all through civilization.

Biotechnology has a multidisciplinary approach that involves various disciplines and sciences. It covers today a wide area of knowledge that arises from Basic Sciences (Molecular Biology, Microbiology, Cell Biology, Genetics, *etc.*), Applied Sciences (Immunological and biochemical techniques, as well as techniques based on Physics and Electronics) and other technologies (Fermentations, Separations, Purification, Computing, Robotics and Process Control). It is a complex network of knowledge where science and technology are intertwined and complementary.

It is necessary to come to the understanding that the development of biotechnology in the Republic of Cuba is one of the gains of the Revolution. Although, there were notable efforts in science in the 19th century on the island of Cuba by world-class figures such as Carlos J. Finlay and Tomas Romay, in 1959, when the Revolution triumphed, the country had more than one million illiterates and the few research groups numbered just above100 dedicated scientists.

In contrast, the country now has more than 600,000 university graduates, and out of this number more than 31,000 are dedicated to research and development. This crop of researchers is working in over 200 Science, Technology and Innovation entities. There are a similar number of professors who carry out their scientific activity in more than 40 universities.

The spectrum of application and development prospects of biotechnology in Cuba presently is wide with its achievements visible in many areas, such as the production of medicines; the creation of new therapies for the treatment of diverse diseases such as cancer, Hepatitis B, meningitis and HIV, as well as in the agro-food and allied sectors, energy, chemistry and even computer science.

The success of Biotechnology in Cuba is not only in the improvement of the quality of life of its people, it has equally been extended to other countries with limited economic resources through export and collaboration with these countries.

## Materials and Methods

Historical - Logical Method: Study of the documents that record the development of science, technology and innovation in Cuba, after the triumph of the Cuban Revolution. In addition, advances in the field of biotechnology and main achievements in this field.

Documentary Analysis: Reports of research and results reported by the Science, Technology and Innovation Entities based in Havana, development of innovations applied by companies.

## Background of Biotechnology in Cuba

The development of biotechnology in Cuba has been based on strategies into the human resources formation, a strong investment process, technological assimilation, creation of new knowledge, expansion of that knowledge, integration of scientific potential, strengthening of the scientific-productive infrastructure and organization of the System of Science and Technological Innovation.

Cuba in 1961, embarked on their massive education development plan inclusive of the Literacy Campaign. The goal of massive education was taken to all nooks and crannies of the country with a view to eradicating illiteracy and establishing the necessary schools. All this facilitated the large training plans for university students, which in turn provided the critical mass needed for the country's scientific development.

The human resources infrastructure for research was one of the high points in the University Reform that began in 1962. The creation of the Academy of Sciences of Cuba as an institution of excellence that would produce experts to manage the institutions marked a milestone in the new dispensation of placing science on the front burner of services to the Cuban population.

The period between 1962 and 1976 witnessed a concerted effort in promotion of science and university development accompanied with increased research output. In 1964, the possibilities of training of technologists were expanded with the establishment of the Technological University of Havana Jose Antonio Echeverria (named initially University City Jose Antonio Echeverria, CUJAE). It improved a program of accelerated development of engineers in various fields such as Process Engineering, Electronics and Industrial Engineering.

The policy to accelerate the development of biotechnology to support the country's social welfare and economic development was formulated in July 1981 with the creation of the Biological Front, which serves as the flagship of the most advanced ideas in the field of Biotechnology. Its purpose is to propose to the directorate of the country the actions to be undertaken to achieve the strategic objectives of being a true key player of Third World medicine and intensify the development of Biology.

The Biological Front worked assiduously in defining the national research priority agendas in health, (Interferon production); Genetic Engineering; the applications of the computer in the neuro physiological diagnosis; Medical Microbiology and Tropical Medicine; the human genetics program; the production of Vaccines and Biosimilars and the application of biotechnology to the treatment of malignant neoplasia.

In the case of agriculture, the priority lines are the development of Tissue Culture techniques and diagnosis of diseases in sugarcane; the production of proteins for human consumption and the development of crop breeding techniques as well as livestock improvement. To this, it was considered necessary to work in the field of biology in order to obtain new products for human consumption, develop the production of medicines, develop plant varieties resistant to diseases and solve the problems of food.

Cuba invested seriously in the necessary state-of-the art infrastructure to promote Biotechnology Program, between 1982 and 1995 especially for research in the health sector. This investment included training of human resources for this nascent industry through synergy between universities and research centers. Research centers created included: the Center for Biological Research; the Center for Genetic Engineering and Biotechnology (CIGB), the Laboratory Animal Production Center, the National Center for Biopreparations, the Center for Immunoassay and the Centro de Inmunología Molecular (CIM). In addition, others such as the Institute of Tropical Medicine Pedro Kouri and the Institute of Vaccines Finlay were remodelled and expanded.

In furtherance of biotechnology promotion since the mid-1980s, biotechnology activities have been taken to several provinces of Cuba outside Havana, with the inauguration of the Center for Genetic Engineering and Biotechnology in Camagüey and the Plant Biotechnology Center of the Central University of Villa Clara. Similar institutions were sited in Ciego de Avila, Sancti Spiritus, Holguin and Santiago de Cuba. At a higher stage of development, in 1991 a new form of organization for the empowerment and integration of resources emerged called the "Scientific-productive Pole of West Havana". The results showed the desirability of extending this form of integration of the scientific-technological potential to the whole country.

## Current Biotechnology in Cuba

The spectrum of application of biotechnology in Cuba is broad and its prospects for development are immeasurable. Its achievements today are visible in multiple industries and sectors in all provinces, as discussed above.

The Biotechnology and Pharmaceutical Industries Group (BioCubaFarma) is a high-tech business organization, a product of the merger between research centers of the western scientific center and pharmaceutical companies. Its function is the production of high technology drugs, equipment and services, based on technical scientific development aimed at improving the health of the people, the generation of export goods and services and advanced technologies for food production.

BioCubaFarma is charged with the responsibilities of promptly developing strategies, technologies, products and assistance for prevention, early diagnosis and treatment of health disorders. It is made up of 31 companies, 8 commercial companies and 64 industries. BioCubaFarma has a total of 21,785 worker force in its facilities which include 6,325 professionals, out of which are 262 with doctorate degree in science, 1170 masters degree in sciences and 719 researchers. The equipment and medicines generated by this business group currently impact all stages of people's lives and constitutes a true strength and evidence of the humanism of the Cuban Revolution.

The Cuban health system has achieved significant social impacts with important contributions from biotechnology and the national pharmaceutical industry, based mainly on the implementation of national scientific and technological programs for the development of prophylactic vaccines for disease prevention; early diagnosis and treatment of pathologies of different types of cancer; treatment of diabetes and its complications, such as diabetic foot ulcers; diagnosis of non-infectious diseases (cardio logical, neurological, *etc.*) with novel medical equipment and the program for the investigation of congenital malformations and hereditary metabolic diseases.

The basic picture of medicines in Cuba has 801, of which 505 are produced by the national pharmaceutical and biotechnology industry. Today, BioCubaFarma has 450 products of research and development programs, and the development of the closed cycle concept is a priority, since the productive forces take off in a cycle of research, production and marketing.

Some achievements of Cuban biotechnology:

- ☆ Vaccine against meningitis type B and C,
- ☆ Polyvalent vaccine against *Haemophilus influenzae* type b,
- ☆ Recombinant vaccine against Hepatitis B,
- ☆ Interferon such as Alpha-Interferon,
- ☆ Recombinant streptokinase to treat acute myocardial infarction,
- ☆ Enzymes for industrial use,
- ☆ PPG.Policosanol to treat atherogenic lipidemias,
- ☆ Diagnostic systems for diseases such as AIDS-HIV,
- ☆ Epidermal Growth Factor (EGF),
- ☆ SUMA. Ultra-Micro Analytical System,
- ☆ Human recombinant erythropoietin (EPOhr),
- ☆ More than one hundred monoclonal antibodies,
- ☆ Medical equipment and software.

The success story of diabetes program Heberprot-P which is the leading drug developed in Cuba which allowed more than 240,000 patients to be treated in 24 countries and more than 55,000 in Cuba and the prevention of more than 12,000 amputations. This program is supported with the production and distribution in national pharmacies of glucometers and biosensors.

Significant are the results in the field of a disease that affects the entire world: cancer. With the application of research in the face of this distressing condition, the incidence of liver cancer was reduced by the Hepatitis B virus, thanks to the specific prophylactic mass vaccination.

In Cuba there is a high incidence of cutaneous cancer, a disease that has as its main trigger factor the excess exposure to the sun. Recently, a new drug called Heberferon has been registered for the treatment of skin cancer, obtained from biotechnological formulations.

The Heberferon is a scientific novelty obtained by the CIGB of Havana after more than 20 years of research and clinical trials. This drug is a formulation where Alfa-Interferon and Gamma-Interferon are combined. The injectable medicine eliminates or reduces non-melanoma skin tumors and can prevent the effect of surgeries in areas of the face, where it is complex to operate.

The Centro de Inmunología Molecular (CIM) addresses the development of biosimilar and innovative products that cover monoclonal antibodies, therapeutic vaccines for cancer and other immune-related non-infectious diseases such as:

Recombinant Human Erythropoietin (EPOhr) for patients with chronic renal failure IRC on dialysis to control anemia and improve their quality of life; NIMOTUZUMAB for the treatment of tumors of head and neck, brain, esophagus and other locations; ITOLIZUMAB for the treatment of Psoriasis and Rheumatoid Arthritis; LEUKOCIM for the treatment of patients with Neutropenia due to the use of cytostatic in Oncology; CIMAVAX-EGF and VAXIRA, two therapeutic vaccines for patients with advanced lung cancer and other diagnostic products.

Other achievements are the elimination of diseases by vaccination such as: poliomyelitis, tetanus, diphtheria, measles, whooping cough, rubella, among others. In addition, meningococcal disease and leptospirosis have been brought under control. A significant finding is that Hepatitis B has been maintained at zerolevel (cases) in children under 5 years of age since 1999, and since 2006 in children under 15 years of age.

In 2015, Cuba became the first country in the world to eliminate mother-to-fetus HIV transmission. In addition, it worked to prevent kidney failure by examining micro albuminuria, which extended to laboratories throughout the country.

The country also has an extensive network of bio-factories for the production of vitro plants in order to improve the agricultural sector. News varieties of crops with resistance to diseases and pests have been developed. These include sugar cane, potatoes, tobacco, bananas, vegetables and citrus fruits. Likewise, there are advances in animal biotechnology, leading to development of veterinary vaccines of new generation and diagnostic means.

## Cuban Biotechnology Activities around the World

As a result of South-South cooperation, Cuba has made technological transfers to several countries, including Brazil, Venezuela, Viet Nam, China, Algeria, India, South Africa and Iran.

In addition, 5 companies have been created:

1. Biotech Pharm in Beijing, China (Monoclonal Antibodies and Therapeutic Vaccines against Cancer).
2. ChangHeber in Changchung, China (Recombinant Proteins).
3. Lukang-Heber in Shandong, China (Biotech products for agriculture).
4. Recombio in Spain (Therapeutic Vaccines against Cancer).
5. Innocimab in Singapore (Monoclonal Antibodies).

Today Cuba's economic model includes foreign investment. An example is the Mariel Special Development Zone with the commercial proposal of 43 biomedical products and 10 agro-biotechnological products.

BioCubaFarma would provide expertise in the design of industrial facilities, a highly qualified staff and the portfolio of generic and innovative products. On the other hand, the foreign partner is required to provide the financial resources for investment in the construction of the Factory and cost of production. Both parties will be in charge of the commercialization of the obtained products.

Currently, more than 200 research-development projects are underway to find new and improved products to continue contributing science and innovation to the health of the population and the country's economy. The products with the greatest potential are:

- ✰ HeberNasVac therapeutic vaccine, with a strong patent position for the treatment of chronic Hepatitis B;
- ✰ A new product under development for the treatment of cardiac infarcts;
- ✰ RituxiMab, a bio similar antibody with clinical evidence of effects on lymphomas;
- ✰ A new peptide to inhibit the tumor cells;
- ✰ Amilovis, diagnostic of Alzheimer's disease;
- ✰ Clinical trial, phase II, of the cholera vaccine.

## Conclusions

1. The Cuban state invests to ensure the development of Biotechnology. The infrastructure for research and production has been created, coupled with the specialized training of human resources.
2. The Cuban health system has achieved significant social impacts with important contributions from biotechnology and the national pharmaceutical industry, based fundamentally on the results of national scientific and technological programs.
3. Development of competitive products made it possible to meet the demands of the Cuban Health System and break new ground in a highly demanding international market.

## REFERENCES

1. Academia de Ciencias de Cuba, 1986. Informe de Balance del Frente Biológico 1981-1985.
2. Anaya, B., Martín, M., Biotecnología en Cuba: origen y resultados alcanzados. Centro de Estudios de la Economía Cubana, Universidad de La Habana.https: //www.nodo50.org/cubasigloXXI/pensamiento/anaya_300410.pdf
3. Cuba patenta nuevo fármaco para el tratamiento de cáncer de piel.
4. http: //www.salud.carlosslim.org/cuba-patenta-nuevo-farmaco-para-tratamiento-de-cancer-de-piel
5. De Armas, I. 2008. *Registran en Argelia medicamento cubano para pie diabético,* Periódico Granma, 13 de septiembre, versión digital, en sitio:
6. http: //www.granma.cubaweb.cu/2008/09/13/cubamundo/artic01.html
7. De Armas, I., 2016. Registra Cuba vacuna terapéutica contra cáncer de pulmón. Periódico Granma, 25 de junio, versión digital:
8. http: //www.granma.cubaweb.cu/secciones/cienciaytec/medicina/medicina28.htm

9. Lage, A., 2007. Biotecnología en Cuba.http: //www.profesionalespcm.org/_php/MuestraArticulo2.php?id=7932
10. Lage, A., 2010. Prueban en Cuba anticuerpo monoclonal contra 11 tipos de cáncer.http: //www.cubadebate.cu/noticias/2010/11/21/prueban-en-cuba-anticuerpo-monoclonal-contra-11-tipos-de-cancer/#.Wd-W2TtZ3IU
11. Lage, A., 2015. Ahora es cuando más necesitamos de la ciencia.www.granma.cu/ciencia/2015-03-13/ahora-es-cuando-mas-necesitamos-de-la-ciencia
12. Lage, A., 2016. Empresa estatal socialista: diez verdades esenciales. http: //www.cubadebate.cu/opinion/2016/09/17/empresa-estatal-socialista-diez-verdades-esenciales/
13. Pestana, L., 2015. Surgimiento y desarrollo del sector biotecnológico en Cuba. www.ipscuba.net/./surgimiento-y-desarrollo-del-sector-biotecnologico-en-cuba
14. Ramón, M., 2015. Biotecnología cubana en 2015: avances que marcaron un año. http: //www.cubadebate.cu/noticias/2015/12/31/biotecnologia-cubana-en-2015-avances-que-marcaron-un-ano/#.Wd-VGjtZ3IU
15. Somoza, J., 2002. Industria biotecnológica y médico-farmacéutica, Estructura Económica de Cuba, Capítulo V, Tomo 1, pg. 236

*Chapter 2*

# The Mathematical Language in Biotechnology: Case Study

*Mostafa M. Abo Elsoud*

*Microbial Biotechnology Department,*
*National Research Centre, EGYPT*
*E-mail: masnrc@gmail.com*

## ABSTRACT

In most industrial biotechnology set ups, the approach for optimization of process conditions is generally done by varying one factor at a time. However, this strategy is laborious and time consuming, especially for a large number of variables and often does not consider interactions among variables. Individual and interactive effects enable each reaction parameter to be optimized in coherence with others. Alternatively, mathematical modelling can be used. Mathematical models are tools that we can use to describe the past performance and predict the future performance of biotechnological processes. They can be applied to processes operating at different levels, from shake flask to the commercial/industrial scale. Mathematical models can be powerful tools in both basic research and applied research and development. Mathematical modelling has become an important tool in understanding and unravelling biological complexities. This paper presents the process of mathematical modelling in biotechnological systems starting from start to obtaining results.

***Keywords:*** *Cells factory, Biotechnology, Metabolic model, Industrial production, Operations research, Mathematical modelling.*

## INTRODUCTION

An increasing number of industrial bioprocesses depend on living cells for production of valuable bio-products. These processes range from production of bulk chemicals in yeasts and bacteria to the synthesis of therapeutic proteins in mammalian cell lines (Almquist *et al.*, 2014). The approach for process optimization is generally done by varying one factor at a time. However, this strategy is laborious and time consuming, especially for a large number of variables and often does not consider interactions among variables (El-Bendary *et al.*, 2016). Furthermore, due to the complexity of microbial metabolism, both due to the large number of interacting reactions and the complex regulation, there has been an increasing focus on the use of statistical design of experiments (DOE) for determining the factors that influence the response and/or their optimum levels (Sunitha and Lee 1999; Soh *et al.*, 2012). It is a collection of mathematical and statistical tools that is powerful in both fundamental research and applied research and development (Almquist *et al.*, 2014).

Industrial biotechnology can benefit from mathematical models by using them to understand, predict, and optimize the properties and behavior of cell factories (Tyo *et al.*, 2010). With valid models, improvement strategies can be discovered and evaluated in silico, saving both time and resources.

The steps of the kinetic modelling procedure are now described briefly, and then followed by elaboration and in-depth discussions on some of their aspects (Almquist *et al.*, 2014):

### Purpose

The first step of modelling is to define the purpose of the model, an important step as it includes the very reason for setting up a model in the first place. Typical questions are: *Why do we model? What do we want to use the model for? What type of behavior should the model be able to explain?*

### Network Structure

The model network structure is the wiring diagram of the model. It defines the network of inter connected elements that are assumed to be important for the modelling task in question.

### Determination of the Mathematical Expressions

Having defined the model network structure, the next step in the modelling process is the determination of the mathematical expressions that define the interactions between the different components. The model network structure already delivers information about which elements should take part in the mathematical expressions.

### Model Structure

When the network structure and the mathematical expressions have been determined, the structure of the model is complete. The model can now be written as a set of equations.

### Parameter Determination

Next, the numerical values of the parameters need to be determined. Parameter values are sometimes established one by one, either from targeted experiments measuring them directly or from other types of a priori information on individual parameter values. In contrast, parameter values can also be determined simultaneously in an inductive way by utilizing the implicit in formation in measurements of other quantities than the parameters themselves, using parameter estimation methods.

## Validation

With the parameter values determined, the quality of the model should be assessed. Such model validation can consist of both qualitative reasoning as well as formal statistical testing. In addition to explaining experimental data used for setting up the model, it is common to further validate the model's predictive power based on new sets of experimental data that was not used previously in the modelling process.

## Usage

When a model has been established it can be used in a number of different ways to answer the questions for why it was created. This involves various types of what–if analysis that explores different scenarios and investigates the impact of model assumptions.

**Table 2.1: Elements of Mathematical Modelling and Description of the Work that they Entail**

| Modeling Element | What It Entails |
|---|---|
| 1. Analyze the situation or problem | • Identify a problem taken from an external context (often from an everyday life context) that must be solved or a situation that must be understood and explained.<br>• Do background research if necessary.<br>• Make sense of the situation or problem and understand the question. |
| 2. Develop and formulate a model | • Determine all given information.<br>• Determine what assumptions are necessary.<br>• Translate the information given in the problem together with the assumptions into a mathematical problem that can be solved.<br>• Use mathematics appropriate for the information given and assumed as well as the students' expertise. |
| 3. Compute a solution of the model | • Solve the mathematical problem stated in the model.<br>• Analyze and perform operations in the model.<br>• Check for correctness. |
| 4. Interpret the solution and draw conclusions | • Interpret the mathematical solution in terms of the original situation.<br>• Draw conclusions that the solution implies about the original situation. |
| 5. Validate conclusions | • Reflect on whether the mathematical answer makes sense in terms of the original situation (e.g., is the answer within a valid range of values?).<br>• If the conclusions are satisfactory with regard to the accuracy needed, report the solution. If the conclusions are not satisfactory or need to be improved, go back to stage 2 ("Develop and formulate a model"). |
| 6. Develop and formulate a new or modified model | • Revise the assumptions made according to what was learned in the first solution and translate them into a new or modified mathematical problem that can be solved.<br>• The type of mathematics in the current model may be different from the previous one.<br>• Go through these stages again: Compute, Interpret, and Validate. |
| Report the solution | • Share your conclusions and the reasoning behind them. |

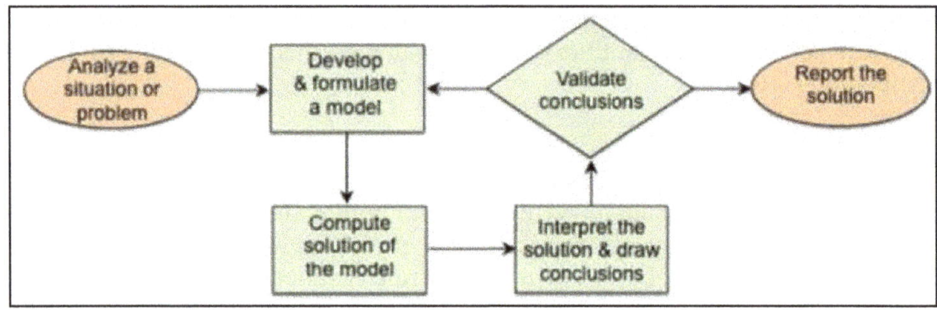


**Figure 2.1: Illustration of the Main Steps of Mathematical Modelling Procedure.**

## Case Study

The following explains a general example that can be replaced by biological, biochemical process or any other complexity regarding the field of study.

### Problem

A factory produces two types of products (x and y). Each unit of x takes 2 hours and costs 3 pounds, while y takes 4 hours and costs 2 pounds for production. If the profit per unit of x and y are 5 and 3 pounds, respectively. What are the number of x and y for maximum profit, if we have only 40 hours and maximum budget of 50 pounds (Taha, 2007).

## Results and Discussion

For solving this problem, we first summarize the data in a table as follows:

**Table 2.2: Summary of Problems' Data**

| | *x* | *y* | *Total* |
|---|---|---|---|
| Time | 2 | 4 | 40 |
| Cost | 3 | 2 | 50 |
| Profit | 5 | 3 | ? |

The summarized data are then converted into mathematical equations as follows:

Maximize $(5x + 3y)$ *Objective*

$$\left.\begin{array}{ll} \text{Equ. 1} & 2x + 4y \le 40 \\ \text{Equ. 2} & 3x + 2y \le 50 \\ \text{Equ. 3} & x \text{ and } y \ge 0 \end{array}\right\} \quad \textit{Constraints}$$

Next, these equations – which are linear equations - are represented and the area of solution is also represented on the graph as follows:

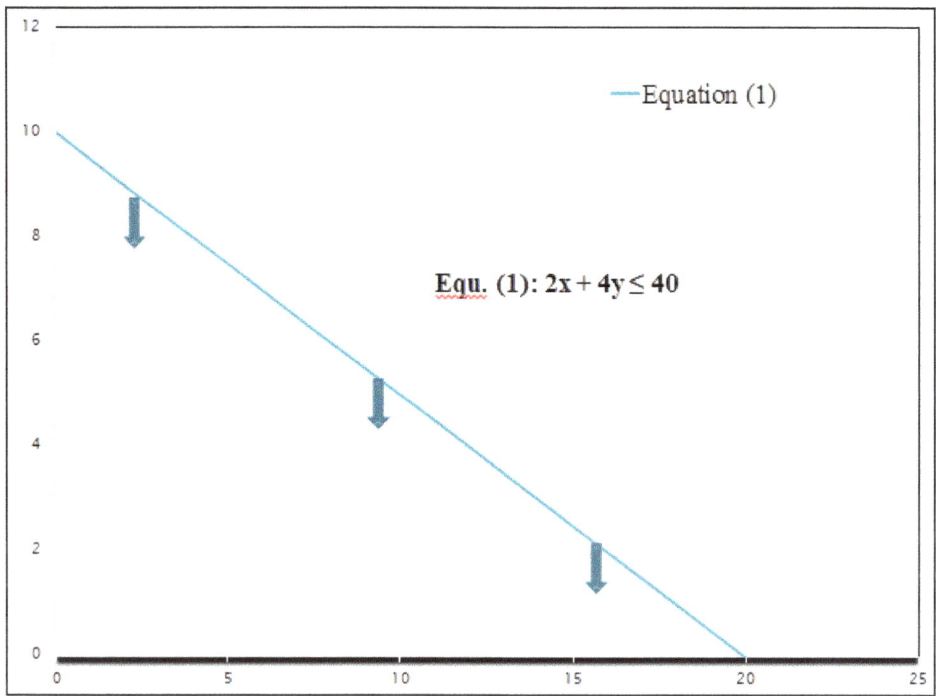


**Figure 2.2: Graphical Demonstration of the First Equation.**

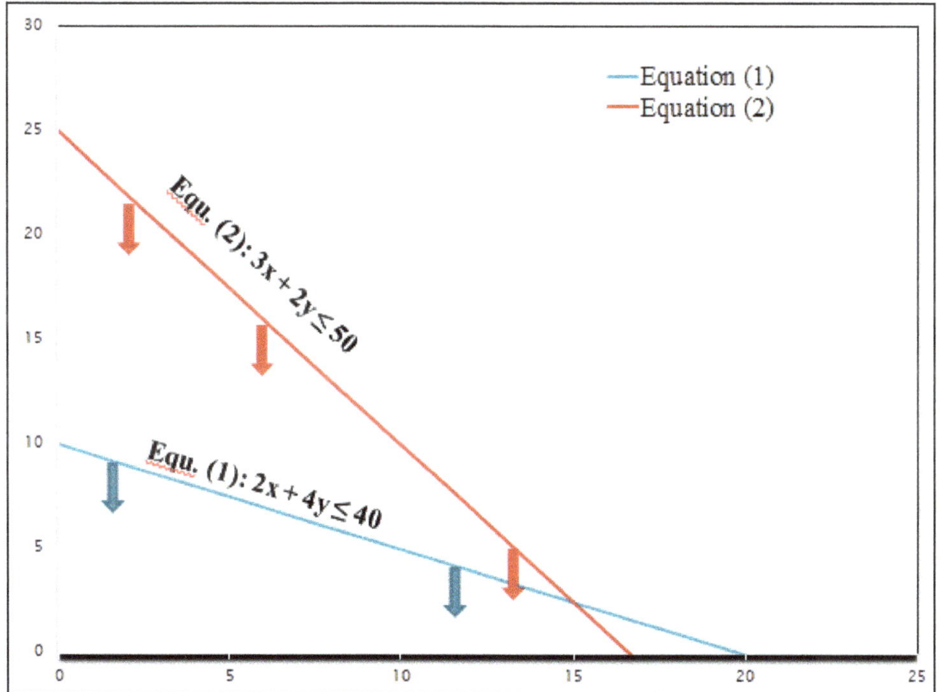


**Figure 2.3: Graphical Demonstration of the Second Equation.**

In Figure 2.2, the arrows represent the direction in which the equation can be solved. Equation (2) can be solved graphically in similar way as equation (1).

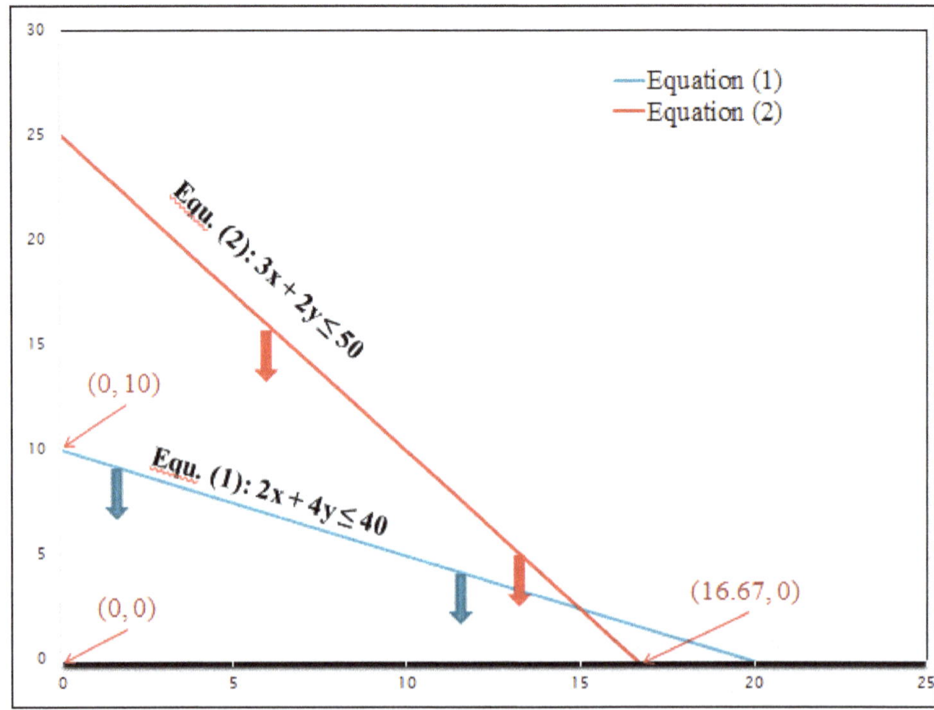


**Figure 2.4: Graphical expected solutions of the mathematical model.**

According to the last constrain, the objective function cannot be solved in the negative area. The solution of the objective function must be one or more of the intersections (vertices) represented in Figure 2.4. These points are: (0, 10), (0, 0), (16.67, 0) and the point of intersection between equation (I and 2). This last point can be obtained as follows:

$2x + 4y = 40$ *Equ[1]*

$3x + 2y = 50$ *Equ [2]*

Multiply Equ (2) X2

$6x + 4y = 100$ *Equ[3]*

Subtract: Equ (3)-Equ (1)

$4x = 60$

$x=60/4=15$

Substitute x=15 in Equ (1)

$30 + 4y=40$

$y= (40-30)/4=2.5$

$(x, y)= (15, 2.5)$

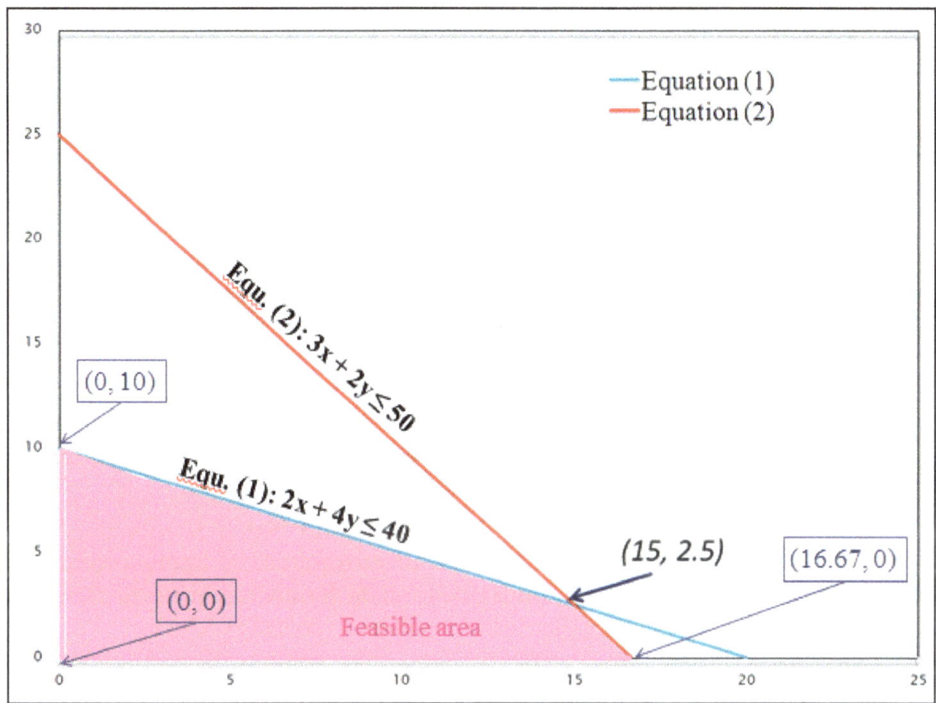


**Figure 2.5: Full Graphical Solutions and Feasible Area.**

In Figure 2.5, the area marked by the points (0, 0), (0, 10), (15, 2.5) and (16.67, 0) is the feasible area (area of solution).

To obtain the maximum profit in the current process, we have to solve the objective function using all the vertices and then select the maximum result for solution.

**Z= Max. (5x + 3y)** *Objective*

**At** (0, 0):

$Z_1 = 0$

**At** (0, 10):

$Z_2 = 0 + 3(10) = 30$

**At** (16.67, 0):

$Z_3 = 5\ (16.67) + 0 = 83.35$

**At** (15, 2.5):

$Z_4 = 5(15) + 3(2.5) = 82.5$

Now, we can conclude that at x=16.67 and y= 0 the profit can be maximum and equals (83.35 pound).

Finally, we should validate these results by application of these conditions and comparing the obtained experimental results with that obtained mathematically.

## Disclaimer

Models are not explanations and can never alone provide a complete solution to a biological problem.

## Conclusions

The use of mathematical models in the field of biotechnology represents a useful tool for saving time, efforts and extra-expenses. In addition, mathematical representation of the biological processes inherits simulation of the current situation and prediction of the future data along with the capability for answering many questions about mechanisms and mode of actions.

# REFERENCES

1. Almquist, J, M. Cvijovic, V. Hatzimanikatis, J. Nielsen and M. Jirstrand, 2014. Kinetic models in industrial biotechnology – Improving cell factory performance, Mini review. *Metabolic Engineering;* 24, 38–60.
2. El-Bendary, Magda A., Mostafa M. Abo Elsoud, Sahar S. Mohamed and Shimaa R. Hamed, 2016.Optimization of mosquitocidal toxins production by Lysinibacillussphaericus under solid state fermentation using statistical experimental design. *Acta Biologica Szegediensis,* Vol 60(1): 57-63.
3. Soh, K.C., Miskovic, L. and Hatzimanikatis, V., 2012. From network models to network responses: integration of thermodynamic and kinetic properties of yeast genome-scale metabolic networks. *FEMS Yeast Res.* 12, 129–143.
4. Sunitha, K. and Lee Jung-Kee TK, 1999. Optimization of medium components for phytase production by *E. coli* using response surface methodology. *Bioprocess Biosyst Eng* 21: 477-481.
5. Taha, H.A., 2007. Operations research: an introduction 8^th^ed. Pearson Prentice Hall, Pearson Education, Inc.
6. Tyo, K.E.J., Kocharin, K. and Nielsen, J., 2010. Toward design-based engineering of industrial microbes. *Curr.Opin. Microbiol.* 13, 255–262.

# *Chapter 3*

# Promotion of Biotech Industry in India

*Keerti Mishra*

***Research Associate,***
***Centre for Science and Technology of the Non-Aligned and***
***Other Developing Countries (NAM S&T Centre),***
***Lodhi Road, New Delhi, INDIA***
***E-mail: keertim033@gmail.com***

## ABSTRACT

With growing population, it has become lucrative for the fast-growing economies, for example, India, to grow well into the sector of Industrial or White Biotechnology and make efforts to prove themselves as the hub of scientific and technological development.

The government of India has taken several policy initiatives in this direction and has created an impressive institutional set-up for the promotion of Biotechnology research and industries in the country. It has stepped up its expenditure to augment the growth of the sector with the aim to spend US$ 3.7 Billion on biotechnology during 2012-17. Industrial Biotechnology sector is one of the sunrise sectors in India which is amongst the top 12 biotech destinations in the world and ranks third in the Asia-Pacific region, accounting for 2 per cent of the market share globally. According to the estimates of the year 2011, Indian Biotechnology market by now must have reached US$11.6 billion in 2017.

Some of the flagship programmes initiated by the government of India in the recent past such as "Make in India", "Skill India", "Start Up India", "E-YUVA", "SPARSH" *etc.* have provisions in their objectives on the promotion of Industrial Biotechnology and nurturing innovation and entrepreneurship. A large number of institutions have been established by the government of India under the administrative control of the Department of Biotechnology (DBT), Department of Science and Technology (DST), Indian Council of Medical Research (ICMR), Council of Scientific and Industrial Research (CSIR) and Indian Council of Agricultural Research (ICAR) that deal with various aspects of R&D and Industrial Biotechnology.

The Department of Biotechnology (DBT), Ministry of Science and Technology is the nodal agency in the government of India for the promotion of large-scale use of Biotechnology in the country including providing support for R&D and manufacturing in biology and human resource development. It has a key role to play in the transfer of technology, validation, licensing and in creation of infrastructure and training for successful commercialisation of technologies emanating from hard-core research with emphasis on translational capacity to be embedded in major research centres and programmes, support for business incubation infrastructure, technology validation and scale-up infrastructure and technology management, professional development and licensing of technologies for successful commercialisation. The National Biotechnology Development Strategy 2015-2020 was launched by DBT to give boost to Industrial Biotech sector and provide an environment for the development of new and innovative biotech products.

Biotechnology Industry Research Assistance Council (BIRAC) has been set up by DBT as a not-for-profit Public-Sector Enterprise in order to stimulate, foster and enhance the strategic research and innovation capabilities of the Indian Biotech industry, particularly start-ups and SME's and for the creation of affordable products addressing the needs of the largest section of society. BIRAC has supported over 618 projects, 850 start-ups, entrepreneurs, biotech companies and organizations and 20 incubators across the country, resulting in over 66 products and technologies and 120 Intellectual property rights being generated.

The steps recently taken by the government of India to promote industrial growth in biotech sector include:

- India has moved forward in the area of IPR regime to provide more impetus to the start-ups.
- India has also relaxed its Foreign Direct Investment (FDI) norms in order to adopt new techniques and to place the country on the top of this sector.
- Exemption in service tax to the Bioincubators under BIRAC.
- Some states like; Andhra Pradesh, Telangana and Gujarat have come out with their specific Biotech policies.
- Total budget allocated to BIRAC in FY 2016-17 is US$ 18713460 for supporting start-ups and promoting innovation in biotech industries.

The government has plans to invest US$ 5 billion to develop human capital, infrastructure and research initiatives to realise the dream of growing the sector into a US$ 100 billion industry by 2025.

## INTRODUCTION

India is moving ahead in the field of Biotechnology. It is one of the sunrise sectors in the world. For a country like India, biotechnology is a powerful enabling technology that can revolutionize agriculture, healthcare, industrial processing and environmental sustainability. This technology has become lucrative for a country like India where productivity of agriculture is facing many stresses as well as decreasing due to increase in natural calamities. India is one of the top biotech destinations of the world and ranks third in the Asia-Pacific region. India has the second-highest number of US Food and Drug Administration (USFDA)–approved plants, after the USA and is the largest producer of recombinant Hepatitis B vaccine. Out of the top 10 biotech companies in India (by revenue), seven have expertise in bio-pharmaceuticals and three specialise in agri-biotech. This sector supports high level of innovation and has growth potential up to a greater extent.

India's biotech industry holds 2 per cent of the global market share. The government of India has provided adequate scope to this sector by providing facilities for Research and Development (R&D) in the field of biotechnology. Various government initiatives like 'Make in India', 'Start Up India', 'Stand Up India', 'Digital India' also support the growth of this sector. India has emerged as a leading destination for clinical trials, contract research and manufacturing activities owing to the growth in the bio-services sector. The high demand for different biotech products has also opened up scope for the foreign companies to set up base in India.

## Materials and Methdos

### Government Initiatives and Institutions

The department of biotechnology (DBT) was formed in 1986 under Ministry of Science and Technology when India realised the need for a separate Biotech department for better growth in this field. DBT along with other government funded institutions such as National Biotechnology Board (NBTB) and many other autonomous bodies representing the biotechnology sector, are working together in order to project India as a global hub for biotech research and business excellence.

Biotechnology Industry Research Assistance Council (BIRAC) has been set up by DBT as a not-for-profit Public-Sector Enterprise in order to stimulate, foster

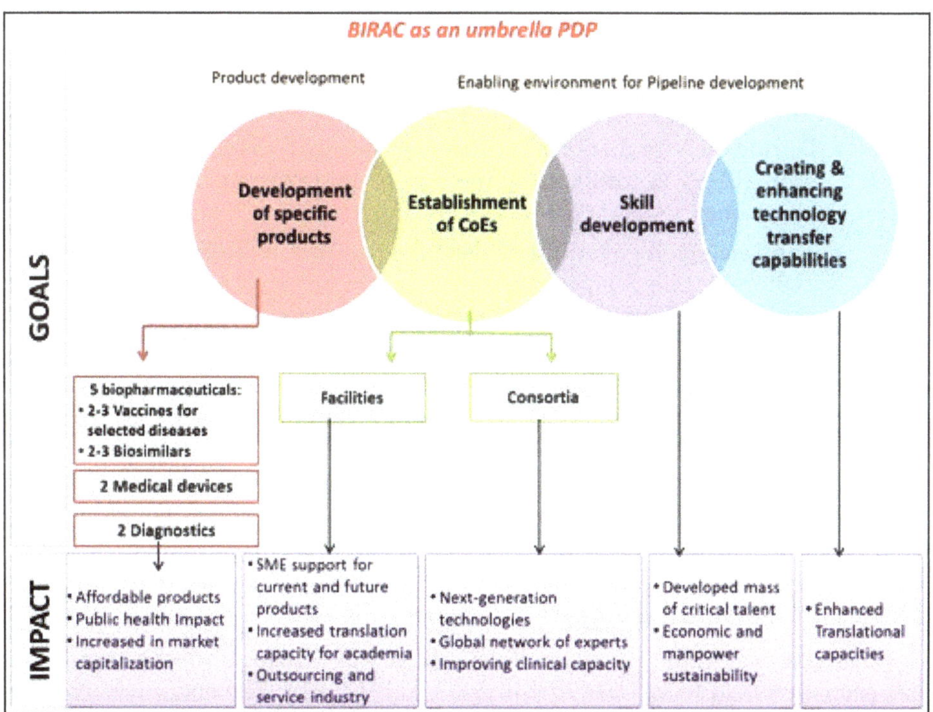


**Figure 3.1**
**[*Source*: DBT, Innovate in India (i3) (http://www.dbtindia.nic.in/launch-national-biopharma/)].**

and enhance the strategic research and innovation capabilities of the Indian Biotech industry, particularly start-ups and SME's and for the creation of affordable products addressing the needs of the largest section of society.

The Department of Biotechnology has established biotech parks in various parts of the country to facilitate product development, research and innovation, and the development of biotechnology industrial clusters.

Operational biotech parks are located at Lucknow in Uttar Pradesh, Bangalore in Karnataka, Kalamassery and Kochi in Kerala, Guwahati in Assam and Chindwara in Madhya Pradesh. Biotech Industrial clusters are located in Bangalore (Bangalore Lifesciences cluster and Bangalore Bio innovation Centre), NCR Faridabad, Pune, Hyderabad and Chennai (Medtech). The parks offer investors incubation and pilot plant facilities for solvent extraction and laboratory and office spaces. BIRAC has funded 15 incubation centers offering a whole host of instrumentation facilities and services. India constitutes around 8 per cent of the total global generics market, indicating a huge untapped opportunity in the sector Hybrid seeds, including GM (Genetically Modified) seeds, represents new business opportunities in India based on yield improvement.

Recently government has taken many crucial steps to provide impetus to this sector. Some of them are:

- In the Union Budget 2017-18, DBT received US$ 333.31 million, an increase of 22 per cent, to continue implementing the department's national biotech strategy and target increasing the turnover from the sector to $100 billion by 2025 from $7 billion in 2016.
- During the Vibrant Gujarat Global Summit-2017, 54 MoUs worth Rs 5,022 crore (US$ 736.1 million) in the biotechnology sector were signed by 37 companies.
- The Telangana government also inked an MoU with PE firm Cerestra to explore a 'Life Sciences Infrastructure Fund' with a corpus of Rs 1,000 crore (US$ 150 million) to create a sophisticated modular plug and play infrastructure for pharma, biotech and medical devices industry.
- A Network of Technology Centres and promotion of start-ups by Small Industries Development Bank of India (SIDBI) are among the steps taken by the Government of India to promote innovation and entrepreneurship in the agroindustry proposed by the Ministry of Micro, Small and Medium Enterprises (MSME) in a new scheme.

## Investment Criteria has been rectified through Tax Incentives since 2016 via the Union Budget

The turnover limit to avail the Presumptive Tax Scheme under section 44 AD, has been increased from USD 153846.2 to USD 307692.3. The tax payers carrying a business will be allowed to avail this scheme for which they will have to declare profit at minimum 8 per cent of the total turnover and they will be exempted from the requirement of maintaining any books of accounts.

New manufacturing companies incorporated on or after 1st March, 2016 to be given an option to be taxed at 25 per cent + surcharge and cess provided on fullment of certain conditions Lower corporate income tax has been proposed for the next financial year of relatively small enterprises 100 per cent deduction of profits for 3 out of 5 years for start-ups setup during April, 2016 to March, 2019.

MAT will apply in such cases 10 per cent rate of tax on income from worldwide exploitation of patents developed and registered in India by a resident Custom single window project have been announced and would be implemented at major ports and airports from the beginning of next financial year.

## Service Tax

Exemption from the service tax on services provided by BIRAC approved biotechnology incubators to incubate with effect from 1.4.2016 Service tax services of assessing bodies empanelled centrally by Directorate General of training, ministry of Skill Development and Entrepreneurship Development with effect from 1st April, 2016.

## Centres of Excellence and Innovation in Biotechnology (CEIB)

The DBT has been implementing a scheme known as Centres of Excellence and Innovation in Biotechnology (CEIB). The scheme provides funding to augment and strengthen institutional research capacity for promotion of excellence in interdisciplinary science and innovation in specific areas of biotechnology. The programme is intended for institutions with a substantial investment in, and commitment to, biotechnology research. The programme provides flexible long-term support for highly innovative research (both basic and translational in nature) in biotechnology, which creates not only high-quality publications and intellectual property but also translational outputs through mid and high-end innovation.

The following three categories of grants are provided under this programme:

**Category I:** Centres of Excellence (CoE) in Biotechnology with a specific thematic focus, that can involve single or multiple institutions

- ✰ The above will provide support, in part or full, research and development activities from very basic or fundamental to translational or applied in areas of health, agriculture, energy, environment, industrial biotech research *etc.*

**Category II:** Outstanding Scientist Research Programme in Biotechnology

- ✰ Meant for providing long-term R&D support to an individual outstanding investigator of high scientific caliber with publications and/or patents record at the highest level.
- ✰ The support is recognition of investigators for their recent performance and planned future work.

**Category III:** Institutional Programme Support (to both single institutional programme as well as multi-institutional programme) to the identified institution(s)/department(s) with multiple investigators in various disciplines

- ✩ To create and strengthen research capabilities at university or institutional level for categorical research by a number of investigators from different disciplines for a joint research effort; or investigators from the same discipline who focus on a common research problem. Support is proportional to size and quality of Ph.D. and Post-Doctoral programmes.

To enable re-design of objectives and research programme to be inter-disciplinary and address specific weaknesses.

BIRAC has several flagship programs for supporting start-ups and SMEs across the biotechnology innovation pipeline including funding (from ideation stage to commercialization), incubation, patent assistance, capacity building through training and mentoring including business and technical mentoring. The total budget from BIRAC in FY 2016-17 for start-ups and innovation research in industries is Rs. 120 crores.

## BIRAC Regional Entrepreneurship Centre (BREC)

Promotion of Bio-entrepreneurship through BIRAC Regional Entrepreneurship Centre (BREC) with an aim to impart bio entrepreneurs with the necessary knowledge and skills required for converting innovative ideas into successful ventures. DBT is setting up 5 Regional Centers in the next 5 years.

## Bio-incubator Support Scheme (BISS)

BIRAC has initiated a scheme for Strengthening and Upgrading of the existing Bio-incubators and also to establish New World Class Bio-incubators in certain strategic locations. These Bio- incubators will provide the incubation space and other required services to start-up companies for their initial growth. The BIRAC Bio-incubator strengthening support is provided to those existing Incubators which have proven experience and competence to run successful Incubators, an existing network for mentoring and hand holding of incubators, and also can provide the enabling services to promote innovation research. Seven existing Bio-incubators across the country have been strengthened and approximately 55,000 sqft of Bio-incubator space has been created to support start up.

## Biotech Industry Partnership Programme (BIPP)

Biotechnology Industry Partnership Programme (BIPP) is a government partnership with industries for support on a cost sharing basis for path-breaking research in frontier futuristic technology areas having major economic potential and making the Indian industry globally competitive. It is focused on IP creation with ownership retained by Indian industry and wherever relevant, by collaborating scientists. BIPP supports the development of appropriate technologies in the context of recognized national priorities in the area of agriculture, health, bio-energy, green manufacturing, when the scale of the problem has serious consequences for social and economic development. (BIPP) is a government partnership program with industries for public support on a cost sharing basis for:

a. Path-breaking research in frontier futuristic technology areas having major economic potential and making Indian industry globally competitive and focused on IP creation with ownerships by Indian industry and where relevant, collaborating scientists.
b. Development of appropriate technologies in the context of recognized national priorities in the area of agriculture, health, bio-energy, green manufacturing for social and economic development.

## Contract Research Scheme (CRS)

The CRS scheme supports the academia-industry interaction between research institutes, universities, public funded research laboratories, governmental organizations, research foundations and companies/industries under the Public-Private Partnership (PPP) mode. The funding is in the form of grant which is given to both the academic as well as the industrial partner. While the industry performs its role as a 'validation partner' and engages on a contractual basis, the IP rights reside solely with the academic partner(s). The Objective of the Scheme is to: (a) Encourage Public and/or Private Universities to validate their translational research that have commercialisation potential (b) Engage with the contract research and manufacturing (CRAM) industry to carry out the validation of a process or a prototype.

## Sustainable Entrepreneurship and Enterprise Development (SEED) Fund

BIRAC has launched SEED Fund of '10 crore for providing financial equity-based support to start-ups and enterprises through bio-incubators for scaling enterprises.

## SPARSH Scheme

Under BIRAC the SPARSH scheme aims at promoting development of innovative solutions to address society's most pressing social problems through biotechnology approaches.

It has two basic components:

I. Product Development
II. Social Innovation Immersion Programme (SIIP)

Under Product Development funding is provided to support innovation towards affordable product development that can bring significant social impact and addresses the challenge of inclusive growth.

SIIP is an immersion fellowship scheme aimed to create a pool of Social Innovators/Entrepreneurs who could identify specific social needs.

### Innovate in India (I3) for Biopharma: Empowering the Biotech Entrepreneurs and Accelerating inclusive Innovation

The mission will focus on development of product leads that are at advanced stages of the product development lifecycle and relevant to the public health need by focusing on managed partnerships to upgrade shared infrastructure facilities and establish them as shared infrastructure for both product discovery/discovery validation and manufacturing, develop human capital by providing specific trainings to address the critical skills gap among nascent biotech companies across the product development value chain, including business plan development, technology transfer, intellectual property registration and market penetration, satisfy surplus demand for start-up incubation space and services (through establishing and strengthening biotech clusters, pertinent consortia and clinical trial networks).

This is a US$ 250 M programme over 5 years to be led by Department of Biotechnology Ministry of Science and Technology, Government of India implemented by Biotechnology Industry Research Assistance Council (BIRAC).

### Guidelines on Similar Biologics- Regulatory Requirements for Marketing Authorization in India, 2016

The new Biosimilar Policy known as the Guidelines on Similar Biologics announced by the Central Drugs Standard Control Organization (CDSCO) in March 2016 addresses the regulatory pathway regarding manufacturing process and safety, efficacy and quality aspects. The 2016 version allows a reference biologic (for which the biosimilar is being developed) not marketed in India, to be licensed in any International Council for Harmonization of Technical Requirements for Pharmaceuticals (ICH) country (*i.e.* EU, Japan, US, Canada and Switzerland).

The guidelines advocate for post-marketing studies within 2 years of receiving marketing permission/manufacturing license. It also provides information on when a confirmatory clinical safety and efficacy study can be waived.

## Skill Development

The DBT and BIRAC have taken multiple initiatives for teaching and training in Biotechnology sector:

- ☆ Indo-Australian Career Boosting Gold Fellowships announced under which it will support researchers to undertake a collaborative research project at a leading science institute or university in Australia for a period of up to 24 months.
- ☆ DBT and Ministry of Science and Technology, India and Russian Ministry of Education and Science (RMES), Russia, have invited joint research proposals in the area of biotechnology. The objective is to broaden and deepen cooperation in science and technology in the field of biotechnology; to encourage industrial R&D and related investment flows, bilaterally and/or regionally in the field of biotechnology and to promote transparency through exchange of information and cooperation among relevant institutions. The total grant earmarked is '7.8 Crore with a maximum of up to '2.6 Crore per project spread over three years.
- ☆ 1600 personnel trained under UG, PG training courses.

- ✰ Under Biotechnology Industrial Training Programme (BITP) minimum 2000 candidates will be trained in biotech industries.
- ✰ IP, Entrepreneurship Development (ED) and Grant Writing Workshops – More than 25 workshops have been organized by BIRAC benefiting 1300 stakeholders.

## Market Structure of Biotechnology Industry in India

The biotech industry included either service driven companies, or product driven companies. The net worth of India Biotech Industry is US$ 11.6 billion in 2017.

The growth is due to a range of positive trends such as growing demand for healthcare services, increase demand for food and nutrition intensive R&D activities and strong government initiatives. The government has to invest US$ 5 billion to develop human capital, infrastructure and research initiatives if it is to realise the dream of growing the sector into a US$ 100 billion industry by 2025. The Indian biotech sector is divided into five major segments:

I. Bio Pharmaceutical Sector
II. Bio Services Sector
III. Bio Agricultural Sector
IV. Bio Industrial Sector
V. Bio Informatics Sector

Biopharma is the largest sector contributing about 62 percent of the total revenue followed by bio-services (18 percent), bio-agri (15 percent), bio-industry (4 percent), and bio-informatics contributing (1 percent).

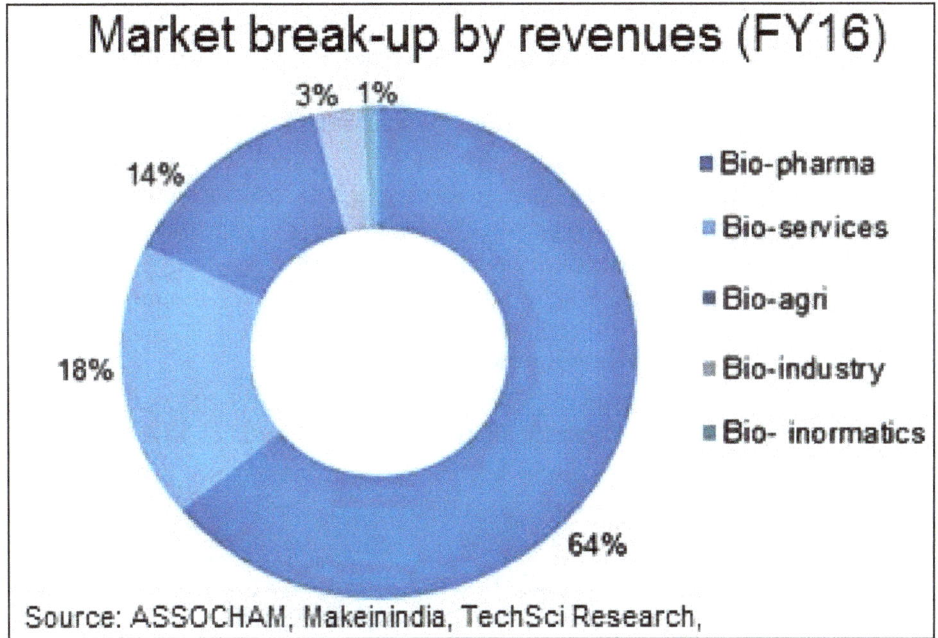

## Major Policy Initiatives of the Government of India

### The Regional Centre for Biotechnology Act, 2016

The Government of India has enacted an Act for the establishment of a Regional Centre for Biotechnology to facilitate transfer of technology and knowledge. The aim is for India to be a biotechnology expertise hub in the Asian region.

### National Intellectual Property Rights Policy 2016 (IPR Policy 2016)

India's National IPR policy was released in May 2016 with an aim to:

- ✰ Generate awareness of IP (Intellectual Property) in the country.
- ✰ To push IPRs as a marketable financial asset this will promote innovation and entrepreneurship in the country.

### National Guidelines for Stem Cell Research 2013

- ✰ The guidelines have been laid down to ensure that research with human stem cells is conducted in a responsible and ethical manner and complies with all regulatory requirements pertaining to biomedical research in general and of stem cell research in particular.
- ✰ These guidelines apply to all stakeholders including individual researchers, organisations, sponsors, oversight/regulatory committees and any other associated with both basic and clinical research on all types of human stem cells and their derivatives

### Guidelines on Similar Biologics-Regulatory Requirements for Marketing Authorization in India 2012

- ✰ The Guidelines on Similar Biologics prepared by the Central Drugs Standard Control Organization (CDSCO) and the Department of Biotechnology (DBT) lay down the regulatory pathway for a biologic claiming to be similar to an already authorised reference biologic.
- ✰ The guidelines address the regulatory pathway regarding the manufacturing process and quality aspects for similar biologics.
- ✰ These guidelines also address the pre-market regulatory requirements including a comparability exercise for quality, preclinical and clinical studies and post-market regulatory requirements for similar biologics.

### National Biotechnology Development Strategy 2015

The National Biotechnology Development Strategy 2015-2020 was launched on December 30, 2015. The Strategy intends to establish India as a world class bio manufacturing hub by:

- ✰ Providing impetus to utilizing the knowledge and tools to the advantage of humanity.
- ✰ Launching a major well directed mission backed with significant investment for generation of new Biotech Products.

- Establishing a strong infrastructure for R&D and Commercialization.
- Creating India as a world class Bio-manufacturing Hub.

**Ease of Doing Business initiatives**

Government has taken several initiatives under ease of doing business to promote the sector:

- Norms for import and export of human biological samples have been relaxed; no license required to import or export biological samples with effect from 4th August, 2016.
- A 'Make in India' Facilitation Cell (Biotechnology) at BIRAC has been established for hand holding investors and to enable dissemination of Government policies.

**FDI Policy**

- 100 per cent Foreign Direct Investment (FDI) is allowed under the automatic route for greenfield pharma.
- 100 per cent Foreign Direct Investment (FDI) is allowed under the government route for brown field pharma in up to 74 per cent FDI is under automatic route and beyond 74 per cent is under government approval route.
- FDI up to 100 per cent is allowed under the automatic route for the manufacturing of medical devices.

**Intellectual Property Rights of Biotechnology: Regulatory Framework in India**

Approval for Manufacture and Marketing (Currently, there are multiple regulators, multiple ministries, lack of coordination, lack of a linear progression in the responsibilities of a regulator and lack of a linear progression in the approval process and committees working outside their areas of expertise).

## Proposals to Streamline the Process

- The Institutional Bio-Safety Committee will monitor all development work (up to 20 liters) and recommend to RCGM for Animal Toxicity Tests (ATT) and Scale Up.
- Review Committee on Genetic Manipulation (RCGM) will evaluate the recombinant technology and grant permission for scale up – R&D, review and approve for pre-clinical animal toxicity tests and evaluate ATT data and recommend to DCGI for Human Clinical Trial (HCT).
- Drug Controller General of India (DCGI) will permit Human Clinical Trials, review Human Clinical Trial Data, grant permission for Manufacture and Marketing of the product and inspect the facility where the product is manufactured.
- Genetic Engineering Approval Committee (GEAC) will review the manufacturing process to ensure that the LMO (Living Modified Organism)

is "inactivated" during the process and send its recommendations to the Drugs Controller General of India within the specified time.

**Key Achievements during the Last Two Years are**

- ☆ Current Good Manufacturing Practices (CGMP) Plant inaugurated at CSIR-IIIM, Jammu in October 2016, has world-class infrastructure for the manufacture of phyto pharmaceuticals.
- ☆ India's first cellulosic ethanol technology demonstration plant developed through indigenous technology was inaugurated on April 22, 2016.
- ☆ A virtual centre was launched across five Indian Institutes of Technology, Mumbai, Kharagpur, Guwahati, Jodhpur, and Roorkee, on September 3, 2015, to develop advance technologies in the area of biofuels.
- ☆ 30 Bioincubators and Biotech Parks supported/established during April 2014 to Sep 2016.
- ☆ The Rotavirus vaccine 'Rotavac' is the first indigenously developed as well as manufactured recombinant vaccine launched in 2015.

## Discussion

With the country offering numerous comparative advantages in terms of R&D facilities, knowledge, skills, and cost effectiveness, the biotechnology industry in India has immense potential to emerge as a global key player.

India constitutes around 8 percent of the total global generics market, by volume, indicating a huge untapped opportunity in the sector. Outsourcing to India is projected to spike up after the discovery and manufacture of formulations. Hybrid seeds, including GM seeds, represent new business opportunities in India based on yield improvement.

India would work towards achieving its target of $100 billion Biotech Industry by 2025 and also capturing 5 per cent of the Global Bio pharmaceutical market share. The Mission will be designed in a manner in which it addresses the key components of the vision outlined in the National Missions –'Make in India' and 'Start up India' and also aims to take forward the commitments made by DBT in the National Biotechnology Development Strategy.

India currently has a marginal share in the global market for industrial enzymes. Hence, there is an opportunity in focused R&D and knowledge-based innovation in the field of industrial enzymes, which can innovatively replace chemical-polluting processes into eco-friendly processes that also deliver environmental sustainability. Another interesting field of study is the area of bio-markers and companion diagnostics, which will enable optimal benefits of biotech drugs.

## REFERENCES

1. Department of Biotechnology 2017. 'Biotechnology: Research Development and Demonstration: Thrust Areas', Government of India, New Delhi.

2. Department of Biotechnology Annual Report 2015-16 and 2016-17. Ministry of Science and Technology, Government of India, New Delhi.
3. Ministry of Science and Technology 2017. National Biotechnology Development Program 'Biotech 2015'.
4. BCIL 2001. Directory of Biotechnology Industries and Institutions in India, Biotech Consortium India Limited, New Delhi.
5. Lall, Sanjay 1992. 'Technological Capabilities and Industrialisation', World Development, 20: 165-186.
6. Ministry of Information and Broadcasting, 2015. Press Information Bureau (PIB), Media Reports and Press Releases, Department of Industrial Policy and Promotion (DIPP), Department of Biotechnology,
7. Ministry of Finance, 2017. Union Budget 2017-18 http: //indiabudget.nic.in/.
8. Biotechnology Achievement Report, 2017. Details available at: http: //www.makeinindia.com/sector/biotechnology.
9. Wahab, Seema 1998. 'Biotechnology and Economic of IPM in India' in Biotechnology and Development Review (BDR), Vol. 2 No.1, October.
10. Kumar, Nagesh 1988. "Biotechnology in India", Development (Special issue on Biotechnology), March.

*Chapter 4*

# The Current Status of Industrial Biotechnology in Nigeria

***Deborah Asabe Ashigye***

*Raw Materials Research and Development Council (RMRDC)*
*No. 17 Aguiyi Ironsi Street, Maitama, PMB 232 Garki, Abuja*
*E-mail: debashig@gmail.com*

## ABSTRACT

The application of biotechnology to industrial processes is not only transforming how we manufacture products but is also providing us with new products that could not even be imagined a few years ago. Because industrial biotechnology is so new, its benefits are still not well known or understood by industry, policymakers, or consumers. This is especially true in Nigeria, where not much progress has been made in the industrial biotechnology sector. The National Biosafety Agency Bill was signed in 2015, which is a milestone in the domestication of modern biotechnology in Nigeria – a giant stride that allows the country to join the league of countries advanced in the use of this cutting-edge technology as another window to boost economic development. The paper analyses the current status of industrial biotechnology in Nigeria through the review of online publications and relevant websites. Activities of the major government agencies involved in value addition and beneficiation in the sector are discussed, these include: the National Biotechnology Development Agency (NABDA); National Biosafety Management Agency (NBMA); Sheda Science and Technology Complex (SHESTCO); and Raw Materials Research and Development Council (RMRDC).

A 2001 Survey of the Status of Agricultural Biotechnology in Selected West and Central African Countries by W.S. Alhassan (IITA) indicated that nearly half of the institutions visited in Nigeria (seventeen) were not considered to have functional biotechnology laboratories due to the lack of stable power supply. Other challenges highlighted in the paper include the inadequate funding and the fact that genetically modified crops/products are not being well accepted by the public.

The paper concludes that Nigeria has a lot to harness from the industrial biotechnology sector in terms of safe, sufficient and environmentally friendly bio-products but a lot of measures have to be put in place to make this a reality.

***Keywords:*** *Biotechnology, Industrial, Agricultural, Genetically modified organisms (GMOs), Biosafety, Raw materials.*

## INTRODUCTION

Industrial biotechnology encompasses the application of biotechnology-based tools to traditional industrial processes ("bioprocessing") and the manufacturing of bio-based products (such as fuels, chemicals and plastics) from renewable feedstock. Microbes, microorganisms, enzymes and their genetic engineering form the basis of a suite of technologies and processes that a diverse group of companies, researchers and scientists are seeking to develop for commercial use.

It is one of the most promising new approaches to pollution prevention, resource conservation, and cost reduction. It is often referred to as the third wave in biotechnology. If developed to its full potential, industrial biotechnology may have a larger impact on the world than health care and agricultural biotechnology. It offers businesses a way to reduce costs and create new markets while protecting the environment. Also, since many of its products do not require the lengthy review times that drug products must undergo, it's a quicker, easier pathway to the market. Today, new industrial processes can be taken from laboratory study to commercial application in two to five years, compared to up to a decade for drugs.

The application of biotechnology to industrial processes is not only transforming how we manufacture products but is also providing us with new products that could not even be imagined a few years ago. Because industrial biotechnology is so new, its benefits are still not well known or understood by industry, policymakers, or consumers. This is especially true in Nigeria, where not much progress has been made in the industrial biotechnology sector, more of the recent advances in biotechnology have been in the agricultural sector.

In 2005, Prof. Turner Isoun, a former Minister of Science and Technology estimated that 15 years from then, 50 per cent of the global economy will be bioeconomy-based, hence, by 2020, any nation which does not align itself economically with biotechnology, may miss out on the rewards of yet another revolution. This statement was made at the 8th international conference of the Nigeria Computer Society (NCS), held in Port Harcourt, Rivers State. Prof. Isoun noted that Nigeria as a nation is endowed with enormous bioresources across all its six main ecological zones, namely mangrove/swamp, rainforests, derived savannah, montane/plateau, savannah and semi-arid. He said that what matters most is how Nigeria uses the new Information Technology (IT) domain of bioinformatics to drive the growth and development of modern biotechnology in the country (Remmy Nweke, 2005).

## Status of Biotechnology in Nigeria

In view of the importance of modern biotechnology, the former president, the National Biosafety Agency Bill was signed in 2015, which is a milestone in the domestication of modern biotechnology in Nigeria – a giant stride that allows the country to join the league of countries advanced in the use of this cutting-edge technology as another window to boost economic development in Nigeria. The bill is expected to create more employment, boost food production that will put a smile on the faces of farmers and elevate hunger if given good attention by government.

The National Biosafety Act is crucial in the management of Modern Biotechnology in the country. Modern Biotechnology has been identified as an important tool that can help countries to achieve food sufficiency/food security, industrial growth, health improvement and environmental sustainability while the Biosafety Act will give the legal framework to check the activities of modern biotechnology locally as well as imported GM crops into the country as well as providing avenue to engage Nigerian scientists/experts from different fields to identify and pursue solutions to our local challenges.

According to Nkechi Isaac (2017) Nigeria marked a number of biotechnology milestones in 2016, and 2017 promises even more advancements. The country's National Biosafety Management Agency (NBMA) approved the general release and marketing of Bt cotton in 2016, as well as confined field trials of Bt maize. The year also witnessed massive enlightenment and awareness workshops that engaged Nigerians on a personal and corporate level. These engagements also saw the highest attendance to date of policy makers at an expert roundtable organized by the National Biotechnology Development Agency (NABDA). The ministers of agriculture; science and technology; defense, and environment attended this roundtable, as well as the minister of state for environment. The highpoint of the year was the endorsement of genetically modified organisms (GMOs) by Nigeria's reputable, science-based professional body, the Nigerian Academy of Science (NAS). The institution declared that GMOs are beneficial for crop improvement, as well as for improving the overall industrial sector.

Stakeholders in the biotechnology sector are also committed to continue their efforts to engage policy makers, government institutions, councils, professional bodies, religious organizations, individuals and academia in the quest to improve public understanding of the science behind GM crops and ways that modern biotechnology can profitably contribute to the economic development of the country.

## Key Agencies Involved in Advancement of Biotechnology in Nigeria

### National Biotechnology Development Agency (NABDA)

In recognition of the importance of biotechnology to national development, the Federal Executive Council on 23rd of April 2001 approved the National Biotechnology Policy, which led to the establishment of the National Biotechnology Development Agency (NABDA) in November 2001. The Agency was established under the aegis of the Federal Ministry of Science and Technology to implement the policy that is aimed at promoting, coordinating, and setting research and development priority in biotechnology for Nigeria. Based on this premise, the programmes of the agency are structured in line with the international standard bearing in mind the development of local technological contents

It was established with the mandate of promotion, coordination and deployment of cutting-edge biotechnology research and development, processes and products for the socio–economic well-being of the nation. NABDA has through its departments, bio-resource centres and zonal centres of excellence actively been developing viable and commercializable biotechnology. It also has on-going collaborations with relevant international and local agencies such as International Centre for Genetic Engineering and Biotechnology (ICGEB), Raw Material Research & Development Council (RMRDC), *etc.*

NABDA also hosts the Open Forum on Agricultural Biotechnology in Africa (OFAB) which is Africa's platform that brings together stakeholders in biotechnology and enables interactions between scientists, journalists, the civil society, industrialists, lawmakers and policy makers. In Nigeria, it is a monthly lunch meeting that provides an opportunity for key stakeholders to know one another, share knowledge and experiences, make new contacts and explore new avenues of bringing the benefits of biotechnology to the African agricultural sector (http://www.ofabafrica.org/about-ofabafrica) (Peace Olaito, 2015).

NABDA committed its first fourteen years to ensuring that the National Biosafety law was passed in Nigeria to enable the existence of an institutional framework for the practice of biotechnology, leading to the establishment of the National Biosafety Management Agency. The controversies surrounding transgenic crops, often called Genetically Modified Organisms (GMOs), called for a need to raise the level of public awareness of Genetic Modification (GM) technology in Africa. This is to be accomplished by educating the public about the potential benefits and risks that may be associated with this new technology. To address this challenge, a press release was issued in January, 2017, the Director General of NABDA, spoke about the current status of GMOs in Nigeria. She stated that there are no Genetically Modified food or products currently released for sale in the Nigerian market, explaining that there are only four GM crops currently undergoing field trials in Nigeria, these are:

- White black-eyed beans known as Maruca Resistant Cowpea (Bt Cowpea)
- African Bio-fortified Sorghum
- Water efficient and salt tolerant Rice
- Bt Cotton trial

## National Biosafety Management Agency (NBMA)

The National Biosafety Management Agency (NBMA) was established by the National Biosafety Management Agency Act 2015, to provide regulatory framework to adequately safe guard human health and the environment from potential adverse effects of modern biotechnology and genetically modified organisms, while harnessing the potentials of modern biotechnology and its derivatives, for the benefit of Nigerians. The Act came into force in April 2015, with the appointment of a Director General and Chief Executive Officer. The UN international agreement known as Cartagena Protocol on Biosafety which Nigeria signed is an environment protocol and it requires members to domesticate the agreement through a law. The Biosafety Act is therefore to domesticate the Protocol and address our National Biosafety requirements.

The National Biotechnology Development Agency is sponsoring a biotechnology bill before the National Assembly. Its mandate is to promote biotechnology development in all sectors of the Nigeria economy. It is to promote indigenous acquisition and development of easy and affordable requisite biotechnology in Nigeria and Indigenous R&D to generate copious innovations in biotechnology as well as for the sustenance and growth of the biotech industry.

The National Biosafety Management Agency regulates modern biotechnology activities and the release into the environment, handling and use of genetically modified organisms which are products of modern biotechnology to prevent adverse impact on the environment and human health. On the other hand, the National Biotechnology development Agency promotes modern biotechnology activities and GMOs.

The National Biosafety Management Agency (NBMA) Act 2015 empowers the NBMA to formulate overall policy guidance on issues concerning Biosafety in Nigeria and to implement the National Biosafety Management Agency Act. The Agency reconciles the need for safety of Genetically Modified Organisms (GMOs) in international and national trade as well as biodiversity conservation in order to enhance a rapidly growing modern biotechnology industry in Nigeria for the enhancement of the Nigerian Economy. Essentially, the Agency is charged with responsibility for providing regulatory framework, institutional and administrative mechanisms for safety measures in the application of modern biotechnology in Nigeria, with the view to preventing any adverse effect on human health, animals, plants and environment.

The Agency in addition to its functions regulates activities of Agencies/ Institutes like the National Biotechnology Development Agency, National Cereal Research Institute, Badeggi, Agricultural Research Institute, Zaria, National Root Crops Research Institute, Umudike, Nigeria Institute for Oil Palm Research, Veterinary Research Institute, Jos, Universities, Local and International Companies and organisations that deal on Genetically Modified Organisms (GMOs) *etc.* The Agency approves and monitors the release of GMOs and ensures safety to the environment and human health.

In order to achieve to create more awareness on biosafety issues, NMBA in collaboration with Raw Materials Research and Development Council (RMRDC) organised the 2nd Annual National Biosafety Conference with the theme '**Biosafety, Food Security and Economic Development in Nigeria**' which was held on 10th November, 2016 at 3Js Hotel Utako, Abuja. The conference was aimed at emphasizing the importance of effective biosafety regulation to food security and socio-economic development in the application of modern biotechnology in Nigeria. It was also organized to create a platform for Scientists, Government Institutions, Non-Government Organizations (NGOs) and other stakeholders within and outside the country to cross-fertilise ideas and foster holistic biosafety in Nigeria.

A few of the recommendations made at the conference include:

- NBMA should create more awareness to educate Nigerians on the safety measures put in place for the adoption of modern biotechnology and GMOs in Nigeria.
- Safe adoption of modern biotechnology in Nigeria is vital for the achievement of the second goal of the Sustainable Development Goals which seeks to end hunger, achieve food security, improve nutrition and promote sustainable agriculture.
- NBMA and other relevant organizations should fund research in the field of biosafety and findings of such research presented at future biosafety conferences to stimulate scientific discussions.

## Sheda Science and Technology Complex (SHESTCO)

The Sheda Science and Technology Complex (SHESTCO) is a parastatal under the Nigerian Ministry of Science and Technology. It is a multidisciplinary research and development establishment located about 70 km from Abuja, Nigeria.

SHESTCO was established by the Federal Government of Nigeria in 1993. The complex has three well-equipped laboratories for biotechnology, chemistry and physics, and a Nuclear Technology Centre with a gamma irradiation plant. Although Nigeria does not yet have any commercial production of biotechnology crops, SHESTCO has the capacity to conduct and apply biotechnology research.

Recently, the Biotechnology Advanced Research Centre of SHESTCO won a grant from the International Centre for Genetic Engineering and Biotechnology (ICGEB) to organise an international training workshop titled "Techniques in Molecular Biology and Genetic Engineering of plants and Bacteria" September 19 – 30, 2016.

The workshop was designed to equip participants with the understanding and skills to carry out techniques in modern day biotechnology and to have practical experience on how to generate transgenic plant and bacteria.

RMRDC also supported the organisers of the workshop and I am glad to say that I was one of the participants.

## Raw Materials Research and Development Council (RMRDC)

The Raw Materials Research and Development Council (RMRDC) is an agency under the Federal Ministry of Science and Technology charged with the mandate of developing Nigeria's raw materials into industrial inputs. Over the years, RMRDC has been a key player in driving value addition and beneficiation of biotechnological Nigeria through its six core programmes as listed below:

**Local Raw Materials Content Development Programme**

- ☆ Raw materials deletion programme
- ☆ National raw materials policy
- ☆ Boosting of agricultural raw materials *e.g.* sesame, sorghum, tomato, *etc.*

**Technology Development Programme**

- ☆ Upgrading indigenous technologies for processing raw materials *e.g.* Kilishi (dried meat), shea butter production, *etc.*
- ☆ Establishment of pilot plants for some successful R&D projects
- ☆ Computer-aided processing equipment design
- ☆ Capacity building for design of process equipment and plants

**International Collaboration**

RMRDC is the focal point for Nigeria in its collaboration with organisation like

- ☆ World Association of Industrial and Technological Research Organisations (WAITRO),
- ☆ Pan African Competitiveness Forum (PACF),
- ☆ Action Committee on Raw Materials (G-77),
- ☆ G 15 Project "Collaboration on the Development and Utilization of Non-Met allic Mineral Raw Materials" and of course NAM S&T Centre.

**National Raw Materials Research and Development Programme**

- ☆ Research and Development projects in all industrial sectors (Grant scheme)
- ☆ Raw materials quality reference laboratories (we are currently equipping a reference laboratory at African University of Science and Technology, Abuja)
- ☆ New and Advanced Materials – an information portal for new and advanced materials is being maintained by the Advanced Materials Division, in addition to on-going R&D researches.

**Raw Materials Processing Clusters Programme**

- ☆ Investment promotion in all industrial sectors using cluster approach
- ☆ Investors fora and brokerage services

**Raw Materials Information Programme**

- ☆ Raw materials information system (RMIS)
- ☆ Raw materials resource centres in each of the 36 States of Nigeria and in Abuja
- ☆ Raw materials update magazine and Journal of raw materials research
- ☆ Techno-economic surveys

Over the years RMRDC has directly or indirectly supported the development of biotechnology in Nigeria through its collaborations. Some of these collaborations have been with sister agencies under the Federal Ministry of Science and Technology. Some examples are:

1. The ICGEB 2016 course tagged "Techniques in Molecular Biology and Genetic Engineering of Plants and Bacteria", September 19 – 30, 2017
2. Inception Workshop of the National Biosafety Management Agency, August, 2015
3. Second National Biosafety Conference in collaboration with NBMA, April, 2016
4. Sensitization workshop on the establishment of microbial culture collection in Nigeria titled "Microbial Culture Collection as a Critical Biological Resource for National Development", October, 2014, in collaboration with NABDA

## Challenges

A 2001 Survey of the Status of Agricultural Biotechnology in Selected West and Central African Countries by W.S. Alhassan (IITA) indicated that nearly half of the institutions visited in Nigeria (seventeen) were considered to have non-functional biotechnology laboratories due to the lack of stable power supply. Of the fourteen laboratories using tissue culture, only five were considered to be functional on the basis of stable power supply and possession of the minimal required equipment. The hardest hits were the university laboratories, none of which qualified for operation under the set criteria. None of the seven institutions whose laboratories do fermentation was regarded to have the minimum facilities for work in this field. The worst hit was the area of molecular biology. Only three of the eleven institutions with molecular biology laboratories were minimally equipped to carry out research in the field as per the established criteria. Thus, for the Nigerian institutions surveyed, only 36 per cent of those working in tissue culture, 29 per cent of those in fermentation, and 27 per cent of those in molecular biology had minimum facilities to qualify in the respective fields. In terms of laboratory infrastructure, the Nigerian situation was easily the worst in the region. In contrast, however, the manpower situation was easily the best in the region.

Unfortunately, this is still the story for most of our institutions. There is constraint of:

- Adequate infrastructure
- Modern Equipment
- In a few cases adequate manpower and the technological knowhow to operate sophisticated equipment

In addition to the above, other constraints include:

- Lack of appropriate policy guiding development of industrial biotechnology

- Inadequacy of funding for biotechnology-related research and development. This is perhaps a reflection of the generally low funding of scientific research
- Inadequate commercialization of research findings
- Genetically modified crops/products are not being well accepted by the public

## Future Prospects

Industrial biotechnology is a key technology for future economic development. It is the application of biotechnology to the eco-efficient production and processing of chemicals, materials and bio-energy. It utilises the extraordinary capabilities of micro-organisms and enzymes, and their diversity, efficiency and specificity, to make products in sectors such as chemicals, food and feed, pulp and paper, textiles, automotive, electronics and, crucially, energy. Many economies recognise this potential; this was made clear during the 2004 meeting of Science and Technology Ministers of the OECD countries plus China and South Africa (OECD, 2011)

The outlook for industrial biotechnology is promising owing to the timely convergence of drivers of industrial biotechnology with the unprecedented progress in the biological sciences. The barriers are many, and they have to be tackled through national, regional and internationally harmonised policy.

Nigeria is obviously lagging behind in the area of industrial biotechnology; more effort has been given to Agricultural Biotechnology. A lot of awareness therefore needs to be created for a more holistic approach to biotechnological development. Everyone has a part to play - government, researchers, industry and private institutions have to catch up with the worldwide industrial biotechnology era.

## Conclusions/Recommendations

In conclusion, I would like to state that Nigeria has a lot of potential to tap from the industrial biotechnology sector in terms of safe, sufficient and environmentally friendly bio-products but a lot of measures have to be put in place (infrastructure, funding, *etc.*) to make this a reality.

It is therefore my humble recommendation that followings steps should be taken:

- The deplorable state of laboratory infrastructure should be addressed forthwith. Recourse to a bilateral or multilateral donor should be made for immediate funding.
- Alongside the donor support, a sustainable funding mechanism, such as commodity levying for research support, should be put in place. Research institutions should also be made to link up with the private sector to commercialize any of their available technology.
- A means of ensuring stable power supply and other infrastructure must be determined.

- Government should adequately fund research in Nigeria so that science and technology can contribute to the economic development of the country.
- The controversies surrounding transgenic crops, often called Genetically Modified Organisms (GMOs), call for a need to raise the level of public awareness of Genetic Modification (GM) technology in Africa.
- Introduce a long-term, stable and transparent policy and incentive framework to promote the bio-economy
- Relevant government agencies and the organised private sector should be engaged to establish industrial biotechnology clusters for rapid development of bio-resources in the country.

## References

1. Ademola A. Alenle, 2011. Response to Issues on GM Agriculture in Africa: Are Transgenic Crops Safe? *BMC Research Notes*, 2011, Volume 4, Number 1,page 1, 8 Oct 2011
2. Alhassan, W.S., 2001. The Status of Agricultural Biotechnology in Selected West and Central African Countries, International Institute of Tropical Agriculture Consultative Group on International Agricultural Research, International Institute of Tropical Agriculture (IITA), www.iita.org, pp 15 – 17, ISBN 978-131-195-9, printed in Nigeria by IITA
3. Brent Erickso, Janet E. Nelson and Paul Winters 2012. Perspective on Opportunities in Industrial Biotechnology in Renewable Chemicals, *BiotechhnolJ*.2012 Feb; 7 (2): 176 - 185
4. Nkechi Isaac, 2017. Nigeria's 2017. Prospects for Biotechnology, published in Leadership Newspaper, Nigeria, Tuesday, January 17, 2017,
5. Peace Olaito, 2015. Nigeria's Agricultural Biotechnology Annual, Lagos Nigeria, 2-12-2015, Global Agricultural Information Network (GAIN) Report, pp 3 - 4
6. Remmy Nweke, 2005. Nigeria's Fate in Biotechnology, *http: //www.scienceinafrica. com*(accessed June 20, 2017)

*Chapter 5*

# The Use of Biotechnology in Zambia

***Lordwell K. Witika and Jonas Mundike***

***University of Zambia, School of Mines,***
***Department of Met allurgy and Mineral Processing, Zambia***
***E-mail: lwitika@unza.zm***

## ABSTRACT

Biotechnology can play an essential role in fostering the economic and social development of developing countries like Zambia. Biotechnology applications are used to enhance cultural and biomolecular processes to develop technologies and products that help improve our lives and health in Zambia. Recent advances in biotechnology are helping us to prepare society's most pressing challenges in developing countries like Zambia. Zambia has embarked on increasing production of biofuels in supplementing fuel needs the using biotechnology. There is an urgent need to invest and benefit from the promise of Biotechnology. Various benefit of the technology include using living micro-organisms for extraction of valuable metals from low grade sulphide ores. In Zambia, this technology has been applied in many areas such as mining, waste management, environmental conservation and in agriculture applications. Bioleaching is an emerging technology with significant potential to add value to the mining industry and other important industries so as to deliver attractive environmental and economic benefits. Biotechnology, can be used in processing various low-grade ores such as copper, lead, gold and other useful materials and minerals. From literature, low grade secondary copper sulphide ores are easily processed using this technology. The geology and mineralization of Zambian Copper Mines have revealed that Zambia has substantial amount of sulphide and oxide mineral ores which can be treated using this technology by way of value addition and hence contribution to the revenue generation in form of foreign exchange for boosting the country's economy.

Zambia has made tremendous progress in using this technology to treat human and animal wastes and natural resources such as hyacinth or Kafue weed, chicken dropping, cow, pig and goat-dung mixture to produce biogas in cone-closed gas collector and has proved to be viable for domestic and industrial use to reduce the heavy dependence on fossil fuels.

Bioleaching is well applied in the pre-treatment of refractory gold ores before they are subjected to the cyanidation process. Lumwana Mine in Solwezi, in North Western Province in Zambia uses this method.

Escalating prices of fuel sources require that alternative forms are explored. The Jatropha seedcake could be a better alternative for charcoal and a good raw material for bio-gas production. Glycerine, as a by-product is a good raw material in the soap and pharmaceutical industries While the bio-diesel derived from jatropha can directly be used in diesel engines (B100) or blended with fossil-diesel.

Palm oil yields are the highest per hectare among all oil plants, far much better than Jatropha. It is both a food and bio-energy crop. Although it requires much better soils and more water than Jatropha, Palm oil plantations could support mixed farming, where livestock may be raised, as they feed on green fodder, grown as a cover crop. The palm kernel oil cake is a protein-rich food suitable for livestock feed and the oil is a more favourable bio-energy crop for the northern regions of Zambia, capable of producing good quality bio-diesel.

Sugar cane is a good substrate possibility for bio-ethanol production in Zambia. It has a high energy ratio, around 8:1, and is both a bio-fuel and a food crop. Mazabuka in Zambia, is host to Zambia Sugar Company which produces the crop and process it in sugar.

Sweet sorghum, finger millet and other related millets have high water-use efficiency due to their drought resistant characteristics, rendering them more suitable for drier regions of the country.

***Keywords:*** *Biotechnology, Jatropha, Palm oil, Sugar cane, Bioleaching, Genetically modified organisms, Bioethanol.*

## INTRODUCTION

Bio-energy comes from any fuel that is derived from biomass. It is the utilization of solar energy that has been bound up in biomass during the process of photosynthesis and is a renewable form of energy. There are four main sources of biomass: forestry and agricultural residues, municipal solid wastes, industrial wastes, and specifically grown bio-energy crops. The common examples of bio-fuels include *bio-gas* produced from biomass by anaerobic digestion, *bio-ethanol* derived from fermentation of mainly sugar and starch crops, *bio-diesel* produced through trans-esterification of plant oil, and *second-generation bio-fuels* produced from cellulosic biomass.

According to Boyle (2004), energy crops have attracted increased attention in recent years, for several different reasons among which include:

(a) The need for alternatives to fossil fuels, to reduce net $CO_2$ emissions
(b) The search for indigenous alternatives to imported oil and
(c) The problem of surplus agricultural land.

Even though Zambia is endowed with renewable energy resources which can sustainably supplement fossil fuels, they have for a long time remained unexploited. The policy is aimed at identifying energy sources which are dependable, at the lowest economic, environmental and social costs. Being a land locked country, transporting either crude oil or refined petroleum products into the country has proved costly for the country.

Presently most of the agricultural resources are under-utilized with only 16 per cent of the estimated 9 million hectares of arable land being cultivated. Zambia has an estimated 25 per cent of the Southern African region's surface water resources. Zambia's agricultural potential can support both food and bio-energy crops, if well planned and managed.

The main potential raw materials of bio-fuels in Zambia are from energy crops like sugar cane, sweet sorghum, palm-oil and Jatropha. Bio-ethanol can be derived from sugar cane and sweet sorghum, while bio-diesel can be derived from palm-oil and Jatropha. All these bio-energy crops can and are being grown in Zambia.

Biotechnology can play an essential role in fostering the economic and social development of developing countries like Zambia. Biotechnology which is based on biology harnesses cellular and biomolecular processes to develop technologies and products that help improve lives and health in Zambia. Zambia needs to invest and benefit from the promise of biotechnology. Recent developments primarily relate to peak oil and the resultant increase in the price of petroleum and also due to environmental concerns (Lewanika and Mulenga, 1995, Kasali, 1993). Jatropha is now at the top of the bio-fuels prospects for Zambia, (Sinkala, 2007). However, sugar cane and sweet sorghum have enormous potential as well, with palm oil becoming more popular in the northern regions of the country.

Experience to date underscores the fact that policies play a critical role in success or failure when expanding bio-energy use (Kimble, *2008*). Bio-fuel policies should address critical issues such as feedstock production methods, transformation technologies, bio-fuel quality standards and testing, pricing mechanism, incentives for bio-fuel usage and favourable tax regimes.

## Jatropha

Jatropha originated from Mexico and Central America, but has spread all over the world and has mostly been used for hedges or live-fencing of gardens in Africa. In the tropics, the plant is widely used as a hedge in fields and settlements. It protects plants against wind erosion and keeps animals out.

In Zambia, its use as a live-hedge or fence was to protect mainly vegetable gardens from domestic animals. As a medicine, it has found its use in treating poisonous snake bites by applying stem sap on the wound. The fruit has been traditionally used for extracting oil, which was used as a hair and body lotion. Jatropha oil can be used for soap making on a small-scale level as well as domestic lighting. The current commercial realization of the potential of bio-diesel potential of Jatropha oil has led to it being considered as an economically viable bio-energy crop.

However, the intended utilization of the plantation may determine the water requirements. Though Jatropha is reported to be drought resistant, its use for oil extraction and ultimately bio-diesel production would require enough water in order to obtain maximum yields with good quality seeds. If Jatropha is meant for hedges or soil erosion control, then directly planted cuttings are the best to use. If however, the plantation is for oil production, then plants propagated by seed are reported to yield much better harvest.

In Zambia small-scale farmers use kraal, chicken and goat manure in their Jatropha fields. The direct use of chemical fertilizer in Jatropha fields is not yet practiced both on small-scale or commercial level.

Although Jatropha is adapted to low fertility sites and alkaline soils, better yields seem to be obtained on poor quality soils if fertilizers containing small amounts of calcium, magnesium, and sulphur are used.

Among small-scale farmers, intercropping Jatropha with food crops is practiced. No specific intolerance with other crops has been reported so far. On the contrary the shade can be exploited by shade-loving herbal vegetable plants such as red and green peppers, tomatoes, *etc.* In Zambia, small-scale farmers inter crop Jatropha with crops like groundnuts, maize, cassava and sweet potatoes. However, shade-intolerant crops like groundnuts and maize may not be suitable for intercropping after Jatropha shrubs have grown and expanded in size.

When the Jatropha pods or fruits turn yellowish-brown, then they are ready for harvest. The fruits are manually harvested by hand, and then sun-dried. The fruits become dark brown and open up to release three seeds, when fully dried. Ripening of Jatropha fruits does not have a specific time. Immediately some fruits show signs of ripening, they should be harvested to avoid them dropping on the ground where they may be spoiled or even germinate.

## Palm Oil

Palm oil originated from West Africa. It is cultivated throughout equatorial Africa where the altitude is below 700 metres and the rainfall high. West and central Africa, from southern Senegal to northern Angola is its production belt. The introduction of palm oil into Central and Southern America and Southeast Asia led to the establishment of large, highly productive plantations, to the point where Malaysia now controls the world palm oil market, (Raemaekers, 2001).

Palm oil nursery for young seedlings requires special skills to grow. It may be difficult for a grower to care for a palm oil nursery. Growers usually buy seedlings from nursery experts where the plants already have four or five leaves. These seedlings are transplanted into the palm oil plantation.

Palm oil grows well in very hot regions where there is enough precipitation. The favourable annual temperature is between 25°C to 28°C. Such temperatures promote the production of many leaves which will result into many clusters of fruit. It is important that the growing point of the palm oil tree should produce many leaves, because there will be a flower at the base of each leaf. If there are many leaves, there will be many flowers, which ultimately will result into many clusters of fruit. Plenty of sunshine promotes adequate photosynthesis as more leaves grow big, while the fruits will ripen well, resulting into more oil in the fruits. Palm oil grows well in deep soils due to its deep root system and therefore favours water retaining soils. If the temperature drops, the palm oil produces fewer leaves and becomes susceptible to disease attacks.

The fruits of the palm oil consist of the pulp, which is yellow and when crushed yields palm oil. Inside the pulp is the seed, and inside the shell of the seed is the kernel. When the kernel is crushed, it yields palm kernel oil as well. The kernel also contains the germ.

According to Raemaekers (2001), industrial plantations are productive for 20 to 25 years, depending on local environmental conditions. Harvesting usually stops when the yield falls to about 60 – 65 per cent of normal yield. The fall in yield is linked to harvesting difficulties because of the trees' height (more than 13 metres tall).

Harvesting itself comprises cutting the palm oil bunches and taking them to the pick-up points along the harvest collection paths. Plantations of selected palm oil begin producing fruit in their fourth year.

There are two main methods of oil extraction from the palm fruits, the traditional method and the oil mill extraction. With traditional methods, a lot of oil is left in the pulp and the kernels. The industrial process involves extraction of almost all the oil contained in the pulp and separating the palm kernel.

## Sugar Cane

Sugar cane is grown as a perennial plant and can be cut 10 times in succession depending upon the fertility of the site and the care with which it is grown. Two to three weeks after harvesting, the stumps shoot again, producing the ratoon crop. In Africa, Nigeria, South Africa, Mauritius, Swaziland, Uganda and Zambia are among the main growers of sugar cane.

In tropical Africa, planting, crop maintenance, cutting and loading are often done by hand and it is only soil preparation, transporting the harvested cane and sometimes fertilization that are mechanized. Sugar cane is reproduced vegetatively from cuttings. These consist of sections of cane stalks 30 – 35 cm in length, which are soaked in water at about 52°C to which a fungicide has been added by way of disease control. To plant a hectare requires about 20, 000 to 24, 000 cuttings, or in other words, from 6.5 to 7.5 tonnes of cane stripped of its leaf sheaths (Raemaekers, 2001).

The water requirements of the sugar cane depend primarily on the climatic conditions and the vegetative growth stage the crop has reached. In tropical areas, the water requirements will be in the order of 1, 500 – 1, 800 mm per year, with monthly values varying between 100 and 150 mm. Sugar cane may tolerate a dry period of 3 to 4 months, but yields may fall appreciably if the crop is still in the vegetative stage. Irrigation is often needed to bridge the dry season and to complement an awkward monthly rainfall distribution, (Raemaekers, 2001). Irrigation is almost not used in sugar cane production when the precipitation is around 2140 mm per year and the evapo-transpiration is 1657 mm per annum, (Smeets, 2008).

The harvest starts at the time of physiological ripeness of the cane, that is, when the sugar content in the stalk is at its peak. A yellowing of the leaves and a swelling of the eyes will serve as a guide to ripeness, but the most reliable criterion for deciding when to cut is still to determine chemically the sucrose and invert sugar content, (Raemaekers, 2001). The cane will ripen somewhere between 10 and 24 months after planting. Harvesting will be done in the course of the dry season. Cane is cut by hand using a machete or mechanically using a cutter loader. According to Smeets (2008), manual cutting of sugar cane has the disadvantage of the emission of $CO_2$ when burning. Therefore, the harvesting without cane burning is the best option. The leaves are burnt in order to clear the thickets and make it easier to cut.

The cane sugar manufacturing process consists in separating the sucrose from all the rest (ligneous material, water and impurities). Several operations are involved, the main ones being, extraction, clarification, evaporation, crystallization and centrifuging, in that order. Both brown and white sugar crystals are used in the food industry commercially and domestically. Molasses may be used as fertilizer due to its high potash content, used in ethanol production, vinegar and acetic acid. It may be used in livestock feed formulations. The bagasse may be used for various purposes, either directly or indirectly as a fuel and as a power source at the sugar refinery factory. It may also be used for enriching and fertilizing the soil, in livestock feed (in combination with molasses and urea) or in fibrous products (paper pulps, wrapping paper, cardboard, fibre-board and chipboard (Raemaekers, 2001).

Ethanol from sugar cane has been proved to be a better fuel than gasoline concerning emissions of Greenhouse Gases (GHGs) and improving air quality in urban centres, (Goldemberg, 2008). Ethanol blended with gasoline reduces or eliminates the use of lead and of aromatic hydrocarbons (such as benzene), and reduces the emissions of sulphur and carbon monoxide (CO).

Ethanol has less energy value per volume if compared with gasoline (33 per cent); however, it has a higher octane number and can be used in motors with a higher compression ratio (12 to 1, versus 8 to 1). The result is a motor 15 per cent more efficient using ethanol than gasoline. This compensates the lower energy content, and in resume, ethanol needs about 20 per cent more volume than gasoline per kilometer, (Goldemberg, 2008).

In best cases scenarios of increasing production of ethanol from sugar cane from different countries, it could replace as much as 10 per cent of all gasoline used in the world in the next 15-20 years, (Goldemberg, 2008).

The output/input energy balance from sugar cane production depends on the technology and methodology applied in its production. In the worst case, with cane burning, the ratio is around 5. With the cogeneration of heat and electricity from sugar cane leaves (barbojo) and bagasse (using gasification process) and mechanical harvesting without burning, this ratio can reach up to 15 (*Smeets, 2008*).

## Sweet Sorghum

Since Sweet sorghum is very similar in appearance and agronomic performance to grain sorghum, it is easy to plant sweet sorghum in many Africa countries, which have a potential production of grain sorghum. Nigeria and Sudan are among the five leading producers of sorghum in the world (ICRISAT media, 2008).

Sweet sorghum is a plant that looks more or less like maize with a height of 8 to 12 feet. It is also very similar in appearance and agronomic performance to grain sorghum. It is one of the many types of cultivated sorghum and is characterized by high sugar content in juice of stem. Sweet sorghum grows rapidly and it takes about 4.5 months, and can be followed by a ratoon crop (natural second re-growth from stubble after the first crop is harvested (ICRISAT, 2007).

Sweet sorghum is mainly grown for its grain and fodder. Its stalks are very important as fodder for cattle and goats. Currently, it is also considered as an ideal new smart bio-fuel crop that insures food security. This is mainly because it can be used as food (human consumption), feed (chicken, goat, cattle) and as bio-fuel crop to produce ethanol (Tamil Nadu Agricultural University, 2003). In general, Sorghum production can be separated into grains (for consumption, livestock feed, ethanol production), sugar juice (extracted from the cane and used for ethanol production), and stover (stalks and leaves) for fodder, for energy production, and plastics) (Michael, 2006).

The process of making ethanol from sweet sorghum is simple. The sorghum stalks are crushed yielding sweet juice that is fermented and distilled to obtain bio-ethanol, a clean burning fuel with a high-octane rating (ICRISAT media, 2008). The crushed stalks, called bagasse, can also be burned to provide energy for the distillery.

Sweet sorghum has positive energy balance, producing about 8 units of energy for every unit of energy invested in its cultivation and production, roughly equivalent to sugarcane but four times more than for maize. Only 0.8 unit of energy is produced in fossil fuel production for every unit of energy invested (ICRISAT media, 2008).

Cassava is widely and increasingly used to produce ethanol and food stuff in Zambia. The crop is now produced in large quantities is Luapula province.

In Zambia trials in making wine from some indigenous fruit such as masuku and mpundu have been carried out (Alian and Musenge, 1977). As these wines can be processed on commercial scale, a study of these wines during fermentation and aging was taken and was found to be very successful. The rate of yeast of the sugar in both fruit has also been determined and was found that the sugars preferred by yeast were much more in the mpundu juice than in the masuku fruit which gave better wine(Alian *et al.*, 1978).

## Discussion

The main challenges with bio-energy crop development in Zambia are land use practices and availability, food price implications of bio-fuels, water demands or requirements, historical dependence on fossil fuels and lack of an organized structure and market in the bio-fuel sector.

According to Jumbe (2007), the persistent petroleum price increases, which have put pressure on foreign exchange resources and slowed down economic development, have in turn stimulated Sub-Saharan African countries to diversify their energy sources to achieve energy independence.

Lack of meaningful development in rural areas could be a drawback in the development of the bio-energy sector. Due to historical dependence on fossil fuels for a long time, there has been lack of an organized structure (production, sales and consumption) in the bio-fuel sector, lack of infrastructure like better roads to farms, and lack of adequate national policies on bio-fuels. However, as Jumbe (2007), reports, "despite the tariffs and other incentives that have been put in place in the developed world to promote bio-fuels, investors from these countries are rushing to the developing countries to invest in bio-fuels production". It is hoped that multi-national companies may drag along development to bio-energy plantations, as they invest in bio-energy crop farms.

Land competition between food and bio-energy crops is a great challenge, which is country specific in nature. Some countries may have available arable land while others may not. In certain instances, land may be available, and yet lacking in both irrigation and adequate precipitation. In Zambia, for example, only about 15 per cent of arable land is in use, while only 5 per cent of irrigatable land is in use (Chizyuka, 2007).

Water requirements of bio-energy crops depend on each particular crop. The water requirements could be satisfied in form of irrigation or precipitation. Where rain is inadequate, irrigation becomes a substitute, but where both are lacking, then it is not viable to grow any bio-energy crop. However, Sweet sorghum water requirements are moderate and flexible, while sugar cane is relatively high and evenly distributed throughout the growing season. Jatropha is more drought resistant in that it can withstand dry spells for at least 2 years. Palm oil grows well in high rainfall regions.

Environmental degradation resulting from use of fossil fuels is a global problem. Bio-energy crops are much safer than fossil fuels in terms of release of greenhouse gases ($CO_2$). According to Smeets (2008), burning a cubic meter of sugar cane before harvesting, releases 500 kg $CO_2$ equivalents per cubic-metre, while the same area absorbs 750 kg $CO_2$ equivalents per cubic-metre, resulting into a net gain of 250 kg $CO_2$ equivalents per cubic-metre. Moreover, the move to bio-fuels will also create opportunities for carbon trading for many African countries like Zambia. According to Abdrabbo (2008), Jatropha is a valuable multi-purpose crop to alleviate soil degradation, desertification and deforestation, which can be used for bio-energy to replace petro-diesel, for soap production and climatic protection, and hence deserves specific attention.

Food price implications of bio-fuels are connected to the fact that the same feed stocks for bio-fuels are the same sources for food products. Sugar cane for example provides sugar for consumption and bio-ethanol as a bio-fuel. According to Jumbe (2007), "since feed stocks for bio-fuel production are also key ingredients for processed foods; products containing refined sugar, high fructose corn syrup, and partially hydrogenated soybean or canola oil, amongst others, these products will become more expensive for food manufacturers to produce which will be transferred to consumers". However, Jatropha is not affected being non-edible and also sweet sorghum, since the grain is separate from the stalk, where bio-ethanol is derived.

Energy output input ratio for bio-fuels should always be positive for the industry to be viable and sustainable. If the energy needed to produce the bio-fuel is higher or equal to the output of energy then that crop is not suitable and profitable. One of the major drawbacks of maize from USA, for example, is that the ratio is closer to 1. On the other hand sugar cane has an average ratio of 8, (Smeets, 2008). Sweet sorghum has a similar ratio to that of sugar cane.

It is hoped and expected that the bio-energy sector will positively impact on income and poverty for the rural farming community in Zambia. In the 2007 report by Jumbe, modern bio-energy in its many forms holds promise for new jobs and income creation opportunities for rural farmers, foresters, and labourers, as well as improved access to quality energy services. Since nearly one-half of the labour force in developing countries is employed in agriculture, this boost to incomes could have significant effects on the purchasing power of rural people; thus the bio-fuels sector could address some of the poverty in developing countries. There are potential benefits for agricultural and rural development, including new jobs and income generation, which would undoubtedly help meet the Millennium Development Goals.

The economic activities from bio-fuels will add value to a chain of other related developments. According to Sinkala (2007), Jatropha can, among other things, contribute to poverty reduction through both the creation of income generation activities for various players along the value chain and the provisions of solutions to local village level or rural energy needs thereby making these communities more productive. It can also contribute to reforestation activities as it is a tree. In addition, according to Jumbe (2007), "a study commissioned in 2003 by *Earth-life Africa* showed that an economy creates more jobs when it invests in the bio-fuels industry than in fossil fuel energy production."

The increased demand for bio-fuels in developed countries holds hope for the economies of Sub-Saharan African countries. According to Christodoulou (2007), the Swedish government for instance, decided to be totally fossil fuel independent by 2020. Furthermore, the cheap African labour market has a comparative advantage in the production of labour-intensive bio-energy crops. Locally, the high population in Africa also assures a ready market for bio-fuels. Ultimately, the promotion and use of bio-fuels in Africa would reduce import bills for energy-deficient countries and offer improved balance of trade and balance of payments.

Production costs for bio-fuels in Zambia are still in their infancy. Since many bio-energy crops are still in the early stages of development and research, the costs are still very high. However, according to Goldemberg (2008), the Brazilian experience shows that in a long-term bio-fuels can be competitive even better than fossil fuels.

## Conclusions

Jatropha can be grown on poor soils, though higher yields can be achieved on better soils. Since Jatropha is a tree that keeps growing for more than 30 years, it can be used to prevent soil erosion from wind and water agents. This is a better way of reducing or minimizing desertification and deforestation. Equally, disused agricultural land can be reclaimed back by growing Jatropha on it. The seedcake resulting from oil extraction can be made into heating pellets, a better replacement for charcoal. It is also a very good substrate for bio-gas production, good as green manure due to its high nitrogen content and may be used as animal feed after detoxification.

Glycerine, a by-product from the process of transesterification, can be used for soap and cosmetic production in the pharmaceutical industry. Being a non-edible bio-energy crop, it does not compete with food crops. During the early years, intercropping can be practiced to boost food security at family level. Its flowers are very attractive to honey-bees. The water requirements of Jatropha can be satisfied through rain from 500 mm, rendering it one of the best bio-diesel crops for Zambia. The bio-diesel can directly be used in diesel engines (B100) or blended with fossil-diesel. It can also be used for domestic lighting as well as in electricity generator sets.

Palm oil is a more favourable bio-energy crop for the northern regions of Zambia, capable of producing good quality bio-diesel. It requires enough precipitation, much more than Jatropha. Its raw oil is both useful in the food industry as well as a raw material for bio-diesel. Palm oil yields are the highest per hectare among all oil plants. Palm oil plantations could support mixed farming, where livestock may be raised, as they feed on green fodder, grown as a cover crop. The palm kernel oil cake is a protein-rich food suitable for livestock feed.

Sugar cane is a good possibility for bio-ethanol production in Zambia. Due to its high water demands for irrigation and the use of chemical fertilizers, production costs are comparatively higher than Sweet sorghum. Another important advantage of this crop is its high energy ratio, around 8:1, and the fact that it can be used both for fuel and food production. It is suitable for commercial or large-scale plantations and is capable of absorbing a lot of workers, reducing unemployment. However, the up-coming bio-ethanol industry in Zambia can learn from the well-established industry in Brazil. Environmentally, mature sugar cane per cubic meter absorbs more greenhouse gas ($CO_2$) emissions than is released during harvesting.

Sweet sorghum can be grown on drier regions with less reliable rainfall or irrigation with a short gestation period of 4 – 5 months. It has rapid growth rate, high biomass production, wider adaptation, and has great potential for bio-ethanol production. It is a multi-purpose crop that can be used as food, animal-feed and fuel. This is mainly because bio-ethanol can be produced from its sugar rich stalk and the by-product from the ethanol production could be a good source of animal feed. This could offer new market opportunities for small-scale farmers without threatening food security at family level, while improving live-stock feed and fodder value. Sweet sorghum has high water-use efficiency due to its drought resistant characteristics, rendering it more suitable for drier regions of the country. It therefore could enable Zambia's drier regions, where poverty is deepest, to participate in the bio-fuels revolution instead of being left behind. Moreover, it has high positive energy balance, producing about 8 units of energy for every unit of energy invested in its cultivation and production which is roughly equivalent to sugar cane. Utilisation of pineapple waste for wine making has also been done (Alian and Musenge, 1976) and found the wine from unboiled waste gave better wine than from the pulp. Production and storage stability of carbonate guava beverage has also been carried out (Sufi *et al.*, 1976). Moral (1991) reported that the concentration of alcohol in untreated palm wine reach maximum between three and four days and then started to decrease. In the presence of metasulphite the decrease on alcohol was no longer recorded. Various fruit have been used to produce wines which are as good as that from grapes.

The way forward to tap Zambia's potential in the sources of bio-fuels is to carefully study each bio-energy crop. The advantages of one crop in one region of the country could be a disadvantage in another region and vice-versa.

Biotechnology and its products can contribute significantly to the economic development of Zambia, especially in the areas of agriculture, health, environment and industry birthing. The need for the country is to realign its priorities to modern biotechnology.

Accordingly, the biosafety and biotechnology policy has been used to promote Zambia evolution to the current position on modern biotechnology.

This is to balance the need to use biotechnology in the country's quest for socio-economic development and the need to protect animal health, the environment and biological diversity. According to the ministry of higher education's policy document, approximately 18 million farmers worldwide planted biotech crops in 2015, of which about 90 percent were small-scale farmers.

These farmers were from 28 different countries, with 20 being developing and 8 industrialized. Vietnam which commercialized the maize with different characteristics in 2015 for the first time and Cuba planted biotech maize in the last two years.

Biotechnology in both circumstances increase drought tolerance and produce insect resistance in one generation while conventional breeding techniques will take several years. In Africa, some countries continue to make general progress on several fronts in biotechnology with countries like Cameroon, Burkina Faso, Kenya, Ghana, Malawi, Nigeria, Sudan and Swaziland conducting confined field trials on cotton to control weeds and prevent insect attack.

Confined field trials are also being conducted on maize in countries such as Kenya, Uganda and South Africa. Other crops being researched on include wheat, rice, bananas, cassava, potatoes, sorghum, and cow peas. The trials focus on traits of high relevance facing the continent including drought, efficiency of nitrogen use, Salt tolerance, Nutritional enhancement and resistance to tropical pests and diseases.

While Genetically Modified Organisms (GMOs) continue to stir controversy in Zambia, other countries are using biotechnology to enhance agriculture and health sectors. Zambia has however, not commenced the production of GMOs. The country has adopted a precautionary principle as required by the Cartagena Protocol on Biosafety of GMOs and products. Through this approach, Zambia developed the biotechnology and biosafety policy of 2003, biosafety act number 10 of 2007 and relevant statutory instruments and guidelines. Genetic modification has to devise new products because the focus has only been on the application of biotechnology on human, animal and environmental protection.

Biotechnology has specifically been applied in disease diagnosis, classification of organisms and in tissue culture. According to the National Biosafety Authority (NBA), the major contributing factor has been the absence of appropriate regulations and guidelines and inadequate human capital, dilapidated research and containment facilities. And for NBA board chairperson Paul Zambezi, biotechnology in Zambia should be used as a practical intervention to sustain a rural dependency on agriculture and forestry. 'Some areas have high acidity levels in the soil and others are experiencing drought but through biotechnology, we can breed crops that are resistant to drought among others. Our people at the grassroots should be helped through biotechnology, forests can also be regenerated through the use of tissue culture from tree bucks, trees and other plants can be manipulated and there is no harm, "he said.

GMOs continue to cause controversy and the stakeholders should address the concerns about biotechnology policies within the context of Zambia's specific development of needs and aspirations.

Biotechnology therefore cannot be ruled out in averting situations that threaten food security.

## REFERENCES

1. Abdrabbo, A, Atta, N. M.M, Kheira, A 2008. Response of *Jatropha curcas* L. to water deficit: Yield, water use efficiency and oilseed characteristics, Biomass and Bio-energy xxx, Elsevier.
2. Allan, A, Chishimba, G. M and Lovelace, C. E. A 1978. A preliminary study of sugar utilisation by yeast cultived in musuku and mpundu juices using radio active tracers, *Zambia Jounal of Science and Technology*, Vol 3 No 2.
3. Allan, A, and Museng H. M. Utilisation of Pineapple waste for wine making 1976. *Zambia Jounal of Science and Technology*, Vol 1 No 1.
4. Boyle, G 2004. Renewable Energy- Power for a Sustainable Future, Oxford University Press, New York.
5. Christodoulou, L 2007. ENERGY-SWEDEN: Wood Cellulose - Alternative to Brazilian Ethanol? Inter Press Service, [online] available at http: //ipsnews.net/news.asp?idnews=39416, [Accessed on 2009-05-27]
6. CJP, Centre for Jatropha Promotion and Bio-diesel 2008. [online] available at www.jatrophaworld.org, [Accessed on 2009-04-14]
7. FAO 2007. Sustainable Bio-energy: A framework for decision makers, Food and agriculture Organization of the United Nations, [online] available at ftp: //ftp.fao.org/docrep/fao/010/a1094e/a1094e00.pdf, [Accessed on 2009-01-12]
8. Food and Agriculture Organisation of the United Nations 2008. Breeding and cultivation of sweet sorghum [online] available at http: //www.fao.org/docrep/t4470e/t4470e05.htm [Accessed 2009-01-11]
9. Food and Agriculture Organization of the United Nations [Online] available at http: //www.fao.org/documents/ [Accessed 2009-09-06]

10. Goldemberg J 2008. The Brazilian bio-fuels industry, Biotechnology for Bio-fuels, [online] available at http: //www.biotechnologyforbiofuels.com/ content/1/1/6 [Accessed on 2009-04-05]

11. Grassi, G 2006. Sweet Sorgum: One of the best world food-feed-energy crop [online] available at http: //www.sseassociation.org/SS per cent 20Publications/lamnet/ [Accessed 2009-05-02]

12. ICRISA Working paper 2007. Pro-Poor Bio-fuels Outlook for Asia and Africa: ICRISAT's Perspective [online] available at http: //www.icrisat.org/Biopower/ Winslow/Propoor Biofuels OutlookMarch2007.pdf [Accessed 2009-04-02]

13. ICRISAT 2008. Sorghum Production Practices - Cultivation of Sweet Sorghum [online] available at http: //www.icrisat.org/vasat/learning_resources/crops/ sorghum/ [Accessed 2009-03-02]

14. ICRISAT media 2008. Sweet Sorghum: A New Smart Bio-fuel Crop that Ensures Food Security [online] available at http: //www.icrisat.org/Media/2008/ media6.htm [Accessed 2009-02-01]

15. Jongschaap, R. E. E, Corre, W. J, Bindraban and P. S, Bandenburg, W. A 2007. Claims and Facts on Jatropha Curcas. L, Plant Research International B.V, Wageningen, [online] available at http: //www.ifad.org/events/jatropha/ [Accessed on 2009-03-14]

16. Jumbe, C and Msiska. F 2007. Report on International and Regional Policies and Bio-fuels Sector Development in Sub-Saharan Africa, Complete Competence Platform on Energy Crop and Agro-forestry Systems for Arid and Semiarid Ecosystems–Africa, Bunda College, Malawi.

17. Kimble, M. Pasdeloup M. Vand Spencer, C 2008. *Sustainable Bio-energy Development in UEMOA Member Countries.* [online] available at (http: //www. global problems-global solutions files.org/gpgs_files/pdf/UNF_Bioenergy/ [Accessed on 2009-02-23]

18. Kasali, G, The role of biogas in the overall energy/supply/demand in Zambia Unpulished report.

19. Michael, H. L 2006. The Economics of Ethanol from Sweet Sorghum [online] available at http: //www.afpc.tamu.edu/pubs/2/446/RR per cent 2006-2.pdf [Accessed 2009-01-07]

20. Lewanika, M. M and Mulenga, K.D 1995. *World Journal of Microbiology and Biotechnology*, Vol. 12.

21. Morah, F. N 1991. Effect of metabisuphites on alcohol production in palm wine., *Journal of Sci. Technol*, Vol 9. No 2.

22. New agriculture 2007. Sweet sorghum for food, feed and fuel. [Online] available at http: //www.new-agri.co.uk/08/01/focuson/focuson7.php [Accessed 2009-01-12]

23. Ntengwe,F, Njovu, L, Kasali, G and Witika, L. K 2010. Biogas Production in cone closed flotqing dome batch digesters under tropic conditions. *International Journal of Chemtech,*. Jan-March.Vol 2, No 1.

24. Sinkala, T and Chitembo. A 2007. An analysis of the Global Jatropha Industry and a Case Study of the local Value Chain in Zambia, International Labour Organization, Swedish International Development Agency and Business Development Services (BDS) Zambia

25. Sufi, N. A. and Kaputo, M. T 1977. Identification and determination of free sugars in musuku fruit, *Zambia Journal of Science and Technology, Vol* 3 No 2.

26. Sufi, N. A., Mwale J. M. and Kaputo, M. T 1977. Production and storage of carbonated guava beverage, *Zambia Journal of Science and Technology,* Vol 3 No 2.

27. Smeets, E 2008. The sustainability of Brazilian ethanol–An assessment of the possibilities of certified production, BIOMASS AND BIOENERGY 32, p. 781 – 813, vailable at http: //www.elsevier.com/locate/biombioe, Elsevier, doi: 10.1016/j. biombioe. 2008.01.005.

28. Tamil Nadu Agricultural University 2003. Sweet Sorghum production technology [online] available at http: //www.tnau.ac.in/tech/swc/ swsorghum.pdf [Accessed 2009-04-06].

29. Raemaekers, R. H 2001. Crop Production in Tropical Africa, Directorate General for International Co-operation, Ministry of Foreign Affairs, External Trade, Goekint Graphics nv, Brussels, Belgium.

*Chapter 6*

# Opportunities of Industrial Biotechnology in the Pharmaceutical and Food and Beverage Industry in Advancement of Zimbabwean Industries: Review

*Travers Chirova, Thamari Sengudzwa and Cephas Mawere*

***Biotechnology Department, Harare Institute of Technology,***
***P.O Box BE277 Belvedere, Harare, Zimbabwe***
***E-mail: traverschirova@gmail.com***

## ABSTRACT

Industrial biotechnology is characterized by the use of living cells or microorganisms to produce products through manipulation of natural systems in the living cells. In the Pharmaceutical industry it can be used to produce antibiotics, insulin, growth hormones and other therapeutic proteins that are important as medicines. The production is mostly hinged on the use of the microorganism as the expression system or the producer of the therapeutic products with or without some manipulation done. Currently in Zimbabwe, little or no production of therapeutic proteins is done here and most of the proteins are imported into the country. This translates increased cost of obtaining the therapeutic proteins and eventually results in high priced medicines to the general public. There are vast opportunities to ensure local production of the therapeutic proteins and ensure a reduction in the cost of medicines to the general public and also ensure revenue generation through possible exportation of the products obtained. The food and beverage industry is one area that has great potential to influence the advancement of industrial biotechnology. In this area, industrial biotechnology has been applied in many respects for example, brewing in Chibuku, Maheu production and Delta production of clear beers and lagers. However, there is great potential to ensure the efficacy of the production processes, which translates to a reduction in the cost of production by effectively applying the biotechnology techniques in these industries. Opportunities also come in the production of some key raw materials used in the industry for example, citric acid, which has vast uses in many various industries including the ones under review. Currently, citric acid is imported from countries like China and obviously this has a high cost. Local production of these products offers lower costs and adds value to the local industries with a great opportunity of eventually being able to export the same. In addition, the biotechnology application in industries also ensures to certain levels, lesser pollution and more eco friendly processes. In conclusion, this paper discusses the prospects into the establishment of industrial biotechnology in Zimbabwe.

***Keywords:*** *Industrial biotechnology, Pharmaceutical biotechnology, Therapeutic proteins, Fermentation biotechnology, Local production.*

## INTRODUCTION

Industrial biotechnology is defined as a technique that uses systems that are biological in nature for production of chemicals, materials and energy, with its main thrust being on biocatalysis and fermentation technology (Soetaert and Vandamme, 2006). Industrial biotechnology is also known as "White Biotechnology" (Soetaert and Vandamme, 2010) and is also defined by Weng and Zhao (2009) as the application of modern biotechnological techniques in sustainably producing chemicals and fuels from renewable sources. It also considered as the third wave of biotechnology. Industrial biotechnology is a multidisciplinary technology and encompasses techniques in areas such as molecular biology, biochemistry, microbiology, bioprocess technology to produce useful products and processes. Industrial biotechnology is believed to have emanated from industrial microbiology but with an addition of the use of biotechnological techniques (Bruno-Bárcena and Siñeriz, (2011); Soetaert and Vandamme, (2006)), Industrial biotechnology. According to Keener *et al.* (2000), the industrial biotechnology improves efficiency and reduces environmental impacts in areas such as textile, paper and pulp and chemical manufacturing due to the techniques that are applied. Industrial biotechnology can be applied in various industries that include food and beverage industry, pharmaceutical industry, chemical manufacturing, textile to mention only a few. In all these areas the multidisciplinary techniques are applied to achieve the goal.

In Zimbabwe, industrial biotechnology is being applied in some industries with particular mention to the food and beverage industry, and also the dairy industry. The applications in these areas are somewhat quite established but still have great room for improvement. Opportunities for application of industrial biotechnology are widespread in Zimbabwe, but of particular focus in this regard is the pharmaceutical industry and the food and beverage industry.

### Industrial Biotechnology in the Pharmaceutical Industry

Most pharmaceutical products that are available in Zimbabwe from local companies are only formulated locally but the raw materials are all imported from outside sources, with most of the pharmaceuticals going towards the treatment

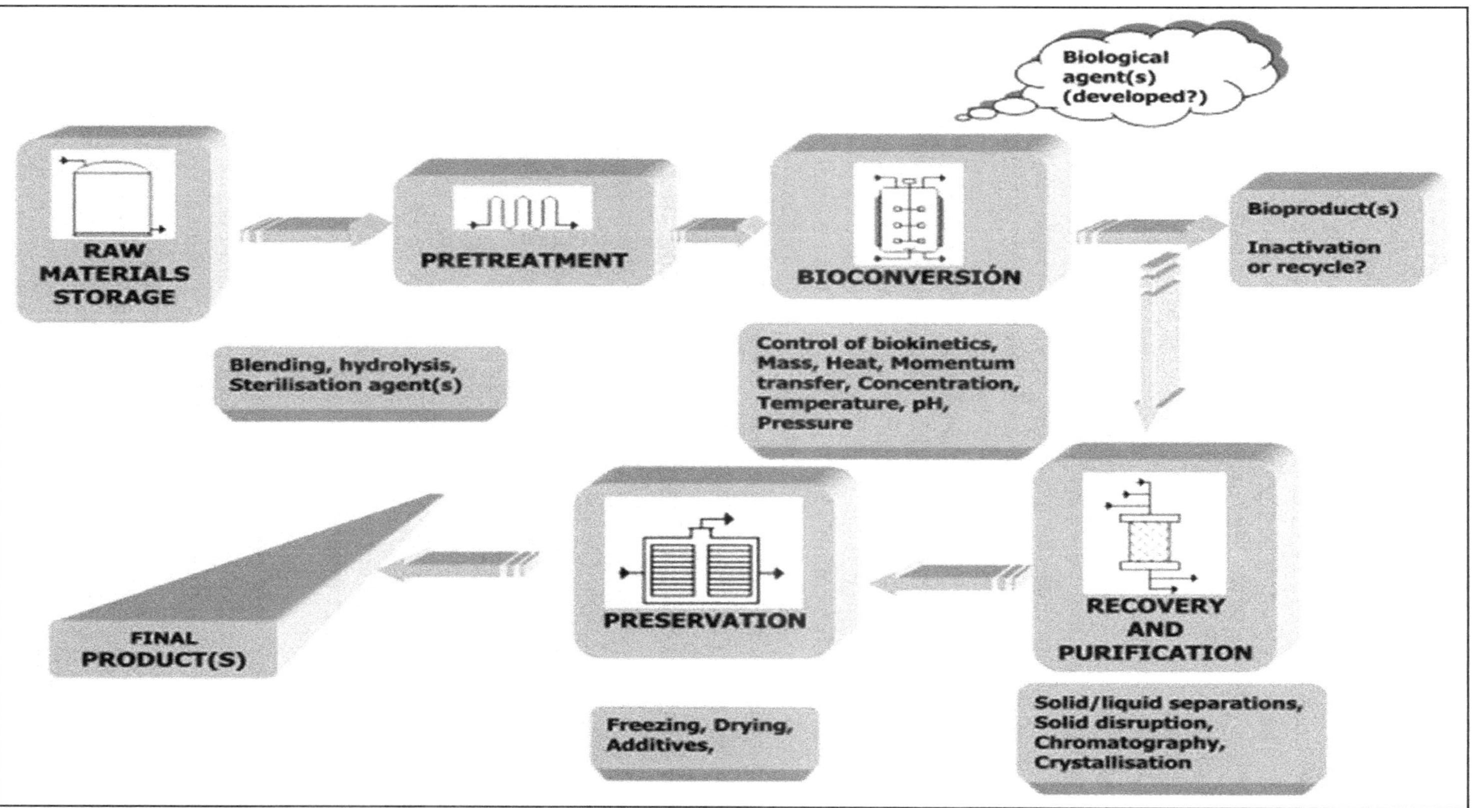


**Figure 6.1: Typical Process in Biopharmaceuticals Production. (*Source*: Bruno-Barcena and Sineriz, 2011).**

of HIV/AIDS, Tuberculosis and Malaria (UNIDO, 2011). Zimbabwe uses about $400 million to import drugs yearly and promises to increase as populations that need the drugs increase, with the major local supplier (CAPS Holdings) no longer functioning enough to satisfy the growing market. Challenges with foreign currency availability are further worsening the situation as suppliers are no longer willing to supply without assurance of getting their payments (The standard, 2015; Daily News 2017). The aspect of importing leads to high prices for the drugs which are too much for a people under the current economy. Of particular concern is the production of therapeutic proteins/biopharmaceuticals which is purely non-existent in our local Zimbabwean industries. Therapeutic proteins or biopharmaceuticals are proteins that are similar to those that are found in normal healthy individuals, for example, insulin, cytokines and growth hormones also fall under that area and these are products of pharmaceutical biotechnology processes. Pharmaceutical biotechnology is defined as the use of biological systems (cells or tissues) or molecules of biological nature (enzymes or antibodies) for or in the manufacture of commercial products that can be used for treatment of diseases or for use in diagnostic kits (Walsh, 2007). Biopharmaceuticals are also defined as therapeutic proteins that are produced by modern biotechnological techniques and most of them being mainly through genetic engineering (Walsh, 2007; Crommelin *et al.*, 2008). Most of these biopharmaceuticals currently being used in Zimbabwe are being imported from other countries (UNIDO, 2011). There is great potential for the production of biopharmaceuticals in Zimbabwe, which can lead to reduced local prices and also be a source of much needed foreign currency through the potential of exporting the locally produced biopharmaceuticals.

## Potential Biopharmaceuticals for Production in Zimbabwe

Industrial biotechnology can be applied to aid in the large-scale production of the biopharmaceuticals to ensure that enough quantities are produced to meet demand and also at affordable prices. The biopharmaceuticals are produced using fermentation technologies to ensure large-scale production (Walsh, 2007). The biopharmaceuticals that can potentially be produced in Zimbabwe include the following:

### Cytokines

These are molecules that are like hormones which control intercellular reactions. They are key in activating immune-systems cells (lymphocytes and macrophages). These cytokines include:

Interleukins which are molecules, that functions as messengers between leukocytes and also involved in the stimulation of lymphocytes. An example is IL-2, aldesleukin (Proleukin), for treating renal cell carcinoma.

Interferons are agents that work against viruses and uncontrolled cell growth (which is the calling card for cancer). Some interferons are being used for the treatment of hepatitis B, genital warts and AIDS related Karposi's sarcoma (Steinberg and Raso, 1998; Newell, 1996)

Granulocytes-colony stimulating factor which functions to stimulate the bone marrow to produce neutrophils (leukocytes that are antibacterial agents) which has some recombinant variants with an example being filgrastim. Granulocyte-macrophage colony-stimulating factor which acts on the bone marrow to produce neutrophils and macrophages and a recombinant product example being sargramostim used in cancer patients (Steinberg and Raso, 1998).

## Insulin

This is a protein that is useful in treatment of diabetics and it was the first recombinant protein to be made and administered to humans after approval by the FDA. The recombinant form of the insulin is produced in non-pathogenic *E. coli* and an example is Lispro (Newell, 1996; Steinberg and Raso, 1998).

## Human Growth Hormone

It a protein used to solve the problem of reduced growth or growth failure in individuals that lack normal human growth hormone production and it is produced by recombinant DNA technology.

## Enzymes

These are proteins that play key roles within the body, with their chief role being to catalyse reactions for them to occur at faster rates, whether in breaking down or building bodily molecules. In this regard, the enzymes (recombinant proteins) produced as biopharmaceuticals are useful in treatment of diseases. Examples include Alteplase a recombinant version of the enzyme plasmin which functions in dissolving blood clots and useful in the treatment of heart attacks, strokes and pulmonary emboli. The enzymes are also known as thrombolytic and fibrinolytic enzymes.

## Clotting Factors

These are necessary in individuals so as to have adequate control of blood loss through bleeding. Haemophilia A and Heamophilia B are conditions in which the individuals minor injuries can lead to prolonged blood loss due to the lack of certain clotting factors. Recombinant forms of the proteins are being made which include antihemophiliac factor (rAHF) and the recombinant factor IX which is produced in milk.

## Vaccines

Vaccines traditionally were produced either as attenuated or killed forms of the organism that causes a particular disease. Recombinant DNA technology now allows the production of what are termed as subunit vaccines. These subunit vaccines are all or part of a surface protein found on the disease-causing pathogen, which are produced and then administered to the patient. The recombinant DNA technology can also be used for production of attenuate vaccine like the Cholera vaccine that has been produced through such means (Crommelin *et al.*, 2008; Newell, 1996, Arakawa *et al.*, 1998).

### Monoclonal Antibodies

These are proteins normally produced by the body in response to an antigen and have the capacity to bind to that antigen and are a product of hybridoma technology (*e.g.* cells of the bone marrow tumor cells fused together with B lymphocytes via biotechnology techniques). These monoclonal antibodies are useful in treatment of immune system rejection of transplants either of heart, kidney and livers. An example is daclizumab (Zenapax) for the prevention of kidney-transplant rejection. They are also useful in diagnostic due to their ability to bind and tag specific proteins, for example diagnosis of hepatitis B (Crommelin *et al.*, 2008; Steinberg and Raso, 1998; Newell, 1996).

### Antibiotics

Antibiotics are molecules that act against diseases caused by bacteria. Biotechnological techniques are being used to enhance the large-scale production of some antibiotics. Bioprocess technology plays a key role in ensuring efficient and meaningful production of the antibiotics. Recombinant DNA technology has been applied to enhance production of the antibiotic amikacin and tylosin (Newell, 1996)

These are some of the biopharmaceuticals that can be produced under the wing of industrial biotechnology and can lead to the availability of local therapeutic proteins which can be cheaper. Inevitably it will lead to employment creation and also eradicate dependency on other countries to supply the medicines to Zimbabwe. Industrial biotechnology has great avenues of opportunity in the pharmaceutical industry in Zimbabwe.

## Industrial Biotechnology in the Food and Beverage Industry

The food and beverage industry have been a key beneficiary of industrial biotechnology in many respects. Fermentation processes have been a key to the production of products in the food and beverage industry and has good use of microorganisms. Mostly yeasts, fungi and bacteria have been widely used in these fermentation processes. Fermentation processes are artificial conditions which allow the biotechnologist to tailor make the growth conditions in the bio-reactor, with the ability to genetically modify the microorganism and direct metabolism to produce desired products. The processes are key because they offer quick growth and product production, use of renewable raw materials, ease of genetic modifications provided by the microorganisms. Microbial fermentation is essential to production of wine, beer, bologna, buttermilk, cheeses, kefir, olives, salami, sauerkraut, and many other products (Glazer and Nikaido, 2007; Soetaert and Vandamme, 2006; Okafor, 2007; Stanburg *et al.*, 1995). Fermentations have two main types which include solid state fermentation and submerged fermentation.

Industrial biotechnology has been applied for many years in the food and beverage sector and the dairy sector. In Zimbabwe, industrial biotechnology has been applied for the production of dairy products that include cheese, yoghurt and other products, with application also being in the food and beverage industry in producing alcohol and some fermented foods. The technology has a lot of room for improvement and enhances the current technologies that are currently being used in

Zimbabwe. There are a number of products that are not being produced that much in Zimbabwe and are being imported yet they play a key role in production of most food products in the Food industry. These have or proffer potential for products that can be produced in Zimbabwe using industrial biotechnology basing on the microbial and fermentation technologies.

## Potential Products in the Food and Beverage Sector for Production in Zimbabwe

### Citric Acid

One key product to mention is citric acid, which is imported from outside sources like China into Zimbabwe and hence becomes expensive to acquire as it is not locally produced. Citric acid is a useful element in the food, beverage, and pharmaceutical, chemical, cosmetic and other industries. Citric acid is used to impart a characteristic tart taste to foods and beverages. It is used in industries for acidulation, anti-oxidation, emulsification, preservation, flavour enhancement and as plasticizer and synergistic agent (Soccol and Vanderberghe, 2003; Chirova *et al.*, 2016). Citric acid is biodegradable and palatable, highly soluble and low/ non-toxic. It is adjudged to be GRAS (Generally Recognized As Safe). Hence, it is one of the most important organic acids produced by fermentation and is the most exploited biotechnological product. It has an annual industrial production of 1.6 million tons (Sauer *et al.*, 2005) with an annual growth demand/consumption rate of 3.5-4 per cent (Nadeem *et al.*, 2010). Local production will be the key to ensure steady availability and also a reduction in the price of the product.

### Pre-digested Foods and Industrial Enzymes

The other area of potential is the production of pre-digested foods using enzymes as the digesters of the food. Industrial biotechnology would play a key role in the production of the enzymes that can be eventually used for the production of pre-digested foods which are usually for consumption by infants. Most enzymes are produced in microorganisms that are generally recognized as safe using fermentation technology. The organisms producing the enzymes are often modified genetically to ensure maximum production of the desired enzyme. The microorganisms include *Aspergillus*, *Trichoderma* fungi, *Streptomyces* fungi imperfecti, and *Bacillus* bacteria of which the enzymes are produced extracellular. Some are obtained from animal sources like pepsin and renin are derived from animal sources like pigs (Soetaert and Vandamme, 2010; Waites *et al.*, 2001). These enzymes can be used in various industries but of focus in this regard, is in the food industry for producing pre-digested foods. In addition apart, from just producing enzymes for the food industry, various enzymes can be produced also for use in other industries like textile, paper, leather and brewing and only to mention a few (Polaina and MacCabe, 2007; Soetaert and Vandamme, 2010).

### Beverage Industry

The food and beverage industry is one area that has great potential to influence the advancement of industrial biotechnology. In this area, industrial biotechnology has been applied in many respects for example, brewing in Chibuku, Maheu production and Delta production of clear beers and lagers. In the beverage industry, industrial biotechnology can be used to enhance the production of alcohol. The interdisciplinary nature of industrial biotechnology becomes useful as it can be employed to genetically modify the microorganisms that produce the alcohol (*S. cerevisiae*) to ensure high production and stability of the microorganisms. This can lead to improved production yield and increased stability of the microorganisms which have been modified.

## Conclusions

The establishment of industrial biotechnology would see the revitalization of the industries in Zimbabwe with the biotechnological techniques playing a key role in the production of products. Local production will lead to cheaper medication (a case of India), improved F and B products and cheaper products, improved economic growth and potential for income generation through export of produced products.

## Acknowledgements

Great appreciation is extended to Biotechnology staff of HIT for their assistance in making the work possible. The key players in industry for their time to direct us in right areas to attend our review research. Above all, we thank the Almighty God for the grace to the work.

## REFERENCES

1. Arakawa, T., Chong, D, K, X. and Langridge, W, H, R 1998. Efficacy of a food plant-based oral cholera toxin B subunit vaccine. *Nature Biotechnology*, (16), pp. 292–298.
2. Bruno-Bárcena, J, M. and Sineriz, F 2011. Industrial biotechnology, Encyclopedia of Life Support Systems, USA, (5), pp. 1-7.
3. Chirova, T, K., Kumar, A. and Panwar, A 2016. Citric acid production by Aspergillus niger using different substrates. *Malaysian Journal of Microbiology*, 12(3), pp. 199-204.
4. Glazer, A, N. and Nikaido, H 2007. Fundamentals of Applied Microbiology, Second Edition, Cambridge University Press, New York, USA.
5. Hugenholtz, J 2013. Traditional biotechnology for new foods and beverages. *Current Opinion in Biotechnology*, Elsevier, Germany, (24): 155–159.
6. Keener, K., Hoban, T. and Balasubramanian, R 2000. Biotechnology and its applications. NC State University, College of Agriculture and Life Sciences, North Carolina, USA, FSR0031, pp. 1-13.
7. Nadeem, A., Syed, Q.,Baig S., Irfan, M. and Nadeem, M 2010. Enhanced Production of Citric Acid by *Aspergillus niger* M-101 using Lower Alcohols. *Turkish Journal of Biochemistry*, 35(1): 7-13.
8. Newell, N 1996. Commercial Biotechnology: An International Analysis (Part 7 of 35). Biological Applications Program.

9. Okafor, N 2007. Modern Industrial Microbiology and Biotechnology. Science publishers, Enfield, NH, USA, pp. 3-31.
10. Pharmaceutical Sector Profile: Zimbabwe. 2011. Global UNIDO Project: Strengthening the local production of essential generic drugs in least developed and developing countries, Vienna, Austria.
11. Polaina, J and MacCabe, A. (Eds.) 2007. Industrial Enzymes: Structure, Function and Applications. Springer, Dordrecht, The Netherlands.
12. Sauer, M., Porro, O., Matlanovich, D. and Branduardi, P 2008. Microbial Production of Organic Acids: Expanding the Markets. Trends in Biotechnology, (26), pp. 100-108.
13. Soccol, C, R., Vanderberghe, P, S., Rodrigues, C. and Pandey, A 2006. New Perspectives for Citric Acid Production and Application. *Food Technology and Biotechnology*, 44(2): 141-149.
14. Soetaert, W and Vandamme, E, J 2006. The impact of industrial biotechnology (Review). *Biotechnology Journal, Germany*, (1): 756-769.
15. Soetaert, W. and Vandamme, E, J. (Eds.) 2010. Industrial Biotechnology: Sustainable Growth and Economic Success. WILEY-VCH Verlag GmbH and Co. KGaA, Weinheim, Germany, pp. 207-223.
16. Stanbury, F, P., Whitaker, A. and Hall, S, J 1995. Principles of fermentation technology, Butterworth Heinemann, MPG Books Ltd, Bodmin, Cornwall, Great Britain.
17. Steinberg, F, M. and Raso, J 1998. Biotech Pharmaceuticals and Biotherapy: An Overview. *J Pharm Pharmaceut Sci, USA*, 1(2): 48-59.
18. Waites, M, J., Morgan, N, L. and Rockey, J, S 2001. Industrial Microbiology: An Introduction. Blackwell Science Ltd, London, United Kingdom, pp. 133-143.
19. Walsh, G 2007. Pharmaceutical Biotechnology: Concepts and Applications. John Wiley and Sons Ltd, The Atrium, Southern Gate, Chichester, England.
20. Weng, L, T. and Zhao, H 2009. Industrial biotechnology: Tools and applications (Review). *Biotechnology Journal, Germany*, (4): 1725-1739.
21. The standard 2015. www.thestandard.co.zw/2015/10/11/zimbabwe-imports-400m-worth-of-drugs-annually/ (Accessed on 01 August 2017)
22. Daily news 2017. www.dailynews/articles/2017/09/14/drug-prices-soar (Accessed on 20 September 2017).

# *Chapter 7*

# Industrial Biotechnology: Then, Now and the Future

*Chenjerayi Kashangura*

*Tobacco Research Board, Kutsaga Research Station,*
*P. O. Box 1909, Harare, Zimbabwe*
*E-mail: ckashangura@kutsaga.co.zw*

## ABSTRACT

The application of scientific discoveries to practical tasks brings about technology. This technology has increasingly become a need driven industry with advances earmarked at addressing pertinent challenges faced by the human (*Homo sapiens*) species in its' endeavours to survive on an evolving planet Earth. Application of living organisms, their parts or processes for the benefit of humankind has been a tradition for eons of times from ancient brewing to modern day production of dairy products such as "Yoghurt" – now utilising recombinant DNA technology-produced starter cultures. The continued existence and evolution of biotechnology at a large and profit-making scale may eventually depend on rapid, directed, precise and accurate genome enhancement of the industrial biotechnology organisms to a postulated extent that those with such capabilities would be able to meet the ever changing demands of the global consumers, regulators and policy makers of industrial biotechnology products. This paper briefly presents the evolution of industrial biotechnology with an emphasis on genome enhancement technology as the potential driving force of penetrating and increasing market share within the ever – evolving global industrial biotechnology sector.

***Keywords***: *Synthetic biology, Genome enhancement, Gene editing, Industrial organism.*

## INTRODUCTION

Technology is the systematic application of scientific knowledge to practical tasks (Reid, 2000). In other words, it is the application of scientific discoveries.

However, not all scientific discoveries can result in technology. Thus, the scientific community has a 'filter' system that removes personal bias, error and dishonesty from primary scientific literature (all published original scientific papers) to secondary literature which is mainly papers cited in review papers, to current textbook material which is considered to be reliable knowledge (Reid, 2000).

The scientific knowledge considered to be reliable knowledge is the one that has potential to evolve into technology when it addresses a challenge faced by the human species (Goldenberg, 1998). Hence, biotechnology is the application of reliable scientific knowledge of living (bio) organisms, their parts or processes to practical tasks, with the practical tasks defined by the needs of the human species (OECD, 2001; Tang and Zhao, 2009).

It then follows that applications of reliable scientific knowledge of living organisms, their parts or processes to a practical task that is not considered to be pertinent by the human species may result in a lack of a market for the biotechnology. Such a scenario is considered, 'good biotechnology' but 'poor industrial biotechnology' due to the lack of the market. In other words, industrial biotechnology is the large-scale, profit making application of biotechnology.

The continued existence and evolution of industrial biotechnology and maintenance of market shares may depend on the ability to rapidly, precisely and accurately enhance the genomes of industrial biotechnology organisms. This paper presents a brief discourse on the potential role genome enhancing technologies (bioengineering technologies) (Kashangura, 2017) have in charting the future market share within the global industrial biotechnology sector.

## Industrial Biotechnology – Then

From ancient time, living organisms especially in the form of microorganisms have been utilised by the human species to produce industrial biotechnology products such as beer, wine, bread and cheese. In these industrial biotechnology processes, the ideal strain is a critical component for success or failure.

The ancients originally left it to chance (the environment) to provide the ideal organism, such as, microbial inoculum in the form of lactic acid bacteria when producing, for example, sour milk. The production of such products as sour milk in this era was left to the micro-evolutionary forces such as mutation which is the original source of variation, natural selection, genetic drift and gene flow to shape the genomes of the industrial biotechnology organisms. Success and the level of profit made heavily dependent on chance isolation of a very productive strain from the natural environment. In this era genome enhancement of the industrial biotechnology organism was left to the micro-evolutionary forces with no human manipulation of the genome.

## Industrial Biotechnology – Now

The current era of industrial biotechnology not only relies on micro-evolutionary forces to improve the organisms, but also employs traditional plant breeding techniques and genome enhancing technologies such as recombinant

DNA technology (genetic engineering). Genetic engineering has produced commercially viable industrial biotechnology enzymes such as cellulase used in the detergent and textiles industry; maltogenic amylase for the starch and baking industries; phytase for the animal feed industry; decarboxylase for the brewing industry and pectin esterase for fruit processing (Waites *et al.*, 2001; Okafor, 2010). In addition, health products such as insulin for diabetes; human growth hormone (somatotrophin) for dwarfism; tumour necrosis factor as an anti-tumour agent, human DNAse 1 for treating cystic fibrosis; lysozyme as an anti-inflammatory agent and erythropoietin for treatment of anaemia and cancers are produced using genetic engineering enhanced industrial biotechnology organisms (Waites *et al.*, 2001; Okafor, 2010).

The current era introduced human manipulation of the genome of the industrial biotechnology organisms. This, enabled the human species to alter the DNA sequence 'paragraphs' of an organism's 'book' to introduce new 'sentences' that instruct for example *Escherichia coli* to now produce insulin. Since the adage 'time is money' reflects on the importance of managing time to result in profits – it implies the technologies that enable the reduction in time in developing an industrial biotechnology organism that addresses the needs of the market will potentially translate to increased market share and higher profits. To this regard, traditional plant breeding techniques which were an improvement from reliance on micro-evolutionary processes, have become superseded by use of modern and rapid genetic engineering technologies in the development of industrial biotechnology organisms that address the human species challenges.

Genetically enhanced industrial biotechnology organisms have been used to produce less harmful products of a better quality, that also result in lower greenhouse emissions such as bread production, detergents, biodegradable plastic films, beverage packaging, cosmetics, vitamin B2 and synthetic rubber (Bang *et al.*, 2009; Tang and Zhao, 2009; OECD, 2011; Erickson *et al.*, 2012).

## Industrial Biotechnology – The Future

Gene editing technologies such as CRISPR and extensive bioengineering technologies such as synthetic biology has potential to bring rapid, directed, precise and accurate genome enhancement of industrial biotechnology organisms (Tang and Zhao, 2009). This is likely to result in better market share and increased profitability for industrial biotechnology stakeholders employing these 'next generation' genome enhancement technologies (BIO, 2013).

The CRISPR technology has potential ability to precisely edit genomes whereas synthetic biology has potential to rewrite the industrial biotechnology organism DNA sequence 'book' to edit existing 'chapters' or even write a 'new book' through development of minimal genomes (Schwille and Diez, 2009; Hutchison III *et al.*, 2016); recoding, redesigning and synthesis of new genomes (Eswelt and Wang, 2012). Thus, theoretically synthetic biology and gene editing technologies have potential to catapult industrial biotechnology to an era where reliance on micro-evolutionary forces, traditional plant breeding technologies and conventional genetic engineering are relegated.

Since synthetic biology attempts to design and rewire the new technological medium of biological components, so as to achieve new functions in a robust and predictable manner (Balmer and Martin, 2008; Erickson *et al.*, 2012; Agustín and Isalan, 2014; Patron *et al.*, 2015), industrial biotechnology potentially can move to a technology era of production of new products that do not exist in nature (Bugaj and Schaffer, 2012; Dragosits *et al.*, 2012; Kashangura, 2017). Stakeholders with such capabilities may potentially have a competitive advantage over other industrial biotechnology stakeholders employing 'older generation' techniques such as conventional genetic engineering through recombinant DNA technology. The potential future of industrial biotechnology is faster, directed, accurate, precise development of industrial organisms with capabilities that address challenges faced by the human species. This possibly can result in a sustainable bio-based economy that uses eco-efficient bio-processes and renewable bio-resources.

## Concerns

The era of application of genome enhancement technologies such as synthetic biology which have potential to rewrite a genome also comes with concerns such as uncontrolled release, bioterrorism and the creation of monopolies (Benner and Sismour, 2005; Balmer and Martin, 2008). Approaches of engineering industrial biotechnology organisms to be dependent on nutrients with limited availability and integration of self-destruct mechanisms that are triggered should the population density become too high can potentially address the uncontrolled release concern (Balmer and Martin, 2008). In addition, robust biosecurity measures (Schmidt, 2008) that includes databases of critical alert sequences will potentially become necessary in the era of widespread genome design and synthesis 'DNA printers era' to effect a counter measure against bioterrorism. The creation of monopolies through patenting of futuristic development of industrial biotechnology organisms that convert biomass into fuels (SEI, 2007) such as ethanol or hydrogen may potentially require an open source movement that will facilitate open scientific research (Bang *et al.*, 2009)

## Conclusions

The potential evolution of genome enhancement technologies may likely result in a new era in industrial biotechnology that result in a sustainable bio-based economy. Stakeholders employing these technologies will possibly have a better market share, wider product portfolio and increased profits in comparison to stakeholders still employing older genome enhancement technologies.

This paper recommends the establishment of national or regional centre(s) of industrial biotechnology research and development to spearhead the embracing of industrial biotechnology in the countries that are still to embrace the modern genome enhancement technologies.

## Acknowledgement

I am thankful to the Tobacco Research Board for facilitating presentation of this training lecture at the 2nd International Training Workshop on Industrial Biotechnology of NAM S&T Centre.

# REFERENCES


1. Agustín- Pavón, C. and Isalan, M 2014. Synthetic biology and therapeutic strategies for the degenerating brain. *Bioessays*, 36: 979-990.
2. Balmer, A. and Martin, P 2008. Synthetic Biology: social and ethical challenges. Institute of Science and Society, University of Nottingham, United Kingdom.
3. Bang, J. K., Follér, A. and Buttazoni, M 2009. Industrial Biotechnology, More than Green Fuel in a Dirty Economy?: exploring the transformational potential of industrial biotechnology on the way to a green economy. WWF, Copenhagen, Denmark. (accessed from www.wwf.dk).
4. Benner, S. A. and Sismour, A. M 2005. Synthetic Biology. *Nature Reviews Genetics*, 6: 533-543.
5. BIO (Biotechnology Industry Organisation) 2013. Current Uses of Synthetic Biology for Renewable Chemicals, Pharmaceuticals and Biofuels.Wahington DC, United States of America.
6. Bugaj, L. J. and Schaffer, D. V 2012. Bringing next-generation therapeutics to the clinic through synthetic biology. *Current Opinion in Chemical Biology*, 16: 355-361.
7. Dragosits, M., Nicklas, D. and Tagkopoulos, I 2012. A synthetic biology approach to self-regulatory recombinant protein production in *Escherichia coli*. *Journal of Biological Engineering*, 6(2): available from http: //www.jbioleng.org/ content/6/1/2.
8. Esvelt, K. M. and Wang, H. H 2012. Genome scale engineering for systems and synthetic biology. *Molecular Systems Biology*, 9: article 641; doi: 10.1038/ msb.2012.66.
9. Erickson, B., Nelson, J. E. and Winters, P 2012. Perspective on opportunities in industrial biotechnology in renewable chemicals. *Biotechnology Journal*, 7: doi 10.1002/biot.201100069.
10. Goldenberg, J 1998. What is the role of science in developing countries? *Science*, 279: 1140-1141.
11. Hutchison III, C. A., Chuang, R., Noskov, V. N., Assad-Carcia, N., Deerinck, T. J. and Ellisman, M. H 2016. Design and synthesis of a minimal bacterial genome. *Science* 351: aad6253 doi: 10.1126/science.aad6253.
12. Kashangura, C 2017. Glance at potential future combating of diseases: bioengineered antimicrobial agents. *Scientific Research and Essays*, 12(5): 51-58.
13. OECD (Organisation for Economic Co-operation and Development). 2001. The Application of Biotechnology to Industrial Sustainability. http: //www.oecd. org/sti/biotechnology (accessed 19 Aug 2017).
14. OECD (Organisation for Economic Co-operation and Development). 2011. Industrial Biotechnology and Climate Change: opportunities and challenges. http: //www.oecd.org/sti/biotechnology (accessed 19 Aug 2017).

15. Okafor, N 2010. Modern Industrial Microbiology and Biotechnology. Science Publishers, Enfield.
16. Patron, N. J., Orzaez, D., Marillonnet, S., Warzecha, H., Matthewman, C., Youles, M. *et al.*, 2015. Standards for plant synthetic biology: a common syntax for exchange of DNA parts. *New Phytologist*, 208: 13-19.
17. Reid, C.P.P 2000. Handbook for Preparing and Writing Research Proposals. EuroLAN, Hungary, pp. 15-22.
18. Schmidt, M 2008. Diffusion of synthetic biology: a challenge to biosafety. *Syst. Synth. Biol.*, doi: 10.1007/s11693-008-9018-z.
19. Schwille, P. and Diez, S 2009. Synthetic biology of minimal systems. *Critical Reviews in Biochemistry and Molecular Biology*, 44(4): 223-242.
20. SEI (Stockholm Environment Institute). 2007. Industrial Biotechnology and Biomass Utilisation: prospects and challenges for the developing world. UNIDO.
21. Tang, W. L. and Zhao, H 2009. Industrial biotechnology: tools and applications. *Biotechnology Journal*, 4: 1725-1739.
22. Waites, M. J., Morgan, M. L., Rockey, J. S. and Higton, G 2001. Industrial Microbiology: an introduction. Blackwell Science, Oxford.

# Specific Biotechnology Efforts — *Agriculture*

*Chapter 8*

# The Application of Biotechnology in Aquaculture Value Addition and Beneficiation: Prospect and Challenges in The Gambia

***Bintou Dibba***

*University of The Gambia,*
*West Coast Region, Brikama, The Gambia*
*E-mail: binsdd@gmail.com, bdibba@utg.edu.gm*

## ABSTRACT

Given the nutritional and economic potentials of the aquaculture sector, the development of subsistence, small-scale and commercial aquaculture is highlighted in The Gambia Aquaculture Strategy 2008. Most fish farms in The Gambia currently are small-scale, distributed within West Coast Region (WCR), Central River Region CRR south, and North Bank Region (NBR). Aquaculture is gradually and steadily growing from infancy status of few trial ponds in 1979 to about 98 small-scale fish ponds in 2016. In The Gambia, aquaculture farms are owned by the Government, communities, private individuals and schools.

Aquaculture in The Gambia is being promoted with the intent to fill the gap between declining fish production from inland resources and the increasing demand for fish proteins from the growing population particularly in urban areas. This makes the need for sustainable management of aquaculture to be high on the national agenda for the Government of The Gambia and the population at large especially the rural population.

Although aquaculture production in The Gambia is believed to have started in 1970s, yet the country has not met domestic production demand for the population. The Gambia is blessed with natural resources such as lands, rivers, streams, reservoirs and lakes but in spite of these great potentials, the country is still unable to bridge the gap in the short fall between total domestic fish production and high population growth. Among the aquaculture establishments in the country, there are two (2) fish farms established for recreational purposes (ornamental fisheries and sport fishing).

The only farm in The Gambia operating aquaculture in large-scale is the shrimp farm, Gambia Shrimp Aquaculture Project (GASAP), which together with its ponds in Pirang, hatchery in Sanyang and other associated facilities, was acquired by the Government in 2015.

Problems with these initial projects include inadequate technical expertise and the inability to co-opt space from rice farmers. Drawing on the experiences documented above, the Government observed the need to diversify the approaches for the development, promotion and adoption of aquaculture in the country through the promotion of the biotechnology for improved performance and to minimize the enormous challenges faced by fish farmers in the country.

***Keywords:*** *Aquaculture, Gambia, Small-scale, Rural, Biotechnology.*

## INTRODUCTION

The word aquaculture, though used rather widely denotes all forms of culture of aquatic animals and plants in fresh, brackish and marine environments (Pillay and Kutty, 2005). Aquaculture is generally considered as a subsector under the Department of Fisheries (DoF) and is still understood by many in The Gambia as culture of fish.

The advent of fresh water aquaculture in The Gambia dates back to late 1970s and early 1980s. The first pond was established in 1979 in Bansang through collaborations between the DoF, the Catholic Relief Services and the United States Peace Corps focusing largely on the introduction of small-scale tilapia farming along the freshwater portions of the river (Rice *et al.*, 2012). Through the joint intervention of the Fisheries Department and its partners, the single earthen pond measuring 20 x 15m was hand excavated. The location of the pond was on a high ground where water supply was through pumping (Jallow, 2014; Rice *et al.*, 2012). This effort was short lived but provided practical experience for The Gambia fisheries officials who participated in subsequent efforts to culture tilapia and other freshwater fish prompting enthusiasm of private rice growers to establish isolated fish ponds in their rice irrigated plots (Rice *et al.*, 2012).

Shrimp farming was introduced in The Gambia in 1986 by Scan Gambia Shrimp Ltd in Pirang. The farm began operations in 1988 with the importation of giant tiger prawn brood stock from Asia. The company ceased operations in 1991 and in 2000 their assets, including ponds, hatchery and processing plant, were acquired by a group of local Gambian investors but later sold to West African Aquaculture Ltd (WAA).

In 1995, a one-hectare poly-culture trial pond was established in Central River Region (CRR) by the DoF for the culture of three indigenous fish species (African Catfish, *Heterotis* and *Tilapia*). The trial did not only prove the cultivability of these species in the country but has raised national awareness of the need to diversify fish production through aquaculture. Government through the DoF solicited funding assistance from the Taiwan Technical Mission (TTM) and Food and Agriculture Organization of the United Nations (FAO) to expand on the gains of the trial resulting in the establishment of more fish ponds in CRR and other parts of the country (Jallow, 2014).

Problems with these initial projects include inadequate technical expertise and the inability to co-opt space from rice farmers. Drawing on the experiences documented above, the Government observed the need to diversify the approaches for the development, promotion and adoption of aquaculture in the country.

Currently the appropriate human resource base needed for achieving the required aquaculture production in The Gambia is not sufficient.

At the DoF, there is an aquaculture unit headed by a Principal Fisheries Officer. There are also other personnel who have some form of training in aquaculture at various levels. Individuals managing aquaculture facilities within various communities also claimed to benefit from in-house training on relevant skills in aquaculture provided by DoF in collaboration with Food and Agriculture Sector Development Project (FASDEP) and Livestock and Horticulture Development Project (LHDP) projects under the Ministry of Agriculture and FAO. However, there are not more than 10 people who studied aquaculture at Masters Level in the country. Therefore, a suitable extension machinery with the appropriate number of adequately trained and experienced extension personnel have to be built up for communities to adapt existing technologies to suit local conditions. These personnel have to be well trained technicians with the necessary logistics, incentives, field experience and proficiency in extension methodologies.

The development of appropriate human resources should form part of the nation's aquaculture development agenda. Since aquaculture is inter-disciplinary by nature, appropriate personnel with specialized knowledge in The Application of Biotechnology in Aquaculture for value addition to aquaculture products are required in The Gambia. These should include preparation of good quality feed and production of quality seed relevant for the development of aquaculture.

The DoF and relevant stakeholders need to undertake training and capacity building activities for aquaculture development in the country. Training needs assessment study should be undertaken in order to identify and recommend appropriate actions for developing human resource capacity in support of aquaculture development in The Gambia. The Government should also emphasize on aquaculture in the school curriculum especially at secondary, vocational and college levels.

A number of aquaculture practices are used in The Gambia in the various water environments for a great variety of cultured species. Freshwater aquaculture is carried out in fish ponds in various communities, schools and private farms. Brackish water aquaculture is done mainly in fish ponds located in coastal areas that are mostly tidally irrigated. Marine culture has not been fully explored in The Gambia. The culture systems in The Gambia are mostly extensive which is almost exclusively oriented towards production for domestic consumption.

The usual practice currently is the stocking of fish of different ages and sexes in the ponds with complete and partial harvesting of small amounts.

Natural resources constitute the basis of The Gambia aquaculture production. Alternative agriculture production has been introduced to some fish farmers. The combination of fish and poultry activities sponsored by LHDP under the Ministry of Agriculture is also being conducted in WCR and NBR.

The main source of pond water is tidal irrigation although few farms employ pump irrigation technologies.

Fish seed are made available by catching from the wild. There seems to be great potential for integrating biotechnology to further develop aquaculture in The Gambia.

In The Gambia where fish ponds are mostly fresh and brackish water, commonly cultured species suitable for those environments include tilapia, catfish, *Heterotis*, eel, carp, mullet, shrimp and oyster. The most cultured species among them are tilapia, catfish and shrimp. However, other species including eel are also being farmed in a poly-culture system in few farms.

Contribution of aquaculture to the national economy is not separated from that of the overall fisheries sector. However, it has been observed that fish farming is a very good source of livelihood improvement through the provision of fish protein and income to the households. In addition to supplying cheap protein for human consumption, aquaculture provides excellent opportunities for employment and income generation, particularly in the rural areas.

Most aquaculture projects in The Gambia are new, designed with intent to meet fully or partly the social and cultural needs of a community. The school ponds are models to increase not only the nutritional requirement of the communities but also to be seen as a potential income generating activity worth imitating by the younger generation.

Though the current situation of aquaculture in The Gambia does not generate any critical environmental review, linkages should be created for sustainability between aquaculture and the application of biotechnology in order to be recognized as efficient contributor to food security. This will require the development of ecosystems approaches and sustainable operating procedures, by incorporating social, economic and environmental context in all aspects of aquaculture development in the country.

## Current Status of Aquaculture in the Gambia

Since the Gambia's aquaculture is still under developed, the introduction of low cost technologies could contribute to greater levels of participation and ownership and thus more sustainable development. This will improve the livelihoods of aquatic farmers through promotion of biotechnology and aquatic resource management related technologies, which could thereby expand aquaculture development to all parts of the country, with the purpose to promote aquaculture production and management on a long-term basis.

The performance of the aquaculture sub-sector in The Gambia is still not well developed due to the types of technologies employed by farmers especially those in the rural areas. Pond culture is the most common in The Gambia. Nearly all the fish farmers in The Gambia are operating either earthen or concrete/cement pond technologies in WCR, CRR south and NBR. There are a total of 98 fin fish ponds in the country operating in small-scale fish farming. 90 per cent of these ponds are earthen ponds impoundments excavated as sunken holes in the ground.

Only 10 per cent of the small-scale fish ponds is concrete or cement ponds constructed by 2 fish farms engaging in recreational ecotourism aquaculture including sport fishing and ornamental fishery practices in Lamin and Bijilo. Unlike the ponds around the estuaries and fresh water zones of the River Gambia which are tidally irrigated, the source of water for the 2 recreational fish farms is borehole.

There is clear need for an improved design capacity with specialized engineers to facilitate the establishment of aquaculture projects in The Gambia. Good site selection is one of the most important factors in fish farm planning along with issues concerning the characteristic of soil, pond lining, and irrigation.

Ponds are fertilized regularly using organic fertilizers like chicken and cow manure to maintain the plankton growth in the ponds. Almost all the ponds are fertilized with these organic materials found locally. This is low cost technology for small-scale farmers with the view to intensify productivity of the aquaculture systems to produce sufficient supplies for local consumption. The fish farmers process organic wastes as feed for the fish as well as fertilizers for the ponds.

Good quality feed production has been observed as the major constraints in aquaculture production in The Gambia. Few of the farmers import feed from outside the country while majority use locally available organic waste such as rice bran, groundnut cake, animal bone, oyster shells and kitchen waste, which are normally obtained and processed locally to enhance production without any specialized or complicated processing techniques and technology.

The application of biotechnology for the production of good quality feed needs to be introduced in order to improve the quality of the products and also to provide efficient services to members in the area of fish feed manufacturing.

Seed quality is an essential attribute for optimizing the potential for aquaculture production (better yield and good returns) and is related to the quality of the brood stock used and the seed produced. Genetic quality and good hatchery/nursery management are among two main factors affecting seed quality. Fish seed supply has been cited as the major constraint to developing aquaculture in the country. The available fish hatchery, situated in Jahally Pacharr was established in 2007 by Taiwan Technical Mission (TTM) in The Gambia. The farm was later handed to the DoF in 2012. The hatchery was producing a relatively low number of fingerlings and because of technical and logistical problems after the Taiwanese left, the farm had no capacity to deploy biotechnology to enhance the quality and quantity of fingerlings' production.

Farmers collect seeds from natural environment such as rivers, estuaries and gutters for stocking. These are the basic principles of acquiring fingerlings for sustaining aquaculture by small-scale fish famers throughout the country.

Seed being the basic input into any aquaculture technologies should be accorded priority in terms of brood stock management, establishment of hatcheries, refinement of induced breeding techniques, rearing and production. Adequate emphasis on the production of quality fish seed should be led by the Government, private sector and development partners to meet the growing requirement of fish producers in the country. Proper and efficient hatchery production of seed is needed to stabilize and ensure regular supply of quality seed. Deployment of biotechnology in the breeding techniques to produce improved seed for better growth and production should be emphasized.

Biotechnology has been observed to have significant impact in all aquaculture practices. The low level of human capital and lack of research establishment is a great barrier for adoption of new technologies by farmers in The Gambia. Players in the fisheries and aquaculture sector have agreed with the fact that, there has to be more emphasis on human resource development to address this need.

A modern aquaculture industry requires well trained biologists and specialized research and technical institutes to be able to address matters such as water and ecosystem control, as well as support the development of an efficient, modern hatchery industry, optimizing feed and treating fish diseases. Therefore, research capabilities and capacity are required in the country's aquaculture technology development plan.

Fish farmers in The Gambia cited harvesting process as the most labor-intensive operation especially in ponds with multiple stocking with different sizes of fish. Fishing nets are the most desired materials used for harvesting.

## Potential of Biotechnology in Aquaculture Techniques in the Gambia

The use of biotechnology in aquaculture in the Gambia has great potential to significantly contribute towards sustained food security, income to rural households, enhance revenue generation for the state through exports, re-enforcement of employment and inward investments. Though the Gambia's aquaculture is in its infant stage, there are opportunities for accelerated and sustained growth through the availability and level of technology, availability of production inputs, support facilities and services amongst others. These are non-negotiable pre-requisites for the development of viable and efficient aquaculture technologies.

The River Gambia has enormous water resources that can sustain various technologies in aquaculture. With the availability of water to grow fish and shrimp, The Gambia aquaculture industry offers more choices and opportunities for the people of the country as well as potential investors.

In any aquaculture technology, the potential environmental effects must be taken into consideration at the planning stage. Aquaculture has been observed to have negative environmental effects. Most of these are related to the destruction of natural ecosystems such as mangrove forest to construct aquaculture farms, the environmental impacts of the effluents on the receiving ecosystems, pollution of water bodies for human consumption, changes on landscape and hydrological patterns as well as introduction of exotic species. Therefore, it is important to choose technologies and techniques for aquaculture development in such a way that the negative environmental effects are minimized.

Most of the fish farms in The Gambia are young about 1-year old and have not had any significant harvest. However, only two (2) situated in Ndemban and Madina Kanuma claimed to have harvested. The products harvested were marketed without putting due consideration on demand. However, there is much concern among fish farmers about competition with wild catch and also the quality of their produce during marketing. It is important for the farmers to tract and anticipates changes that can affect the marketing of their production.

The products harvested are transported by bicycle and sold to the village local market and their surroundings villages. Since most farms in The Gambia are about 1-year old and have not had any significant harvest, the focus now should be to increase production by the application of biotechnology.

The fish harvested from the farms were sold fresh without the application of any specialized processing technique. Frozen and smoked fish processing techniques can be envisaged in the Gambia aquaculture industry in the long-term. Frozen fish offers convenience, guarantee quality and conservation and provides a means for the farmer to sell fish at a better price. This could also enhance the availability of fish to the consumers.

Since the fish harvested are destined for human consumption, the fresh fish are distributed to the markets and surrounding villages with the use of bicycles as a means of transportation. Market linkages in The Gambia are insufficient which may lead to disruptions in supply of aquaculture products. Therefore, biotechnology in the preservation of aquaculture products can reduce post-harvest losses and meet the demand of the growing population.

## Conclusions

The applications of biotechnology in the Development of Aquaculture in The Gambia are highly needed to satisfy the country's growing demand for seafood. Biotechnology approaches in the health, safety and sustainable conservation of the environment and resources is also necessary in order to manage aquaculture and the environment on which the sub-sector depends. Among the potential areas of the application of biotechnology in aquaculture in The Gambia include fish health management, fish nutrition and seed production. These will help in solving the numerous challenges faced by Gambia in its effort to enhance aquaculture output, create employment for youth and women, reduce the impact of aquaculture production on the environment and improve public perception in aquaculture.

## Abbreviations

**CRR:** Central River Region
**DoF:** Department of Fisheries
**FAO:** Food and Agriculture Organization of the United Nations
**FASDEP:** Food and Agriculture Sector Development Project
**GASAP:** Gambia Shrimp Aquaculture Project
**LHDP:** Livestock and Horticulture Development Project
**NBR:** North Bank Region
**R&D:** Research and Development
**TCP:** Technical Cooperation Program
**SWOT:** Strengths, Weaknesses, Opportunities and Threats
**TTM:** Taiwan Technical Mission
**UN:** United Nations
**UNDP:** United Nations Development Program
**WAA:** West African Aquaculture Ltd
**WABSA:** West African Birds Study Association
**WCR:** West Coast Region

## REFERENCES

1. Edward P., Little D.C., and Demaine H 2002. Rural Aquaculture. CABI Publishing, UK. pp. 1-357
2. Jallow, A 2009. History of Aquaculture in The nation. The Gambia Daily Observer. 1st December, 2009.
3. Jallow, A 2014. Aquaculture Training Manual. Department of Fisheries.
4. National Environmental Agency 2010. State of the Environment Report – The Gambia. 2nd Edition.
5. Pillay T.V.R and Kutty M.N 2005. Aquaculture: principles and practices, 2nd Edition. Blackwell Publishing Company. pp. 3-624.
6. Rakocy E 1989. Tank culture of tilapia. Southern regional aquaculture centre. University of Virgin Island. SRAC Publication no. 282
7. Rice A.M., Darboe S.F., Drammeh O., Kanyi B 2012. Aquaculture in The Gambia. University of Rhodes Island. pp. 29-71.
8. UN 2014. United Nations Conference on Trade and Development Enhanced Integrated Framework. United Nations Publication, UN. pp. 1-54.
9. UNDP 2013. TRY Oyster Women's Association, The Gambia. Equator Initiative Case Study Series. New York, NY. pp. 1-12.
10. http: //www.mof.gov.gm/publication/2014 cited 2016

*Chapter 9*

# The Use of an *In vitro* Derived Seedling in Indonesian Cocoa Replanting Programme

*Taryono*

*Faculty of Agriculture and Research Centre of Biotechnology, Universitas Gadjah Mada*
*Bulaksumur, Yogyakarta, INDONESIA*
*E-mail: tariono60@gmail.com, tariono60@ugm.ac.id*

## ABSTRACT

It has been realized since in the 80's that Indonesia's economic growth could not be based only on the fossil fuel, and so agriculture must also play a major role in national development. Due to long experience in exploring estate crops as big private plantations for export purpose, the government then introduced some estate crops as the recommended perennial crops for growers through Nuclear Estate Smallholders (NES). In this system, farmers as growers grew estate crops with the supervision of public and national big plantations. By such national program, Indonesia for example, is considered as the third world biggest cocoa production with plantation area more than 1 million ha, however since 2008 production has been on the decline due to pest infestation, and improper cultivation system. Government therefore introduced the National Cocoa Program for Production and Quality Improvement as big as 450,000 ha with 70,000 ha for replanting, 235,000 ha for rehabilitation and 145,000 ha for intensification. Theoretically, by 2.5 × 2.5 m plant spacing, a replanting required 70 million seedlings in three years. Nevertheless, the conventional seed multiplication system is not able to produce the high quantity of seedlings rapidly. Therefore, a simple biotechnological strategy by *in vitro* culture is supposed to be implemented. The Indonesian Coffee and Cocoa Research Institute (ICCRI) assisted by Nestle have been able to produce a large quantity of cocoa seedlings through somatic embryogenesis. Hence, *in vitro* culture has been chosen as a proper biotechnological approach to fulfill the seedling multiplication requirements.

In 2009, nearly 20 million of cocoa *in vitro* derived seedlings were produced and grown in farmers' fields in nine provinces of the eastern part of Indonesia. In some areas, *in vitro* derived seedlings grew well. Thus, many growers worked diligently to manage their lands. A study in 2011 reported that in general, the *in vitro* derived trees produced normal dense flowers and as a result, growers looked very enthusiastic. Growers estimated that *in vitro* derived trees would be able to reach a good yield. Unfortunately, when pods matured, they were predisposed to pest and the seeds evaluated, tend end to be small in size. Such findings informed growers' lack of interest in the cultivation technology. Furthermore, growers did not manage the cocoa trees properly, and even some growers gave out their land. A study in 2014 showed that the cocoa growers were not in favour of growing *in vitro* derived seedlings and in 2011 as much as 30,000 ha was not well-managed. The study in 2014 also found that the productivity of cocoa *in vitro* derived trees was very low due to pest attack and improper production management system. Based on such experience, growers must be empowered to use simple industrial biotechnology.

***Keywords:*** *Cocoa, Somatic embryogenesis, Replanting.*

## INTRODUCTION

Cacao (*Theobroma cocoa* L.) is a crop of the humid lowland tropics and one of the essential crops in the world since its beans are the main ingredients for the manufacture of drinking cocoa and chocolate. Many developing countries across tropical Africa, Latin America, and Asia grow cacao. Also, more than 95 per cent of cocoa produced globally is grown by small holders farmers who cultivate only a few hectares and usually rely on family labor (Neilson, 2010).

Indonesia, Cote d'Ivoire and Ghana are among the largest cocoa producing countries in the world (Meulemans *et al.*, 2002). Indonesia accounts for 13 per cent of the global cocoa production mainly bulk cocoa based on Forestero hybrid and becomes the most valuable cocoa producers in Asia. (Johnson *et al.*, 2004).

Indonesia was historically recorded as the earliest centre of cocoa cultivation in the world. The cocoa was introduced to Celebes (now Sulawesi) in 1560, and the success of this introduction extended the cultivation area to Java during Dutch colonization with a high yielding flavoured variety. In 1880, cocoa had become an extremely profitable crop in Java. Then, in 1888, there were early attempts to develop new varieties and later succeeded producing the hybrid in 1892 (Bloomfield and Las, 1992). Indonesian cocoa area gradually declined from the 1920s due to the fast and uncontrollable spread of pests especially cocoa pod borer.

The new Indonesian cocoa boom production has begun since the 1980s (Li, 2002). Sulawesi island is central of small holders cocoa farmers (Johnson *et al.*, 2004), who work in areas ranging from 0.5 – 1.5 ha produce over 80 per cent Indonesia cocoa (Abbate, 2007). It underwent several stages, *i.e.*, the early stage from 1980 to 1989, the developing stage from 1990 to 2000, and transition into industrialisation from 2000 onwards (Li, 2002).

In the early stage, the new massive area opened for cocoa cultivation and sharply increased in production. Between 1980-1990 the cocoa cultivation area reached almost 350,000 ha from only 40,000 ha. The driving factors were speculated by Indonesia migrant workers initiatives (Jamal and Pomp, 1998), Indonesian Government Programs such as PRPTE (Program of Rehabilitation and Expansion of Export Crops) in 1980, and PDSA (Plantation Development in Special Areas) in 1990 due to the availability of suitable land, low production cost and competitive markets (Abbate, 2007).

The second stage was due to the economic crisis in 1998 followed by the devaluation of Indonesian currency. The cocoa price rose almost three times, and farmers discovered that export crops such as cocoa were more valuable than food crops. Since the 2000s, Indonesia has maintained the position as the third world cocoa producers. Cocoa is grown throughout the nation with two large production regions, *i.e.*, Sulawesi and Sumatra. As a result, cocoa became the fourth most valuable agricultural export commodities of the country after palm oil, rubber, and coconut. The small holder farmers played an important role as the engine of Indonesia cocoa boom (Akiyama and Nishio, 2006) with bean yields ranging from 400 to 800 kg/ha. In 2004, the productivity reached 1,189 kg/ha, but suddenly declined over time to only 820 kg/ha in 2009.

The main challenge of Indonesia cocoa is low quality, and productivity due to cocoa pod borer attack, low knowledge of farming practice and unproductive old cocoa trees. The damaged cocoa fields in 2008 were estimated to reach 450,000 ha. The national cocoa production therefore dropped to only 700,000 ton a year. The Indonesian Government tried to restore the cocoa boom production with better bean quality by introducing the Cocoa National Program on Production and Quality Improvement, which started from 2009 to 2012. In this program, a huge amount of planting materials is expected. Thus, industrial plant biotechnology through somatic embryogenesis must be investigated.

## Cocoa National Program for Production and Quality Improvement

The Indonesian Government started to pay attention to cocoa as from 1975s at the time when Public Plantation Company succeeded increasing productivity by the use of hybrid technology. This crop further developed fast in the 1980s due to PRPTE project. At that time, the government sought and developed non-fuel export commodities to cope with the reduction of natural energy production and export. The cocoa area grew tremendously in the 1990s and led Indonesia to become the third largest cocoa world exporter.

In 2008, it was reported that approximately 70,000 ha cocoa fields showed aging, damage and unproductive due to heavy pest attack, 235,000 ha seem unproductive due to medium pest attack, and 145,000 ha depict improper cultivation management. The main cocoa pest and disease are pod borer and Vein Streak Dieback (VSD) which can decrease the domestic cocoa productivity by 25.6 per cent. Such pest and disease also declined the bean quality. Since cocoa plays a prominent role in Sulawesi economy, the local government attempted to cope with pest problem by introducing some measures to save the farmers cocoa condition. The Government of South Sulawesi for instance in 2007 launched "Cocoa Production and Quality Recovery Movement" with the objectives to increase the production, productivity, and quality through improving cultivation methods, plant protection, and better post-harvest. As a result, on 31 July 2007, the Government of West Sulawesi declared "Cocoa Renewal Movement" to improve the community welfare and eradicate poverty through the improvement of cocoa productivity, quality, and profitability.

However, the impact of such measures did not seem so optimal. Consequently, the vice President of Indonesia on 6 August 2008 proposed the need for Cocoa National Movement for Production and Quality Improvement and on 10 August 2008, the Vice President declared as "Cocoa National Program for Production and Quality Improvement". This Program involved destruction of old unproductive cocoa replanting, rehabilitating unproductive rescuable cocoa, and nurturing those with low yield to optimal level. Such program was in line with Government Development Policy that must be Pro-Growth, Pro-Job, Pro Poor and Pro Environment.

One of the targets of the National Program for Production and Quality Improvement is cocoa crop improvement as big as 450,000 ha, which consists of 70,000 ha replanting, 235,000 ha rehabilitation, and 145,000 ha intensification. In the case of replanting, by the assumption that cocoa spacing is 2.5×2.5 $m^2$, each ha requires at least 1,000 seedlings. Hence, at least 70 million seedlings must be produced in 3 years (Table 9.1). No conventional cocoa seed producers can provide such a huge amount of planting materials. New technology such as *in vitro* culture therefore must be introduced, and somatic embryogenesis is averred as the most feasible technology.

**Table 9.1: The Target Area of Indonesia Cocoa Replanting Programme 2009-2011**

| *No.* | *Year* | *Target Area (ha)* | *Planting Material Requirements (seedlings)* |
|---|---|---|---|
| 1 | 2009 | 20,000 | 20,000,000 |
| 2 | 2010 | 22,600 | 22,600,000 |
| 3 | 2011 | 27,400 | 27,400,000 |
| **Total** | | **70,000** | **70,000,000** |

*Source*: Ministry of Agriculture, 2009.

## Somatic Embryogenesis as an Appropriate Propagation Method

The high performance of planting materials is an important aspect in a sustainable cocoa intensification. Cocoa can be multiplied through sexual and asexual methods. Seeds are the product of sexual reproduction where fertilization of a female gamete by a male gamete is necessary to produce a zygote (Lockwood, 2015) and can be produced in the seed garden through manual hand or natural pollination. A seed garden system can be an efficient and economic way to supply high quality of planting materials in large quantities, yet it was hindered by cash investment, availability of suitable land in favourable agro-climatic zone, production of heterogeneous plant due to flower morphology and incompatibility. The asexual method of vegetative propagation has been used as a potential means of recovering cocoa production in different countries (Rudgard *et al.*, 1993). Also, various conventional vegetative propagation techniques may be utilized by placing bud or graft materials from improved clones onto seedling rootstock in the nursery or onto plants already grown in the field, and even using rooted cutting of improved materials (Laliberte and End, 2015). Nonetheless, there were some disadvantages related to current methods of vegetative propagation including low propagation rate and undesirable growth pattern (Figueira and Janick, 1995). Clonal propagation using modern biotechnology of micro-propagation provided the advantage of reducing time in the scaling-up of elite planting material (Chantrapradist and Kanchanapoom, 1995). Micropropagation can be done through organogenesis such as shoot bud proliferation, adventitious shoot production, and somatic embryogenesis (Bonga and Durjan, 1987). Clonally propagated by *in vitro* culture has the potential to produce plant at a competitive cost and in the large number needed to meet the demand (Smith and Aynsky, 1995). *In vitro* cultured plants are in general free from fungal and bacterial and even virus diseases (Debnath *et al.*, 2006). The main advantages of cocoa *in vitro* culture include the rapid generation of a vast number of genetically uniform plants, producing the orthotropic plants with normal dimorphic architecture, disease free materials and as a tool for germplasm conservation (Maximova and Guiltinan, 2015).

Somatic embryogenesis refers to the process by which haploid or diploid somatic cells develop into a differentiated plant through characteristic embryological stages without fusion of gametes. (Williams and Maheswaran, 1986). There were two general patterns of somatic embryo development, *i.e.*, direct and indirect embryogenesis (Evans *et al.*, 1981). Indirect embryogenesis requires redetermination of differentiated cells, callus proliferation and the development of the embryogenically determined state, whereas direct embryogenesis occurs from embryos originated from tissue characterized by the absence of callus proliferation. Somatic embryos obtained by direct embryogenesis seems less numerous than embryos derived from indirect embryogenesis (Dulas *et al.*, 2007). The choice of the technology depends on the species of interest, the available technology and the cost (Venkateswarlu and Korwar, 2005), but indirect somatic embryogenesis is probably the only efficient possible approach for mass clonal micro-propagation. The main advantages of somatic embryo production included the possibility of rapidly generating asexually propagated uniform seedlings with orthotropic dimorphic architecture and taproot formation (Maximova *et al.*, 2002). Somatic embryo and plantlet production have been achieved in a significant number of genotypes (Li *et al.*, 1998). The use of *in vitro* propagation method through embryo production therefore can potentially contribute to the effort of crop improvement and rapid distribution of new improved planting materials (Maximova *et al.*, 2008).

Cocoa somatic embryogenesis process begins with the immature flowers especially the staminodes, which are grown in sterile laboratory conditions using solid nutrient media containing various mixtures of plant growth regulators. Proper mixtures of plant growth regulators trigger a reprogramming of somatic cells to de-differentiate initiating the embryogenesis developmental programme. During such developmental programme, a single or group of somatic cells begin to divide and form embryogenic calli or pro-embryonic structure then followed by further development to produce mature embryos (Maximova and Guiltinan, 2005). These

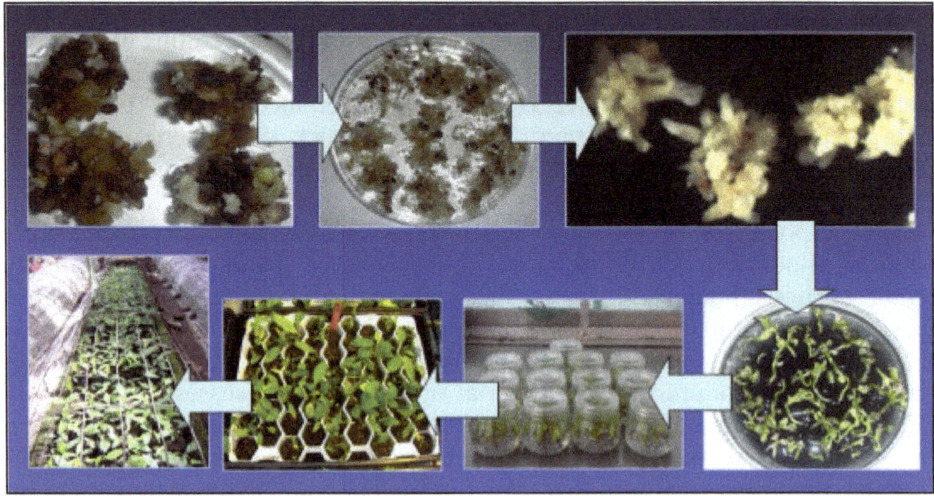

**Figure 9.1: Process Flow of Cocoa Somatic Embryogenesis. (*Source*: ICCRI, 2009).**

mature embryos later can be *in vitro* germinated into plantlets; and plantlets are acclimatized to a greenhouse to produce seedlings (Figure 9.1).

The process flow of somatic embryo production can be detail classified into four stages, *i.e.* (1) the induction of embryogenic calli followed their identification and selection by physical isolation, (2) multiplication of embryogenic cells, (3) a regeneration of a large number of embryo, and (4) conversion of the immature embryo to generate plantlets (Dulas *et al.*, 2007).

## Industrial Plant Biotechnology for Scaling Up Somatic Embryo Production

Industrial biotechnology refers to the application of biotechnology based tools to a traditional industrial process for commercial purposes (Erikson *et al.*, 2012). Moreover, industrial biotechnology can be a key to the future strategies for viable economic growth (Murugan and Wins, 2010). Besides, it can provide a cheaper option to achieve industrial sustainability than the traditional process.

Somatic embryogenesis enables rapid and massive vegetative propagation of elite genotypes, and so it is widely accepted as the promising approach for capturing genetic gain quickly through rapid and large-scale dissemination of elite individuals (Etienne *et al.*, 2000). Furthermore, somatic embryogenesis process has been reported to be successfully applied on an industrial scale such as in Loblolly pine, oil palm, and coffee for which annual production goes up to several million plants annually.

Industrial feasibility of somatic embryogenesis can be fitted to different stages of its process flow such as embryogenic tissue production, multiplication of embryogenic calli and embryo differentiation, embryo maturation and germination (Etienne *et al.*, 2000). However, multiplication of embryogenic calli is the bottle neck

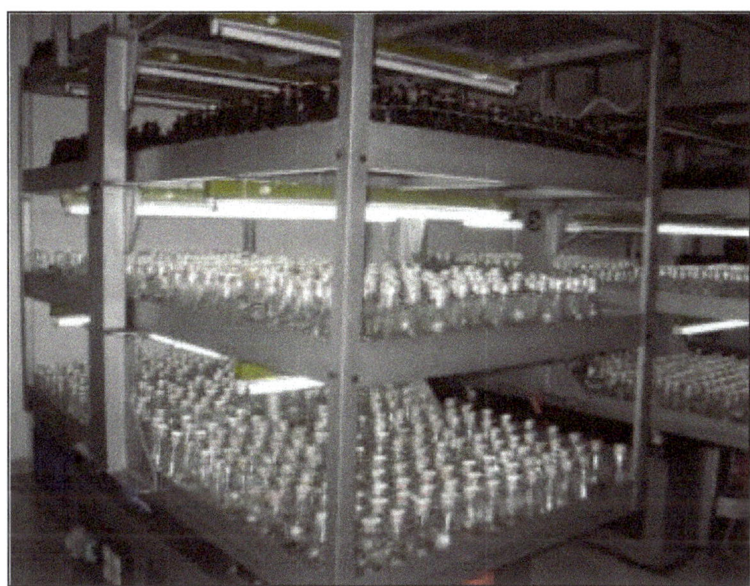

**Figure 9.2: Multiplication of Embryogenic Calli in Liquid Media.**

of the massive production of mass propagation. Embryogenic calli can be multiplied on the semi solid medium or liquid culture (Figure 9.2). Additionally, multiplication on semi solid medium is costly due to intensive manual manipulation (Paek *et al.*, 2001, Ziv, 2005). Hence, adapting liquid media is favourable due to the ease of scaling up (Preil, 1991). The use of liquid culture can provide rapid proliferation and separation (Aitken-Christie *et al.*, 1995), therefore scaling up of plant regeneration in a liquid medium is easier than on a semi solid one (Okamoto *et al.*, 1996).

By the combination of semi solid and liquid media with about 250 laboratory workers, ICCRI (Indonesian Cocoa and Coffee Research Institute) is the most successful institution in scaling up the cocoa somatic embryogenesis technology for commercial purposes by establishing a tissue culture laboratory to produce up to 50 million plants per year (Maximova and Guilitinan, 2015).

## The Performance of Somatic Embryo Derived Cocoa Plant at the Farmer Field

There were five cocoa clones, which can be multiplied using *in vitro* culture though somatic embryogenesis. They are different in flush leaf colour, yield potential and seed size (ICCRI, 2010). ICCRI developed ICCRI-03 and ICCRI-04. The flush leaf colour can distinguish both of them. ICCRI-03 has reddish flush whereas ICCRI-04 has green flush colour. Sca-6 was introduced from Kew Garden, England with a green flush, small seed size, and many flowers. On the other hand, Sul-01 and Sul-02 were difficult to distinguish based on flush colour only because the flush colours look similar.

**Table 9.2: Cocoa Clone Flush Leaf Color, Yield Potential and Seed Size**

| *No.* | *Clone* | *Clone Characteristic* | | |
|---|---|---|---|---|
| | | *Flush Leaf Color* | *Seed Size (g)* | *Yield Potential (ton/ha/year)* |
| 1. | ICCRI-03 | Reddish | 1.280 | 2.09 |
| 2. | ICCRI-04 | Green | 1.270 | 2.06 |
| 3. | Sca-6 | Green | 0.725 | 1.54 |
| 4. | Sul-1 | Reddish | 1.100 | 2.15 |
| 5. | Sul-2 | Reddish | 1.000 | 2.27 |

*Source*: Ministry of Agriculture, 2011.

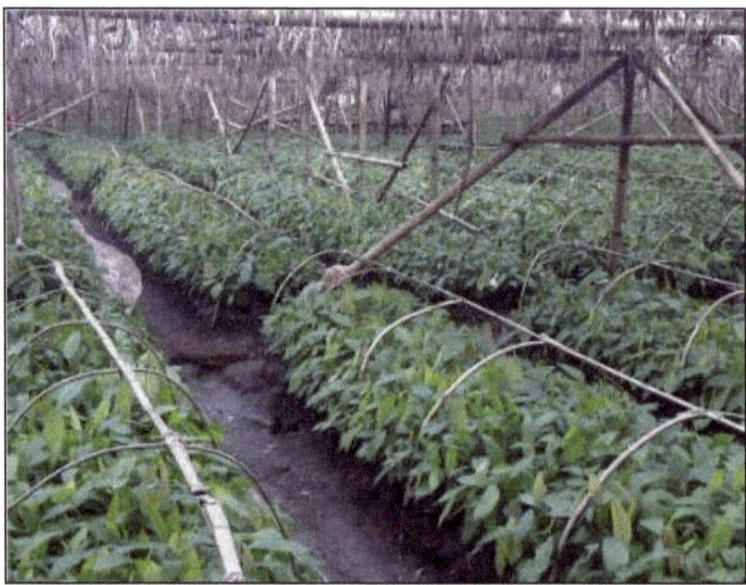

**Figure 9.3: Seedling Performance at the Nursery.**

Table 9.3 presents the realization area and planting material requirements from 2009 to 2012. A total of 82 million somatic embryos derived seedlings were distributed to farmers around the nation especially in the eastern part of Indonesia. Also, a thorough field evaluation has been carried out to 20 million somatic embryos derived seedlings grown in 2009 since the time of the distribution. The growth of somatic derived seedlings at the nursery looked normal and homogeneous in the morphology (Figure 9.3).

Field monitoring and evaluation were carried out by the Government through the involvement of 3 universities as independent researchers every year from 2009 – 2012. Field evaluation was done in 5 selected provinces by observing 100 plants of 5 farmer samples. General evaluations were also executed in 2011 and 2013. Seedlings distributed in 2009 were cultivated in early 2010 due to water availability

**Table 9.3: The Realization Area of Indonesia Cocoa Replanting Programme 2009 -2012**

| *No.* | *Year* | *Target Area (ha)* | *Planting Material Requirements (Seedlings)* |
|---|---|---|---|
| 1 | 2009 | 20,000 | 20,000,000 |
| 2 | 2010 | 14,920 | 22,600,000 |
| 3 | 2011 | 42,700 | 27,400,000 |
| 4 | 2012 | 4,900 | 4,900,000 |
| **Total** | | **82,520** | **74,900,000** |

*Source*: Ministry of Agriculture (2013).

that is normally enough during wet season. Field monitoring was done in September 2010. The seedlings have been grown successfully in the farmer field, and jourgette was normally formed (Ministry of Agriculture, 2010). Further field evaluation was also carried out in 2011 when the plant was between 12 – 15 months old. The plant thrived with dominant green flush color, started flowering and potentially produced more than 1-ton dry seeds/ha based on the number of pods per plant, yet the bean size was considered too small. The bean count is found more than 100 (Ministry of Agriculture, 2012). The small size is probably due to the dominance of Sca-6 cocoa plant in the farmer field or initial pods. ICCRI mentioned that initial pods tend to produce small seeds. Further observation in 2012 yielded lower seed weights, which were disappointing to farmers (Ministry of Agriculture, 2012). Good quality seed found in 2011 have influenced the farmer's behaviour to manage their field as they previously failed to manage their field properly. Farmers left the cocoa good agricultural practices such as pruning, fertilizer application, weeding, pest control and even sanitation. The cocoa farmers' field looked contemptible with high weed growth. Some pests started to attack pods and roots. Pod borer, *Helopelthis* severely disturbed the pod's growth and root disease attacked some cocoa plants that caused plant collapse and death.

ICCRI evaluated the performance of SE derived plants in 5 provinces, *i.e.*, Central Sulawesi, West Sulawesi, South Sulawesi, South East Sulawesi and Bali in 2012, It was concluded that 19.6 per cent showed low vigor, especially those found on poorly managed farms, low fertility soil with improper drainage, and no shading. Somatic embryo derived plant exhibited an early prominent flowering, however different results have been reported by Pardomuan and Taylor (2012) based on the survey in West and South Sulawesi. They found that a significant percentage of somatic embryo derived plant were unhealthy with poor root structure and suffering from pest and diseases.

Farmers should be empowered so that they apply good agricultural practices. Intensive empowerment was able to improve the seed weight in 2013, though the pest attack could not be controlled. Consequently, the national evaluation done at the end of 2013 showed that the productivity on the farmer field only reached 350 kg/ha/year. Demonstration plot supervised by ICCRI yielded up to 500 kg/ha/year. Proper field maintenance tended to yield high productivity. Consequently, the government introduced a new program to improve the performance of SE derived cocoa through intensification program which was implemented between 2015-2016.

## Factor Determining the Yield Performance of Somatic Embryo Derived Cocoa Plant at the Farmer Field

Field observation in 2015 was carried out in two provinces, *i.e.* Central and South-East Sulawesi. It was found that the SE derived cocoa in South East Sulawesi looked better than Central Sulawesi. Taryono *et al.* (2017) surveyed to know the agronomic factors determining yield performance in South East Sulawesi. Two districts with dominant SE derived cocoa farms were surveyed on the agricultural practices done by farmers in 2015 and the influence to the productivity. Data were collected from 120 respondents, though only 111 data can be analysed. Correlation analysis was employed to determine factors determining yields.

**Table 9.4: General Cocoa Agronomical Practices in Indonesia**

| *No.* | *Agronomical Practices* | *Farmers Response (per cent)* | | *Frequency* | | *Correlation to Yield (r)* |
|---|---|---|---|---|---|---|
| | | *No* | *Yes* | *Interval* | *Average* | |
| 1. | Deadditsch excavation | 1.80 | 98.20 | 0 - 5 | 1.80 | -0.291* |
| 2. | Fertilizing | 2.72 | 97.30 | 0 - 2 | 1.66 | 0.205* |
| 3. | Weeding | 3.60 | 96.40 | 0 - 12 | 5.18 | 0.211* |
| 4. | Pruning | 4.50 | 95.50 | 0 - 34 | 5.33 | 0.042 |
| 5. | Pest and disease control | 6.31 | 93.69 | 0 - 36 | 14.41 | -0.077 |
| 6. | Sanitation | 2.70 | 97.30 | 0 - 9 | 0.95 | 0.028 |
| 7. | Harvesting | 0 | 100.00 | 1 - 56 | 3.80 | -0.093 |

It is believed that input intensification can increase cocoa productivity. Table 9.4 showed that more than 90 per cent farmers applied a proper good agricultural practice, although not all agricultural practices affected the yield. Fertilizer application and weeding contributed a positive impact on yield, which was similar to the report of Tothmihally and Ingram (2017). Fertilizer can increase cocoa yield since many soils can not supply enough nutrient during cocoa development (Noordiana *et al.*, 2007). The application of fertilizer is beneficial to boost cocoa production (Agbeniji *et al.*, 2010). Opeyemi *et al.* (2005) reported that an efficient fertilizer application would result in not *only improving the yield but also profitability, seed quality, and environment. The* application of fertilizer should be considered as a key factor for maximizing cocoa production because fertilizer can boost cocoa productivity (Ogunlade *et al.*, 2009).

Although nitrogen is one of the most critical yield limiting factor (Ribeiro *et al.*, 2008), the majority of farmers (87.39 per cent) prefer to use NPK compound to improve the nutrient availability. Besides, only 8 per cent of farmers solely apply nitrogen, either in the form of urea or ammonium sulphate as a source of nitrogen. The use of NPK compound is believed better than nitrogen alone because Fasina *et al.* (2006) mentioned that adequate and balanced fertilizer is not only profitable, but also sustain and build high yield over time.

The effect of fertilizer does not only depend on the cocoa tree requirement, but also on current nutrient availability from the soil, and also other environmental condition, the presence of pest and disease, and the management of shade trees including pruning of the cocoa (Van Vliet *et al.*, 2015). Although the frequency of pest and disease control did not significantly influence the yield, the existence of pest and diseases significantly decreased the yield (r= -0.217*). Pest and diseases attacked almost all pods (99.00 per cent), and *Helopelthis* pest significantly decreased bean yield. The attack of *Helopelthis* in the early pod phase inhibited bean development, and it seemed that almost all pods produced by SE derived cocoa trees were sensitive to it.

Good quality of seedlings produced massively by modern biotechnological approach should be cultivated at a suitable land and handled properly with care, so that cocoa can grow properly and yield bean optimally.

## Conclusions

Based on Indonesian experience of using a modern approach to overcome the seedling needs to intensify and extensify the plantation area, it is inferred that:

1. *In vitro* culture through somatic embryogenesis can be used to produce the best quality of crop seedling,
2. Industrial plant biotechnology can be used to scale up the seedling productions for commercial purposes,
3. SE derived cocoa seedlings perform vigorously in the farmers' field at the vegetative phase,
4. SE derived cocoa plants produce enough number of flowers and pods although pods can be attacked by pest and disease, and
5. Fertilizer application is an important input to maintain seed yield of SE derived cocoa trees.

Due to the severe pest and disease attack, SE derived cocoa plants must be grown in suitable land and handled with care from the beginning at the farmers' field while ensuring good agricultural management implementation. In addition, farmers must be intensively empowered.

## Acknowledgements

I gratefully acknowledge the Ministry of Agriculture of the Republic of Indonesia for financial support and the invitation to me to get involved in the long-term evaluation and monitoring on the use of somatic embryogenesis technology for cocoa planting material production. I also would like to thank Mr. Benny Satria from the University of Andalas, Mr. Arifin Noor from the University of Brawijaya, Mrs. Isnainar from University Tadulako in Central Sulawesi as well as Mr. Hamirul Hadini from the University of Haluleo in South East Sulawesi for their collaboration.

## REFERENCES

1. Abbate, M. 2007. The "Sweet Desire" cocoa plantation and its knowledge transfer in Central Sulawesi, Indonesia. George-August-University, Gottingen, Germany.
2. Agbeniji, S. O., M. O. Ogunlade., K. A. Okuyole. 2010. Fertilizer use and cocoa production in cross river state, Nigeria. *ARPN Journal of Agricultural and Biological Science* 5: 10–13.
3. Aiken-Christie, J., T. Kosai, M. A. I. Smith. 1995. Automation and Environmental Control in Plant Tissue Culture. Kluwer Acad. Pub. Dordrecht.
4. Akiyama, T., A. Nihio. 1997. Sulawes's cocoa boom: lessons of small-holders dynamism and a hands-off policy. *Bulletin of Indonesian Economic Studies* 33: 97–121.
5. Bonga, J. M., D. J. Durjan. 1987. Cell and Tissue Culture in Forestry. Martinus .Nijhoff Publ. Dordrecht.
6. Boomfield, E. M., R. A. Lass. 1992. Impact of Structural Adjusment and Adoption of Technology on Competitiveness of Major Cocoa Producing Countries. Working Papaer 69. Paris.
7. Chantrapradist, C., K. Kanchanapoom. 1995. Somaic embryo formation from cotyledonary culture of *Theobroma cacao* L. *Journal of Science Society, Thailand* 21: 125–130.
8. Debnath, M., C. P. Malik, P. S. Bisen, 2006. Micro propagation: a Tool for the Production of High Quality Plant Based Medicines. *Current Pharmaceutical Biotechnology*, 7: 33–49.
9. Dulas, J-.P., C. Lambot, V. Peliat. 2007. Bioreactors for coffee mass propagation by somatic embryogenesis. *International Journal of Plant Developmental Biology* 1: 1–12.
10. Erickson, B., J. E. Nilson, P. Winter. 2012. Perspective on opportunities in industrial biotechnology in renewable chemicals. *Biotechnology Journal* 7: 176–185.
11. Etienne, H., B. Bertrand, A. Ribas, P. Lashermes, E. Malo, C. Montagnon, E. Alpizar, I. Jordan, F. Georget. 2000. Current application of coffee (*Coffea arabica*) somatic embryogenesis for industrial propagation of elite heterozygous materials in Central America and Mexico. ***In***: Proceedings of Advances in Somatic Embryogenesis of Trees and Its Application for Future Forest and Plantation. KFRI.Suwon, Republic of Korea. 59–67.
12. Evans, D. A., W. R. Sharp, C. E. Flick. Growth and behavior of cell cultures: embryogenesis and organogenesis. ***In***: Plant Tissue Culture, Methods and Application in Agriculture (Thorpe, ed.). Academic Press. New York. 45–113.
13. Fasina, A. S., O. S. Shittu, S. O. Omotolo, A. P. Adenikinya. 2006. Response of cocoa to different fertilizer regime on selected soils in Southtern Nigeria. *Agricultural Journal*, 1: 272–276.

14. Figueira, A. J. Janick. 1995. Somatic embryogenesis in cacao (*Theobroma cacao* L.) ***In***: Somatic Embryogenesis in Woody Plant (Jain *et al.*, eds.). Kluwer Academic Publisher. The Netherlands. 291–310.

15. Indonesian Cocoa and Coffee Research Institute. 2009. The Development and Application of Somatic Embryogenesis Technology for High Yielding Cocoa Planting Materials Multiplication (Research Report in Indonesian Language).

16. Jamal, S., M. Pomp. 1993. Smallholder adoption of tree crops: a case study of cocoa in sulawesi. *Bulletin of Indonesian Economics Studies* 29: 69–94.

17. Johnson, G. I., A. Iswanto, J. Ravusiro, P. J. Keane, N. Hollywood, S. V. Lambart, D. I. Guest. 2004. Linking Farmers with Markets: the Case of Cacao. In: Agriproduct Supply Chain Management in Developing Countries (Johnson and Hoffman, eds.). ACIAR.Laliberte, B., M. End. 2015. Supplying New Cocoa Planting Materials to Farmers: a Review of Porpagation Methodologies. *Biodiversity International*, Rome, Italy.

18. Li, Z., A. Trope, S. N. Maximova, M. J. Guiltinan. 1998. Somatic embryogenesis and plant regeneration from floral explants of cacao (*Theobroma cacao* L.) using thidiazuron. *In vitro Cellular and Developmental Biology–Plant* 34: 293–299.

19. Li, T. M. 2002. Local histories, global markets: cocoa and class in upland Sulawesi. *Development and Change*, 33: 415–437.

20. Lockwood, R. 2015. Propagation by Seeds. In: Supplying New Cocoa Planting Materials to Farmers: a Review of Porpagation Methodologies (Laliberte and End, eds.). *Biodiversity International*, Rome, Italy.

21. Maximova, S.N., M. J. Guiltinan. 2015. Tissue Culture. In: Supplying New Cocoa Planting Materials to Farmers: a Review of Porpagation Methodologies (Laliberte and End, eds.). *Biodiversity International*, Rome, Italy.

22. Maximova, S. N., L. Alemano, A. Young, N. Ferriere, A. Traore, M. J. Guiltinan. 2002. Efficiency, genotypic variability and cellular origin of primary and secondary somatic embryogenesis of *Theobroma cacao* L. *In vitro Cellular and Developmental Biology-Plant*, 38: 252–259.

23. Maximova, S. N., A. Young, S. Pisak, C. Miller, A. Traore, M. J. Guiltinan. 2005. Integrated system for propagation of *Theobroma cacao* L. IN: Protocol for Somatic Embryogenesis in Wopdy Plants. (Jain, eds.). Kluwer Pub., Dordrecht, the Netherlands. 1–14.

24. Maximova, S. N., A. Young, S. Pishak, M. J. Guiltinan. 2008. Field performance of *Theobroma cacao* L. Plants propagated via somatic embryogenesis. *In vitro Cellular Developmental Biology–Plant*, 44: 487–493.

25. Meulemans, C. C. E., U. Surapati, A. Tjatjo. 2002. Colometric measurement of cocoa beans (*Theobroma cacao* L.). *Indonesian Journal of Agricultural Science*, 3: 52–57.

26. Ministry of Agriculture of the Republic Indonesia. 2009a. General Overview of National Cocoa Programme for Quantity and Quality of Cocoa Production. (Research Report in Indonesian Language).

27. Ministry of Agriculture of the Republic Indonesia. 2009b. Monitoring and Evaluation of the Possibility of the Existence of Somaclonal Variation among Somatic Embryo Derived Seedlings (Research Report in Indonesian Language).
28. Ministry of Agriculture of the Republic Indonesia. 2010. Monitoring and Evaluation of the Possibility of the Existence of Somaclonal Variation among Somatic Embryo Derived Seedlings (Research Report in Indonesian Language).
29. Ministry of Agriculture of the Republic Indonesia. 2011. Monitoring and Evaluation of the Possibility of the Existence of Somaclonal Variation among Somatic Embryo Derived Seedlings (Research Report in Indonesian Language).
30. Ministry of Agriculture of the Republic Indonesia. 2011. Evaluation of the National Cocoa Program for Improving Quantity and Quality of Bean Yield (Research Report in Indonesian Language).
31. Ministry of Agriculture of the Republic Indonesia. 2013. Evaluation of Bean Yield and The Possibility of the Existence of Somaclonal Variation Among Somatic Embryo Derived Cocoa Trees (Research Report in Indonesian Language).
32. Ministry of Agriculture of the Republic Indonesia. 2013. The Impact of National Cocoa Program for Improving Quantity and Quality of Bean Yield 2009-2012 (Research Report in Indonesian Language).
33. Ministry of Agriculture of the Republic Indonesia. 2015. Bean Yield Quantity and Quality of Somatic Embryo Derived Cocoa Trees (Research Report in Indonesian Language).
34. Murugan, M., J. A. Wins. 2010. Industrial biotechnology–a sustainable future. *International Journal of Pharma and Bio Science*, 1: 1–3.
35. Neilson, J. 2007. Global markets, farmers and the state: Sustaining profits in the Indonesian Cocoa Sectors. *Bulletin of Indonesian Economics Studies*, 43: 227–250.
36. Noordiana, N., S. R. Syed Umar, J. Shamshuddin, N. M. NikAzziz. 2007. Effect of organic-based and foliar fertilizer on cocoa (*Theobroma cacao* L.) grown on an oxisol in Malaysian. *Malaysian Journal of Soil Science*, 11: 29–43.
37. Ogunlade, M. O., K. A. Okuyole, P. O. Aikpokpodion. 2009. An evaluation of the level of fertilizer utilization for cocoa production in Nigeria. *Journal of Human Ecology*, 25: 175–178.
38. Okamoto, A., S. Kishine, T. Hirosawa, A. Nakasomo, 1996. Effect of oxygen enriched aeration on regeneration of rice (*Oryza sativa* L.) cell culture. *Plant Cell Report* 15: 731–726.
39. Opeyemi, A. A., O. A. Fidelis, B. Adenola, O. Phillip. 2005. Quality management practices in cocoa production in South Western Nigeria. Conference on International Research on Food Security, National Resource Management and Rural Development.
40. Paek, K. Y., E. J. Hahn, S. H. Son. 2001. Application of bioreactors of large-scale micropropagation system of plants. *In vitro Cellular and Developmental Biology–Plant*, 37: 149–157.

41. Pardomuan, L. M. Taylor. 2012. Indonesia's "Frankentrees" turn cocoa dream into nightmare. Reuters 15, October. http: //reu.rs/1Fso0we.
42. Preil, W. 1991. Application of Bioreactors in Plant Propagation.In: Micropropagation (Deberg and Zimmerman, eds.). Kluwer Acad. Pub. Dordrecht.
43. Ribeiro M. A. Q., J. O. Da Sila, M. M. Aitken, R. C. R. Machado, V. C. Baligar. 2008. Nitrogen use efficiency in cocoa genotypes. *Journal of Plant Nutrition* 31: 239–249.
44. Rudgard, S. A., T. Andebrahan, A. C. Maddison, R. A. Smith. 1993. Disease Management: Recommendation. In: Disease and Management in Cocoa: Comparative Epidemiology of Witch Broom (Rudgard *et al.*, eds.). Chapman and Hill. London.
45. Smith, R. J., J. S. Aynsky. 1995. Field performance of tissue culture date palm (*Phoenix dactyfera*) clonally produced by somatic embryogenesis. *Principles* 39: 47–52.
46. Taryono, H. Hadini, T. Alam. 2017. The Evaluation of Cocoa Intensification Programme in South East Sulawesi (Research Report in Indonesian Language).
47. Tothmally A., V. Ingram. 2017. How can the production of Indonesian cocoa farms be increased?.Global Food Discussion Paper 103. University of Gottingen.
48. Williams, E. G., G. Maheswaran. 1986. Somatic embryogenesis: factors influencing coordinated behavior as an embryogenic group. *Annals of Botany* 57: 443–462.
49. Van Vliet, J. A., M.S. Lingerland, K. E. Giller. 2015. Mineral Nutrition in Cocoa: a Review. Wageningen University and Research.
50. Venkateswaru, B., R. Korwar. 2005. Micropropagation Technology for Multipurpose Trees: From Laboratory to Farmers Field. CRIDA, Hyderabad.
51. Ziv, M. 2005. Simple bioreactors for mass propagation of plants. *Plant Cell, Tissue, Organ Culture* 81: 277–285.

*Chapter 10*

# Development of an Affordable, Rapid, Sensitive and Specific Field Based PCR Assay for Detection and Quantification of Newcastle Disease (NCD)

*Willis A. Adero[1], K.G Tirumurugaan[2] and G. Dhinakar Raj[3]*

*[1]Research Scientist,*
*Kenya Agricultural and Livestock Research Organisation (KALRO),*
*Biotechnology Centre, P.O. Box 14733-00800, Westlands, Nairobi, KENYA*
*E-mail: aderoabwao@yahoo.co.uk*
*[2]Programme Head, [3]Project Director*
*Translational Research Platform for Veterinary Biologicals,*
*Centre for Animal Health Studies,*
*Tamil Nadu Veterinary and Animal Sciences University,*
*MMC, Chennai-51 Tamil Nadu, INDIA*

## ABSTRACT

We have evaluated a diagnostic system based on the loop-mediated isothermal amplification (LAMP) assay for the rapid, simple, and sensitive detection of Newcastle disease virus (NDV) directly from culture isolates as well as clinical samples. By using one set of specific primers targeting the intragenic regions between the fusion and the matrix gen the LAMP assay rapidly amplified the target gene within 1h. In this study, we have come up with a two-step method which requires only sample processing involving the extraction of the nucleic acid and subsequent performance of the LAMP assay making the process faster than the conventional reported methodology and its application in NDV detection. The methodology also has been evaluated and an advantageous comparison of its sensitivity and specificity to other conventional methods has been established. We have also optimized a single tube assay that involves only two steps from the sample (namely RNA isolation and LAMP assay) with sensitivity equivalent to that conventionally applied RT-

PCR and qRT-PCR. The study used viral nucleic acid extracted from positive allantoic fluid and serial dilution of the RNA to be used in LAMP assay. The detection limit of the LAMP assay was 8pg of viral nucleic acid which is equivalent to that of conventional RT-PCR and qRT-PCR.The results of the LAMP assay could be detected visually by inclusion of HNB at a concentration of 120µM in the LAMP mix and detection limit was equivalent to that of agarose gel electrophoresis. The single tube RT-LAMP assay is quick (requires 1hr and 30 min from sample processing to the end result), sensitive and specific.

## INTRODUCTION

Newcastle disease (ND), an enzootic and contagious disease of poultry except in few countries, is caused by an avian paramyxovirus 1 (APMV1) of the *Avulavirus* genus in the subfamily of *Paramyxo virinae*. The virus is known to infect almost more than 241 species of birds [Kaleta and Baldauf, 1988] exhibiting a key feature of differential virulence depending on the pathotype of the virus and the species it infects. Presently, this disease is still widespread in many countries. The infecting strains can be classified into three categories: highly virulent (velogenic), intermediate (mesogenic), and avirulent (lentogenic) based on their pathogenicity in chickens. The major contributor to the virulence of Newcastle disease virus (NDV) is the formation of an active fusion (F) protein upon cleavage of a precursor and the number of basic amino acids at this cleavage site termed the fusion protein cleavage site (FPCS) [Scheid and Choppin, 1973; Pritzer *et al.*, 1990]. The virulence of NDV is classified based on its pathogenicity in chicken (intra-cerebral pathogenicity index) that ranges from 0.0 (lentogenic viruses) to 2.0 (very virulent viruses).

Due to the wide variety of avian hosts that are susceptible to NDV, diagnosis gains importance in migratory birds which can serve as potential carriers. In addition, NDV also must be differentiated from other respiratory pathogens of human importance like influenza viruses. The isolation of APMV-1 virus is performed by the gold standard method of inoculating embryonated chicken eggs which require 5 to 10 days. However, rapid diagnosis of APMV-1 RNA is carried out by real-time reverse transcription polymerase chain reaction (rRT-PCR) targeting the matrix gene which requires around 3 – 5 hrs from receipt of the sample (Kim *et al.*, 2008). This is used as a screening assay in many diagnostic laboratories world-wide and following positivity additional tests are performed to determine the virulence of the virus with greater specificity except for some Class I and pigeon paramyxovirus (Kim *et al.*, 2006). Developing and optimizing rapid single tube or one-step single enzyme based diagnostic assays working on isothermal conditions would be reducing the turnaround time to less than 1-2 hrs. upon receipt of a sample for screening purposes.

In this context, strand displacement based nucleic acid amplification techniques like loop mediated isothermal amplification (LAMP) (Notomi *et al.*, 2000) gained significance and has been applied for diagnosis of infectious diseases [Dhama *et al.*, 2004]. A LAMP methodology has been reported for detection of NDV targeting the fusion protein [Pham *et al.*, 2005] however the methodology is a three-step protocol which requires sample processing for nucleic acid extraction, complementary DNA synthesis and the LAMP methodology. In this study, we report here an optimized two-step method which requires only sample processing to extract the nucleic acid and directly perform the LAMP making it quicker than the conventional reported methodology. The methodology also has been evaluated for its sensitivity and specificity to the conventional method of RT-PCR targeting the Matrix gene for detection of NDV.

# Materials and Methods

## Newcastle Disease Virus Strain

In this study, we used a velogenic Newcastle Disease Virus (NDV) strain which had been isolated from a pigeon in 2000 from the repository of Dept. of Animal Biotechnology, MVC and maintained at the repository of TRPVB, TANUVAS; NDV-2K3/Pi/2000/IND – GenBank Acc. No.FJ986192, for optimization of the LAMP assay. The virus was revived by inoculating aseptically in to 9-10-day old chicken embryos using standard procedure; allantoic fluid collected aseptically, aliquoted and frozen for use in the study to optimize the protocols. The presence of the virus was also confirmed by hem agglutination (HA) test using chicken RBC's [OIE, 2012]. The titre of the viral stock ($10^{8.25}$/ml) was also determined in embryonated chicken eggs (OIE, 2000).

### Viral Titration

The titre of the viral stock of NDV-2K3 was determined by inoculating serial 10-fold dilutions of the virus in 9-10 day old embryonated chicken eggs through allantoic route. The eggs were candled every day for their viability and upon death of the eggs, they were chilled and the allantoic fluid collected to determine the presence of NDV by HA tests. The data were tabulated and the Reed and Muench method was employed to quantify the amount of infectious virus in the suspension and expressed as $EID_{50}$.

$$EID_{50} = \frac{\text{Per cent infected at dilution immediately above 50 per cent} - \text{50 per cent}}{(\text{Per cent infected at dilution immediately above 50 per cent}) - (\text{per cent infected at dilution immediately below 50 per cent})}$$

## RNA Extraction and cDNA Synthesis

The RNA from the NDV allantoic fluid stock for the study was extracted using High Pure Viral Nucleic Acid Method (Roche Life Sciences, India) according to the manufacture's instructions. The RNA from the tissue/suspected samples were extracted using Trizol reagent (Invitrogen, India) The RNA concentration and purity were determined using the Nanoquant plate in Tecan Infinite 200 Pro Multi-plate reader. The samples were measured in duplicates and the average values were obtained. The RNA sample were converted in to cDNA or stored at -80°C until use.

### Synthesis of Complementary DNA

The extracted RNA samples were converted into cDNA using High Capacity cDNA Reverse Transcription Kit (Thermo Fisher Scientific, India). Briefly RNA of approximately 1-2 µg in a total volume of 10 µl was incubated at 65°C for 5 min. The RNA sample was snap cooled on ice for 5 min and equal volume of 2x RT master mix was added, mixed well and incubated at 25°C, 37°C for 3hrs and 85°C for 5 min. The converted cDNA was stored at -20°C for further experimental procedures.

## Oligonucleotide Primers Used in this Study

The study utilized different primers targeted for different approaches. Identification of the viral stock and the quantitative real-time PCR was performed using a pair of degenerate primers (NDV-FP and NDV-RP) that targeted the 3′ end of Matrix and 5′ end of fusion protein gene (NDV genomic position 4331 to 5090 which also included the fusion protein cleavage site (FPCS)) (Table 10.1). The primers used for RT-LAMP were designed using Primer 3 plus software(http://www.bioinformatics.nl/cgi-bin/primer3plus/primer3plus.cgi/) as described by Notomi *et al.* (2000) with the inner primers of LAMP connected by a TTTT spacer (Table 10.1). The conventional RT-PCR was performed using the LAMP outer primer pair (F3/B3) for comparison of the sensitivity of the reported RT-LAMP method (Table 10.1).

**Table 10.1: List of Oligonucleotide Primers Used in this Study**

| *Type of Primer* | *Sequence (5'-3')* | *Genome Position* |
|---|---|---|
| NDV FP | 5' GAG GTT ACC TCY ACY AAG CTR GAG A 3' | 4331 - 4356 |
| NDV RP | 5' TCA TTA ACA AAY TGC TGC ATC TTC CCW AC 3' | 5090 - 5061 |
| LAMP outer primer (F3) | CGCCCACTCACCCAGATCAT | 4363 - 4382 |
| LAMP outer primer B3 | GCAAGAGGCCTGCCATCAAT | 4592 - 4611 |
| LAMP loop primer F1P (F1C+F2) | TGGAGCCCATCTTGCACCTGGAGTTTTT AAGATTCTGGATCCCGGTTGGCG | 4486-4508 TTTTT 4461-4483 |
| LAMP loop primer B1P (B1C+B2) | TGCTGACTATCCGGGTTGCGCTGTTTTT GGCCTGCCATCAATGGAGTTTGC | 4539-4561 TTTTT 4583-4605 |
| M4100 | 5'-AGT GAT GTG CTC GGA CCT TC-3' | 4100 - 4120 |
| M-4220 | 5'-CCT GAG GAG AGG CAT TTG CTA-3' | 4220 - 4119 |

The Genome position of the primers are indicated based on Lasota genome (KJ563940).

## Optimization of the LAMP Methodology and Visual Detection

TheRT-LAMP PCR in this study was optimized using *Bst* 3.0 DNA polymerase (New England Biolabs, MA) the new version of the isothermal and strand displacement enzyme with improved reverse transcription (RT) activity, strong strand displacement activity and lacks both the exonuclease activity. The LAMP reaction included LAMP buffer, MgSo4, Betaine, LAMP outer primer pair (F3/B3 at 10pmol each), LAMP inner primer pair (FIP/BIP at 20 pmol each), dNTP mix, RNA template and nuclease free water. The optimization of the LAMP reaction was performed with respect to the MgSo4 concentration, reaction temperature and reaction time. Due to the above inherent improved RT activity the optimized diagnostic protocol could be completed in a time span of less than two hours. The optimized RT-LAMP was performed in the presence 120 µM of Hydroxynaphthal blue (HNB) in the LAMP assay mix with a positive amplification resulting in change of the violet color to blue. The amplification was also assessed by electrophoresing the products in a 4 per cent agarose gel.

### Reverse Transcription PCR (RT-PCR) and Quantitative Real-time PCR (qRT-PCR)

For RT-PCR the synthesized cDNA was amplified using the primer pair NDVFP/NDVRP and TAQ DNA Polymerase Master Mix Red (Ampliqon, Denmark). The PCR cycle for the RT-PCR included The cycling reaction for F3 (10 pmol) and B3 (10 pmol) were 94°C for 3 min and then 35 cycles consisting of denaturation at 94°C for 20 s, annealing at 50°C for 30 s and extension at 72°C for 30 s was run up to 30 cycles with one final extension at 72°C for 7 min. For qRT-PCR the synthesized cDNA was amplified using the primer pair M4100 and M4220 primer pair and SYBR Premix Ex Taq (TliRNase H Plus) (Takara Bio USA, CA). The qRT-PCR conditions included amplification condition of 94°C for 3 min and then 35 cycles consisting of denaturation at 94°C for 10 secs, annealing at 54°C for 10 sec and extension at 72°C for 10 secs with one final extension at 72°C for 7 min cycle was run up to 30sec. The RT-PCR and qRT-PCR was performed as a conventional detection methodology and compared with LAMP to assess the efficiency.

### Sensitivity of the Optimized RT-LAMP

The optimized RT-LAMP assay was compared with the routinely used RT-PCR and qRT-PCR to determine its sensitivity for viral detection. For this purpose, the viral nucleic acid was extracted from a known volume of NDV allantoic fluid stock (with a titre of $10^{8.25}$/ml) and the RNA quantified. For RT-LAMP assay, serial dilutions of the above RNA sample were used, however, in the case of RT-PCR and qRT-PCR a known RNA concentration used in the RT-LAMP assay was converted into cDNA and then serial diluted for use in both tests. The specificity of the RT-LAMP methodology was determined by extracting nucleic acids from field samples of other virus infecting chicken namely infectious bronchitis virus (IBV) and Chicken anemia virus (CAV) (Figure 10.4).

## Results

### Optimized RT-LAMP Assay

The LAMP reactions were carried out in a total volume of 25 µL with optimization in the concentration of MgSo4, temperature and time period for amplification. The final optimized concentration of the different components includes 10 pmol each of F3 and B3 primers and 40 pmol each of FIB and BIP primers, 250µM of each of the dNTPs, 0.8M of Betaine, 6mM of $MgSo_4$, 3µl of RNA as template and 8U of Bst 3.0 DNA polymerase with 1X Isothermal buffer (NEW England Biolabs, MA) in the RT-LAMP assay (Figure 10.1). An incubation temperature of 62°C for 60 min was found to be optimum for a single-tube two step RT-LAMP assay for detection of NDV using the above conditions (Figure 10.2).

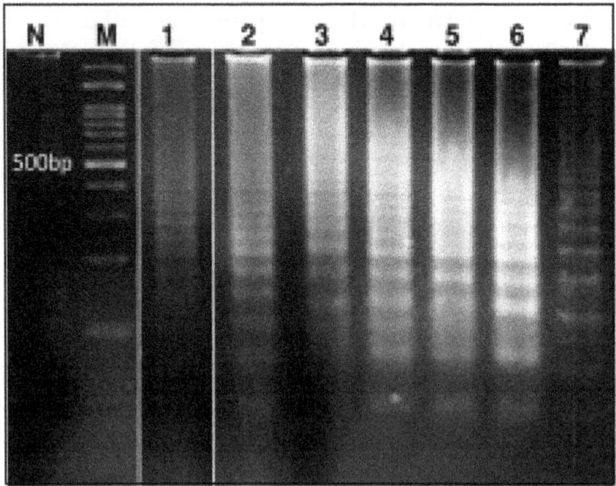


**Figure 10.1: Determination of the Optimal Concentration of MgSo4 in LAMP Concentration was Determined from 2Mm-12Mm in Lane 1-7 Respectively Lane N-NTC and 100Bp Ladder was Used. 8Mm was found to be optimal for the lamp assay since it resulted in a good distributed of the ladder pattern.**

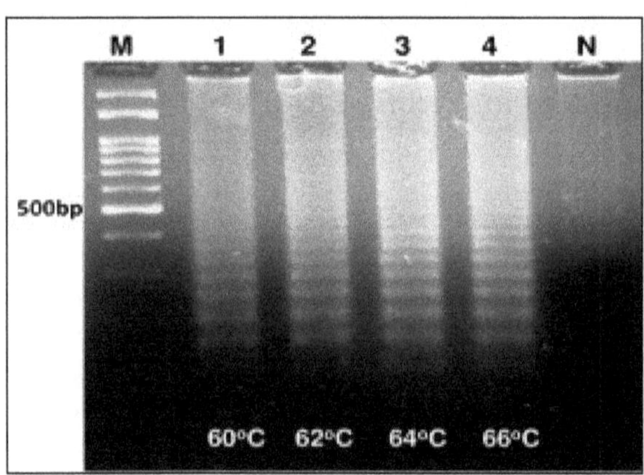


**Figure 10.2: The Assay was Performed at 60°C, 62°C, 64°C and 66°C using Extracted RNA and Nuclease Free Water was Used as Negative Controls. The temperate of 62°C was found to be optimum with improved amplification efficiency.**

## Analysis of LAMP Products

The products of the RT-LAMP assay were analyzed by both the conventional agarose gel electrophoresis and visual detection method (Figures 10.4 and 10.5). The positive RT-LAMP PCR assay resulted in a typical ladder-like pattern because of the stem-loop DNA and other related structures upon gel electrophoresis. The visual assay was performed by adding 120 µM of Hydroxynaphthal blue (HNB) in the RT-LAMP assay mix prior to amplification followed by visual detection. Following RT- PCR a positive sample resulted in a specific size of an amplicon by

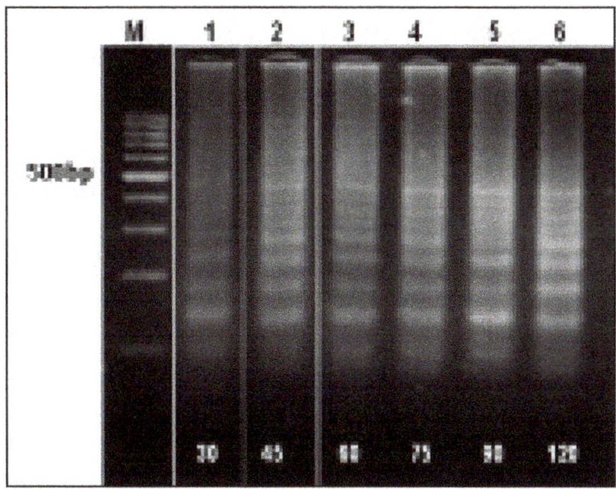


**Figure 10.3: Optimization of the LAMP Assay Time. M-100bp Marker; 1-30 min; 2-45 min; 3-60 min; 4-75 min; 5-90 min; 6-120 min. An appreciable amplification could be observed at the minimum time point of 60 min which was chose for subsequent work.**

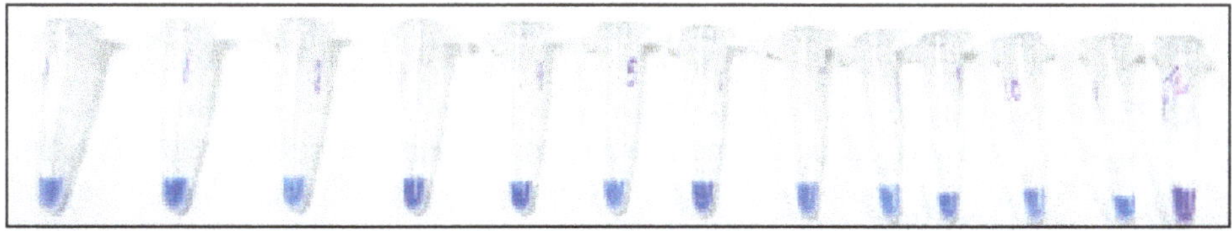

**Figure 10.4: Visual Detection of LAMP Products by Addition of HNB Dye, Lanes: 1-12 positive reaction and NTC: No Template Control. The tube 1 is with a strarting concentration of 834ng of RNA template and the tube 12 is with a starting concentration 8pg and a clear difference in NTC indicating the visual detection of LAMP products could be achieved even at a low template concentration of 8 pg.**

agarose gel electrophoresis while the visual detection resulted in the change of the color from violet to blue. Both the visual detection by HNB addition and agarose electrophoresis could detect amplification until 8pg of the RNA template indicating the utility of the HNB dye for visual detection of LAMP products (Figure 10.4).

## Analytical Sensitivity of the RT-LAMP Assay

To study the limits of virus detection, titrations of NDV was done and titre was calculated by Reed and Muench (1938) method. After calculating the titre, total RNA was isolated from the 250µl of 10-fold serially diluted infected allantoic fluid NDV. The LAMP and PCR reaction were done on the total RNA. The limit of detection for NDV RT-LAMP, qRT-PCR and RT-PCR was found to be 0.1, 2 and 3 TCID50/ml respectively. The sensitivity of RT-LAMP was found to be higher than the RT-PCR and equally sensitive as the qRT-PCR (Figure 10.3).

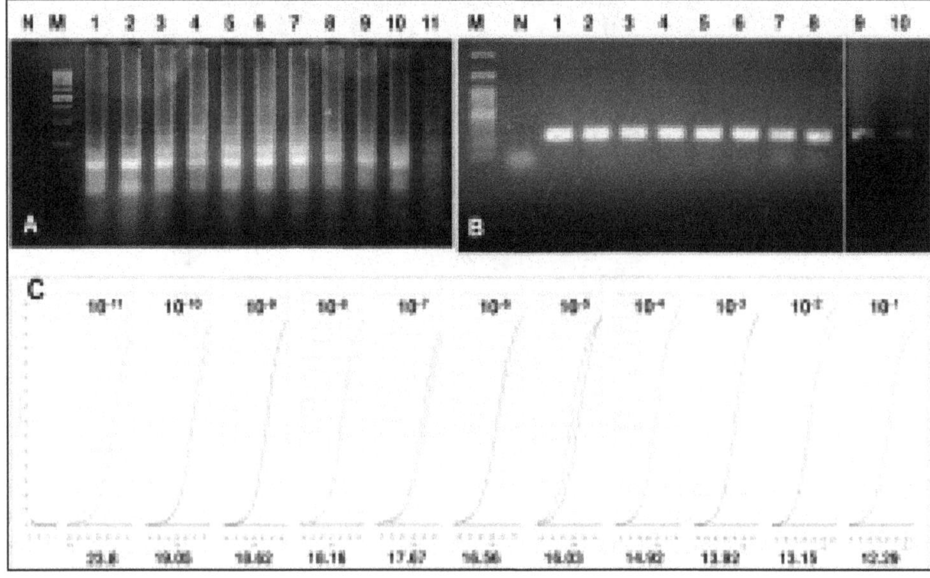


**Figure 10.5: Analytical Sensitivity of RT-PCR. All the assays compared could detection template concentrations until 8pg in this study. However, it is to be noted that the LAMP assay was performed with RNA as template while the other two required the RNA to be converted to cDNA before the same is used providing the LAMP assay with an advantage to be used as a two-step (RNA extraction and PCR). A: Lamp assay; B: RT-PCR and C: qRT PCR.**

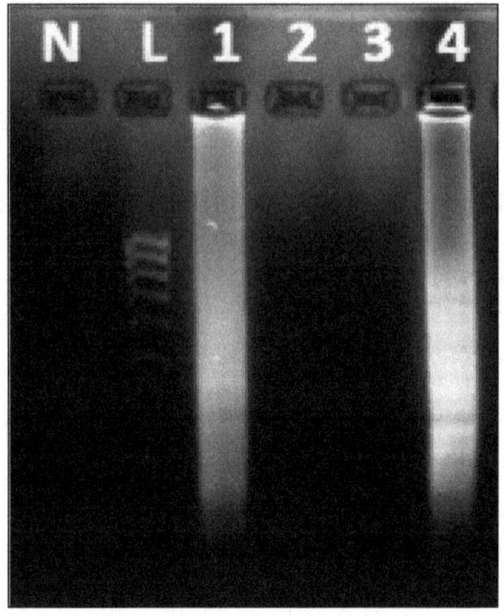


**Figure 10.6: Specificity of LAMP Assay in Detecting NDV for Suspected Samples; N: NTC; L: 100 bp; 1: NDV Positive Control; 2: IBV, 3: CAV, 4: NDV suspected samples.**

## Specificity of the RT-LAMP Assay

The RT-LAMP was carried out under optimal reaction conditions with templates prepared from other viruses like Infectious bronchitis virus (IBV) and Chicken Anaemia Virus (CAV). The template was RNA in the case former while it is DNA in the later. The optimized LAMP assay resulted in a specific ladder like pattern only in NDV positive sample and not with the other two viruses tested in this study (Figure 10.6).

## Discussions

Newcastle disease always has been a threat to poultry worldwide and in addition the disease is complicated due to the report of different strains and also the hypothesis that the currently available vaccine viruses do not provide complete protection against circulating strains of NDV. The routine detection methodologies applied in most of the laboratory include the use of hemagglutination test, ELISA, virus isolation in embryonated chicken eggs and molecular detection (Alexander and Jones 2001). Modification of the molecular methodologies to provide rapid and specific detection is always warranted from diseased birds so that appropriate control measures could be adopted.

In this study, we have optimized a single tube assay that involves only two steps from the sample (namely RNA isolation and LAMP assay) with sensitivity equivalent to that of the conventionally applied RT-PCR and qRT-PCR. The study used viral nucleic acid extracted from positive allantoic fluid and serial dilution of the RNA to be used in LAMP assay. The detection limit of the LAMP assay is 8pg of viral nucleic acid which is equivalent to that of conventional RT-PCR and qRT-PCR. The results of the LAMP assay could be detected visually by inclusion of HNB at a concentration of 120μM in the LAMP mix and detection limit was equivalent to that of agarose gel electrophoresis. Our results indicate that the LAMP is also highly specific in that nucleic acids from IBV and CAV did yielded negative results. This stresses the fact that, as similar to that of a conventional PCR, the design of LAMP primers is crucial as well as optimization of the conditions for the assay. We had designed two sets of primers that target six different regions of the genome (encompassing the 3′ end of matrix gene and 5′ end of fusion protein gene). The novelty in the methodology in study is the use of a newer version of the strand displacement enzyme the *Bst* 3.0 DNA polymerase which also possesses a high reverse transcriptase activity. In addition, the positivity of the reaction could be visually appreciated with greater sensitivity with the pre-addition of HNB in the LAMP mixture (Goto *et al.*, 2009) which results in a sky blue and the time required for the whole protocol from extraction of the nucleic acid to detection is only 1 hr and 30 min. The use of the conventional virus isolation approach needs almost 3-4 days to confirm the presence of the virus.

The single tube RT-LAMP assay described in this study is a quick (requires 1 hr and 30 min from sample processing to the end result), specific, sensitive and cost-effective method and avoids the need to convert the RNA into cDNA before application of the nucleic acid amplification method thus will be a potentially valuable tool in the clinical diagnosis and surveillance of NDV.

## Acknowledgements

I would like to acknowledge my supervisor; Dr K.G Tirumurugaan for the wonderful endless and tireless work considering his commitment, technical and constructive guidance during this research work. I would also wish to acknowledge the NAM S&T center for offering me this fellowship to pursue my research project. My Gratitude also goes to the TANUVAS (Tamil Nadu University of Animal sciences) for offering me an opportunity in their University where the research work was curried not to forget the entire staff at TRPVB Platform for their kind and unforgettable hospitality and technical advises during the entire period. Not to forget my employer and organization KALRO for their support.

## REFERENCES

1. Alexander D, Senne D. Newcastle disease and other avian paramyxovirus and Pneumovirus infection. In Diseases of Poultry 2008; 12$^{th}$ edn, Saif YM, ed. (Blackwell Publishing Ltd, Oxford): pp.75-115.
2. Alexander, D. J., and R. C. Jones. 2001. Paramyxoviridae, p. 257–272. In F. Jordan, M. Pattison, D. Alexander, and T. Faragher (Eds.), Poultry diseases, 5th ed. W. B. Saunders, Harcourt Publishers Ltd., London, United Kingdom
3. Alexander, D.J., Senne, D.A., 2008. Newcastle disease, other avian paramyxoviruses, and pneumovirus infections. In: Saif, Y.M., Fadly, A.M., Glisson, J.R., McDougald,L.R., Nolan, L.K., Swayne, D.E. (Eds.), Diseases of Poultry. Iowa State University Press, Ames, pp. 75–116.
4. Dhama K, Karthik K, Chakraborty S, Tiwari R, Kapoor S, Kumar A, Thomas P. 2004. Loop-mediated isothermal amplification of DNA (LAMP): a new diagnostic tool lights the world of diagnosis of animal and human pathogens: a review. *J. Clin. Microbiol.*
5. Goto, M., E. Honda, A. Ogura, A. Nomoto, and K.-I. Hanaki. 2009. Colorimetric detection of loop-mediated isothermal amplification reaction by using hydroxynaphthol blue. *Biotechniques* 46: 167-172.
6. Kaleta KF, Baldauf C. Newcastle disease in free living and pet birds. *Developments in Veterinary Virology* 1988. 8: 197-246.
7. Mori, Y., K. Nagamine, N. Tomita, and T. Notomi. 2001. Detection of loop-mediated isothermal amplification reaction by turbidity derived from magnesium pyrophosphate formation. *Biochem. Biophys. Res.*
8. Notomi, T., H. Okayama, H. Masubuchi, T. Yonekawa, K. Watanabe, N. Amino, and T. Hase. 2000. Loop-mediated isothermal amplification of DNA. *Nucleic Acids Res.* 28: E63.
9. Pritzer E, Kuroda K, Garten W, Nagai Y, Klenk H-D. 1990. A host range mutant of Newcastle disease virus with an altered cleavage site for proteolytic activation of the F protein. *Virus Res.*, 15: 237-242.

10. Goto M, Honda E, Ogura A, Nomoto A, Hanaki K 2009. Colorimetric detection of loop-mediated isothermal amplification reaction by using hydroxynaphthol blue. *Biotechniques*. 46: 167-72. 10.2144/000113072.
11. Goto, M., E. Honda, A. Ogura, A. Nomoto, and K.-I. Hanaki. 2009. Colorimetric detection of loop-mediated isothermal amplification reaction by using hydroxynaphthol blue. *Biotechniques* 46: 167-172.
12. Jakhesara SJ, Prasad VVSP, Pal JK, Jhala MK, Prajapati KS, Joshi CG. Pathotypic and Sequence Characterization of Newcastle Disease Viruses fromVaccinated Chickens Reveals Circulation of Genotype II, IV and XIII and in India. *Transboundary and Emerging Diseases* 2014.
13. Kaleta KF, Baldauf C 1988. Newcastle disease in free living and pet birds. *Developments in Veterinary Virology*, 8: 197-246.
14. Kapczynski DR, King DJ 2005. Protection of chickens against overt clinical disease and determination of viral shedding following vaccination with commercially available Newcastle disease virus vaccines upon challenge with highly virulent virus from the California 2002 exotic Newcastle disease outbreak. *Vaccine*, 23: 3424-3433.
15. Khan ST, Rehmani, Rue C, Miller P, Afonso CL 2010. Phylogenetic and pathological characterization of Newcastle disease virus isolates from Pakistan. *J. Clin. Microbiol.*, 48: 1892–1894.
16. Kho, C. L., M. L. Mohd-Azmi, S. S. Arshad, and K. Yusoff 2000. Performance of an RT-nested PCR ELISA for detection of Newcastle disease virus. *J. Virol. Methods* 86: 71–83.
17. Kim LM, King DJ, Suarez DL, Wong CW, Afonso CL 2007. Characterization of class I Newcastle disease virus isolates from Hong Kong live bird markets and detection using real-time reverse transcription-PCR. *J. Clin. Microbiol.*, 45: 1310–1314.
18. Krishnamurthy, S. and Samal, S. K 1998. Nucleotide sequences of the trailer, nucleocapsid protein gene and intergenic regions of Newcastle disease virus strain Beaudette C and completion of the entire genome sequence. *J. Gen. Virol.*, 79: 2419-24.
19. Miller PJ, Decanini EL, Afonso CL 2010. Newcastle disease: evolution of genotypes and the related diagnostic challenges. *Infect. Genet. Evol*, 10: 26-35.
20. Mori, Y., K. Nagamine, N. Tomita, and T. Notomi 2001. Detection of loop-mediated isothermal amplification reaction by turbidity derived from magnesium pyrophosphate formation. *Biochem. Biophys. Res.*
21. Nagamine, K., T. Hase, and T. Notomi 2002. Accelerated reaction by loopmediated isothermal amplification using loop primers. *Mol. Cell. Probes.*
22. Notomi, T., H. Okayama, H. Masubuchi, T. Yonekawa, K. Watanabe, N. Amino, and T. Hase 2000. Loop-mediated isothermal amplification of DNA. *Nucleic Acids Res.*, 28: E63.

# Chapter 11

# Study on the Antifungal Activities of Effective Fungi as a Control of Plant Pathogenic Fungi

*Win Min Than[1], Khaing Nwe Nwe Oo[1], Nann Miky Moh Moh[1], Kyi Pyar Win[1], Ei Mon Myo[1], Myat Phyu Khine[1], Ko Ko Lwin[1], Win Htun Yin[1] and Aye Aye Khai[2]*

*[1]Mycology Lab., Biotechnology Research Department, Kyaukse, Myanmar*
*[2]Biotechnology Research Department, Kyaukse, Myanmar*
*E-mail: aakhai@gmail.com, hladaw@gmail.com*

## ABSTRACT

Effective fungi (7 strains) were isolated by direct culture and serial dilution methods. According to colonial morphologies and microscopic morphologies, the isolated fungi (BIF-3, BIF-5, 2-OF and C-1) were *Penicillium* spp. whereas the other three strains (BIF-6, ROF and C-4) were unidentified spp. After that, the indigenous plant pathogenic fungi (OR-3, OR-3.2, S-1 and S-2) were isolated from the infected roots and leaves of commercial crop plants such as orange and sesame. Colonial morphology, cultural characteristics and microscopic morphology of the isolated fungi were studied. Antifungal activities of the isolated effective fungi against *Phythium* sp. and the isolated plant pathogenic fungi were tested by using dual culture method and well diffusion assay. *In vitro* screening, the isolated effective fungi had the antifungal activities. Among them, strain BIF-3 showed the significant antifungal activities against the plant pathogenic fungi tested. The cultural conditions of the effective fungi (BIF-3 and 2-OF) were also determined in surface and submerged cultures. Dextrose is the best carbon source. In addition, 18 per cent and 12 per cent of Dextrose sugar was the best for the growth of BIF-3 and 2-OF, respectively. The optimum pH for the growth of BIF-3 and 2-OF was pH 5 and pH 3, respectively. However, the maximum antifungal activities showed at pH 9 and pH 10 for BIF-3 and 2-OF in course of fermentation, respectively. This research was focused on the potential of biofungicides to control fungal plant pathogens.

***Keywords:*** *Effective fungi, Antifungal activities, Plant pathogenic fungi, Cultural conditions.*

# INTRODUCTION

Humans label as "pests" any plants or animals that endanger their food supply, health or comfort. Many agricultural losses are due to plant diseases, insect pests and herb pests. These pests inflict heavy damage to crops leading to reduce productivity. Because Myanmar is an agricultural country, it is very important to be successful in agriculture. To manage these pests, pesticides are needed.

Generally, these pests have been fought by synthetic agro-chemicals. Environmental degradation and harmful consequences of indiscriminate usage of chemical pesticides are being increasingly documented. These concerns have led to the search of environmental friendly and safer pesticides.

Biopesticide has become a tendency for and goal of global pesticide development because of its relatively low side effects and friendliness to environment. Biopesticides refer to products made from natural sources such as animals, plants and microorganisms.

Spore forming beneficial microbes are used as a fungicide in agriculture. When applied to seeds, the microbes colonizes the developing root system of the plants and then competes with and suppresses plant pathogenic organisms. The microbes continue to live on the root system and provide protection throughout the growing season. Because beneficial microbes form spores, pesticidal products containing these microbes are stable. Thus, even if treated seeds are stored for prolonged periods, the microbes stay alive and then grow and multiply after the seeds are planted. In addition, beneficial microbes produce surfactin, chitinase, iturin, *etc.* which have biopesticidal activity. So, biopesticidal products are now used in agriculture by producing such components from beneficial microbes.

The objectives of the present research are to isolate and identify beneficial microbes by direct culture and to apply the isolated beneficial microbe as biofungicide in agriculture directly with spores solution or indirectly by producing the bioactive compound from it to protect common plant pathogens.

## Materials and Methods

### Sample Collection

Alkaline soil (pH 11–12) was collected from Sakhanthar village, Sagaing Region, Myanmar. Onion was collected from Myittharr, Mandalay Region in Myanmar. The infected Sesame plants were collected from the field of Myat Hnar Ban village, Sagaing Region, Myanmar.

## Isolation of Effective and Plant Pathogenic Fungi

Effective fungi and plant pathogenic fungi were isolated from the collected samples with direct culture method and serial dilution method.

### Direct Culture Method

The sample was checked under a stereo-microscope for a fungal sporulating structure and labeled. Under a stereo-microscope, the fungal sporulating structure was picked up with a sterile needle and transferred into a drop of sterile water on a sterile glass slide. The conidial suspension was checked under a compound microscope to ensure the identity. Then, the conidial suspension was picked up with a sterile wire-loop and streaked on a medium plate (Potato Dextrose Agar with 0.5mg/L streptomycin sulfate). Plates with fungal conidia were incubated at 25°C for 24-48 hours and periodically checked under a stereo-microscope for germination. When the germination occurred successfully, a small plug of agar with the germinated conidia was picked up and transferred on PDA medium plate. At least 5-10 isolates of each species were selected and transferred to ensure that these isolates were identical. Pure isolate was finally transferred to grow on a PDA (Potato Dextrose Agar) medium plate and incubated at 25°C for 3 days. After incubation, the plates were maintained at 4°C for further study.

### Serial Dilution Method

Alkaline soil (1g) was dissolved in 9ml of normal saline in a test tube. Then, the sample was diluted with 10-fold serial dilutions. The diluted sample (100µL) was streaked on a medium plate (Potato Dextrose Agar with 0.5mg/L streptomycin sulfate). Plates with fungal conidia were incubated at 25°C for 24-48 hours and periodically checked under a stereo-microscope for germination. When the germination occurred successfully, a small plug of agar with the germinated conidia was picked up and transferred on PDA medium plate. At least 5-10 isolates of each species were selected and transferred to ensure that these isolates were identical. Pure isolate was finally transferred to grow on a PDA (Potato Dextrose Agar) medium plate and incubated at 25°C for 3 days. After incubation, the plates were maintained at 4°C for further study.

## Studying Effective and Plant Pathogenic Fungi

The sample or plate was checked under a stereo-microscope for a fungal sporulating structure. Under a stereo-microscope, the fungal sporulating structure was picked up with a sterile needle and transferred into a drop of lactophenol on a glass slide and then covered with a cover slip. Slides were examined and photographed under a compound microscope (40x).

## Screening the Antifungal Activities

The antifungal activities of the isolated fungi were tested with dual culture method and well diffusion assay and then selected the best strains.

## Dual Culture Method

*i.* ***Preparation of Plant Pathogenic Fungi.*** *Phythium* sp. and the indigenous plant pathogenic fungi (OR-3, OR-3.2, S-1 and S-2) were sub-cultured and incubated at 25°C for 5-days to get fresh inoculum.

*ii.* ***Preparation of Effective Fungi.*** Effective fungi (7 strains) were sub-cultured and incubated at 25°C for 5-days to get fresh inoculum.

*iii.* ***Determination of Antifungal Activities.*** The antifungal activities of the effective fungi (7 strains) against the plant pathogenic fungi were screened by dual culture method. A minute piece of each plant pathogenic fungus agar plug was taken with a sterile needle under stereo-microscope and then put onto the center of each PDA medium plate. After that, a minute piece of each effective fungus agar plug was picked up with a sterile needle under stereo-microscope and then put onto each PDA medium plate at the side of each plant pathogenic fungus agar plug about 1.5cm distance. Each PDA medium plate containing one plant pathogenic fungus and two effective fungi. Then, they were incubated in BOD incubator at 25°C. The antifungal activities were checked sequentially about 30 days and photographed.

## Well Diffusion Assay

*i.* ***Preparation of Potato Dextrose Broth.*** Potato Dextrose Broth (39g/L) was dissolved in distilled water (1L). Each PDB medium (20 ml) was put into each conical flask (100 ml). Then, they are sterilized by autoclaving at 121°C for 15 min and then cooled.

*ii.* ***Preparation of Culture Filtrate*** A minute piece of each selected effective fungus agar plug was taken with a sterile needle under stereo-microscope and then put into each conical flask containing PDB medium (20 ml). Then, they were incubated in a shaking incubator at 25°C, 150 rpm for two weeks. After incubation, each fungal broth was harvested and then filtered. Each filtrate was collected for testing the antifungal activity of each effective fungus.

*iii.* ***Preparation of Fungal Inoculum*** A minute piece of *Phythium* sp. agar plug was taken with a sterile needle under stereo-microscope and then put into each test tube containing PDB medium (10 ml). Then, the test tubes were incubated in a shaking incubator at 25°C, 150 rpm for three days.

*iv.* ***Determination of Antifungal Activities.*** Fungal broth of *Phythium* sp. was swabbed onto PDA medium. Wells were made on each standard PDA medium plate containing *Phythium* sp. Each collected cultural filtrate (100 µL) was put into each well with micro-pipette. Then, they were incubated in a BOD incubator at 25°C for 5 days. After incubation, the plates were taken out and examined the antifungal activities by measuring the inhibition zone diameters for strain selection.

v. ***Determination of Cultural Conditions.*** Cultural conditions of the selected effective fungi-*Penicillium* spp. (BIF-3 and 2OF) were determined in surface and submerged cultures.

## Growth pH

PDA media with various pH (3 – 12) were used to test the optimum pH for the growth of selected effective fungi.

i. ***Preparation of Agar Plates.*** Potato Dextrose Broth (39g/L) and agar (20g) were dissolved in distilled water (1L) and then adjusted to various pH (3 to 12). They were sterilized by autoclaving at 121°C for 15min. Each sterile medium (15 ml) with various pH was put into each plate and then cooled until solidify.

ii. ***Determination of Growth pH.*** A minute piece of each selected effective fungus agar plug was taken with a sterile needle under stereo-microscope and then put onto the center of each PDA medium plate with various pH (3 – 12). Then, they were incubated in a BOD incubator at 25°C. The growth of each selected effective fungus was studied by measuring the colony diameters daily.

## pH for Antifungal Activities

PDB media with various pH (3 – 12) were used to determine the optimum pH for antifungal activities of selected effective fungi.

i. ***Preparation of Potato Dextrose Broth.*** Potato Dextrose Broth (39g/L) was dissolved in distilled water (1L) and then adjusted PDB media to various pH (3 to 12). Each PDB medium (20 ml) with various pH was put into each conical flask (100 ml). They are sterilized by autoclaving at 121°C for 15 min and then cooled.

ii. ***Preparation of Culture Filtrate at Various pH.*** A minute piece of each selected effective fungus agar plug was taken with a sterile needle under stereo-microscope and then put into each conical flask containing PDB medium with various pH (3 – 12). Then, they were incubated in a shaking incubator at 25°C, 150 rpm for two weeks. After incubation, each fungal broth was harvested and then filtered. Each filtrate was collected for testing the antifungal activities in order to determine the optimum pH for antifungal activities.

iii. ***Determination of Antifungal Activities.*** The antifungal activities of cultural filtrates were determined by well diffusion assay.

## Preparation of Fungal Inoculum

A minute piece of *Phythium* sp. agar plug was taken with a sterile needle under stereo-microscope and then put into each test tube containing PDB medium (10 ml). Then, they were incubated in a shaking incubator at 25°C, 150 rpm for three days.

## Well Diffusion Assay

Fungal broth of *Phythium* sp. was swabbed onto PDA medium. Wells were made on each standard PDA medium plate containing *Phythium* sp. Each collected cultural filtrate was put into each well by using micro-pipette. Then, they were incubated in a BOD incubator at 25°C for 5 days. After incubation, the inhibition zones diameters were measured and recorded.

## Selection of Carbon Sources

Sugars (Dextrose, Glucose, Starch and Sucrose) were used as carbon sources in order to select the best carbon source for the growth of selected effective fungi.

i. ***Preparation of Potato Infusion.*** Potatoes were washed thoroughly with tap water, sliced and boiled. The potato (200g) was unpeeled with distilled water (1L) for 30 min. After that, they were filtered through cheesecloth. The effluent was collected as potato infusion.

ii. ***Preparation of Agar Plates.*** The potato infusion (1L) was mixed with 15g of each sugar (Dextrose, Glucose, Starch or Sucrose) and agar (20g) and then boiled to dissolve. After boiling, they were sterilized by autoclaving at 121°C for 15 min. Each sterile medium (15ml) was put into each plate and cool until solidify.

iii. ***Study the Growth of Effective Fungi on Various Carbon Sources.*** A minute piece of each selected effective fungus agar plug was taken with a sterile needle under stereo-microscope and then put onto the center of four types of medium plate prepared containing Glucose, Dextrose, Starch or Sucrose. Then, the plates were incubated in a BOD incubator at 25°C. The growth of each selected effective fungus was studied and measured the colony diameters daily. The best carbon source was selected based on the growth of selected effective fungi in various carbon sources.

## Determination of Dextrose Concentration

Various Dextrose concentrations (2, 4, 6, 8, 10, 12, 14, 16, 18, 20, 22 g/L) were used as carbon sources in order to select the best carbon source concentration for the growth of selected effective fungi.

i. ***Preparation of Agar Plates.*** The potato infusion (1L) was mixed with various concentration of Dextrose (2 – 22 g/L) and agar (20g) and then boiled to dissolve. After boiling, they were sterilized by autoclaving at 121°C for 15 min. Each sterile medium (15 ml) was put into each plate and cool until solidify.

ii. ***Study the Growth of Effective Fungi on Various Dextrose Concentrations.*** A minute piece of each selected effective fungus agar plug was taken with a sterile needle under stereo-microscope and then put onto the center of medium plates prepared containing various concentrations of Dextrose. Then, the plates were incubated in a BOD incubator at 25°C. The growth of each selected effective fungus was studied by measuring each colony diameters daily. The best Dextrose concentration was selected based on the growth of selected effective fungi in various Dextrose concentrations.

## Results

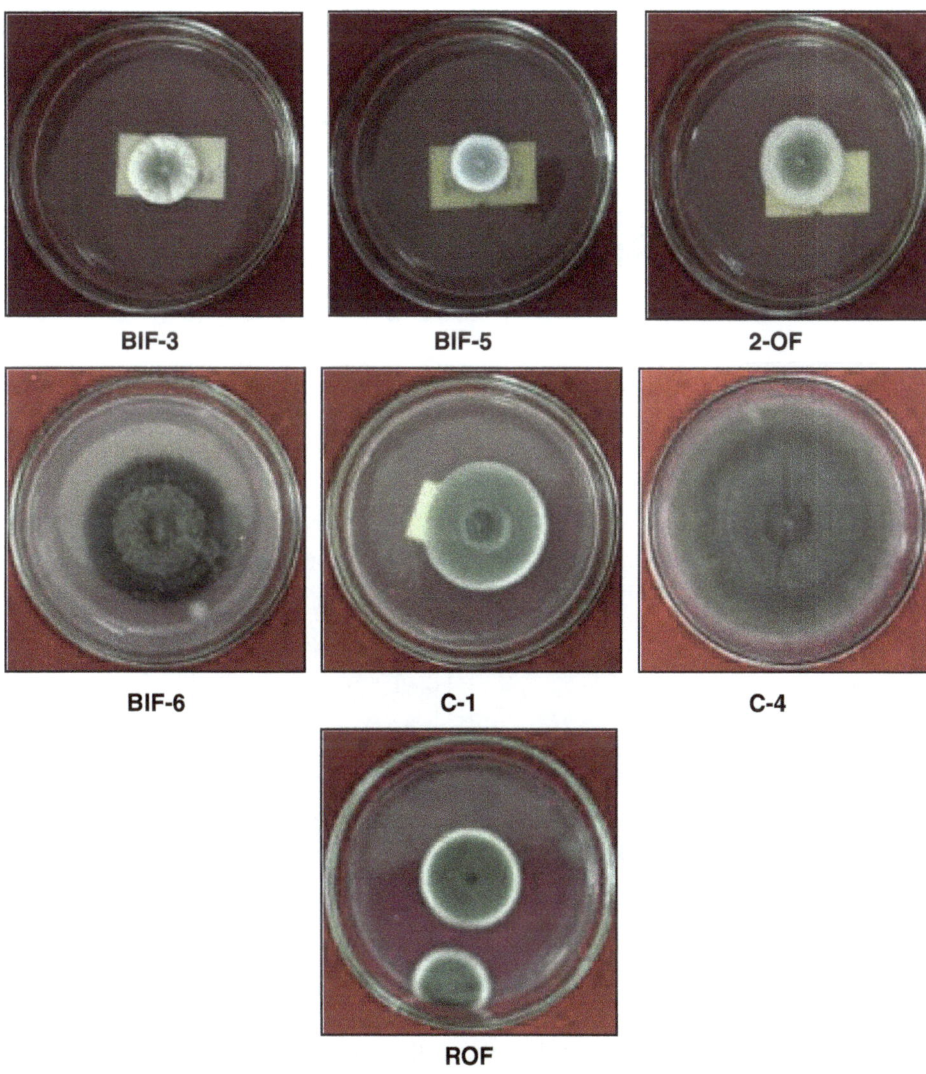


**Figure 11.1: Colonial Morphologies of Effective Fungi on PDA Media.**

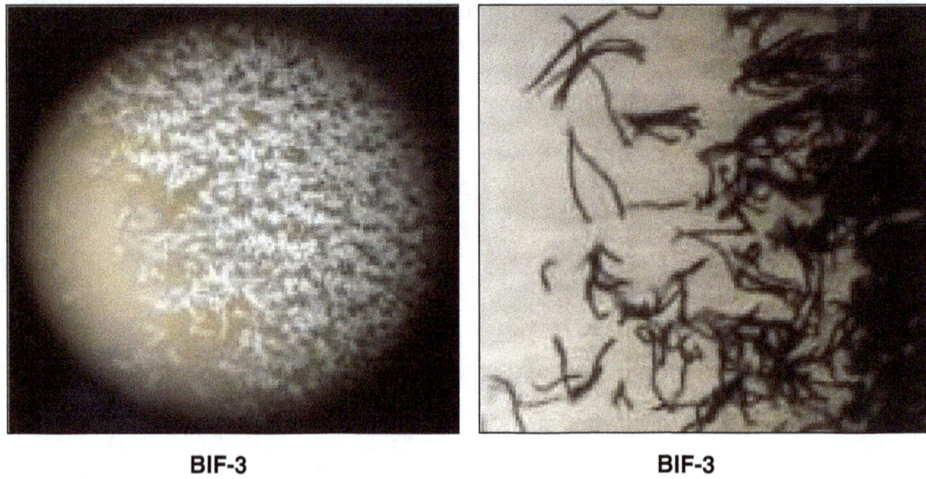


**Figure 11.2: Sporulating Structures of Effective Fungus – *Penicillium* sp. (BIF-3) under Stereo-microscope.**

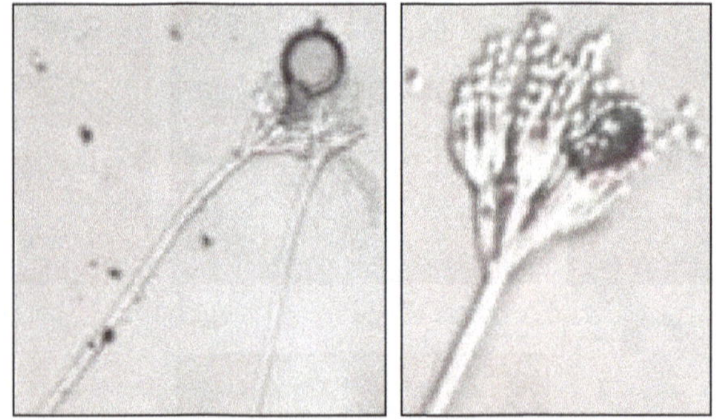

**Figure 11.3: Microscopic Morphology of Effective fungus – *Penicillium* sp. (BIF-3) under Compound Microscope.**

## Discussions

In this research work, the effective fungi (7 strains) were isolated by direct culture method. Colonial morphologies, sporulating structures and microscopic morphologies of the isolated fungi were studied. Among them, four strains (BIF-3, BIF-5, 2-OF, C-1) were *Penicillium* spp. according to their colonial morphologies, sporulating structures and microscopic morphologies. However, the other three strains (BIF-6, ROF and C-4) were unidentified species. In addition, plant pathogenic fungi (S1 and S2) were also isolated from infected roots and leaves of sesame plants. The identification of isolated plant pathogenic fungi was ongoing process. The common plant pathogenic fungus (*Phythium* sp.) was collected from Department of Biotechnology, Mandalay Technological University, Mandalay, Myanmar.

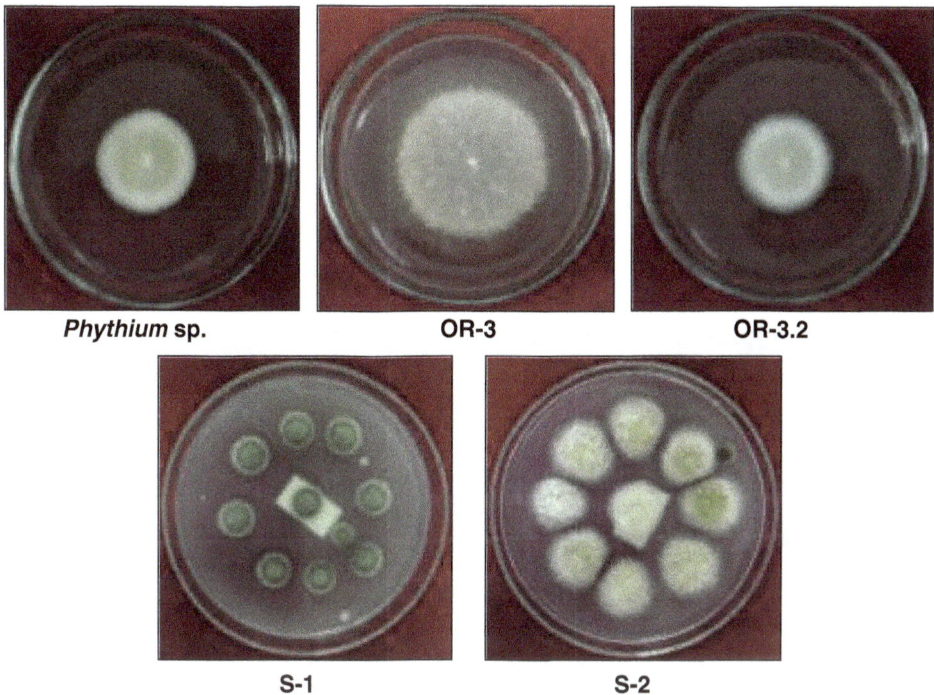


**Figure 11.4: Colonial Morphologies of Plant Pathogenic Fungi on PDA Media.**

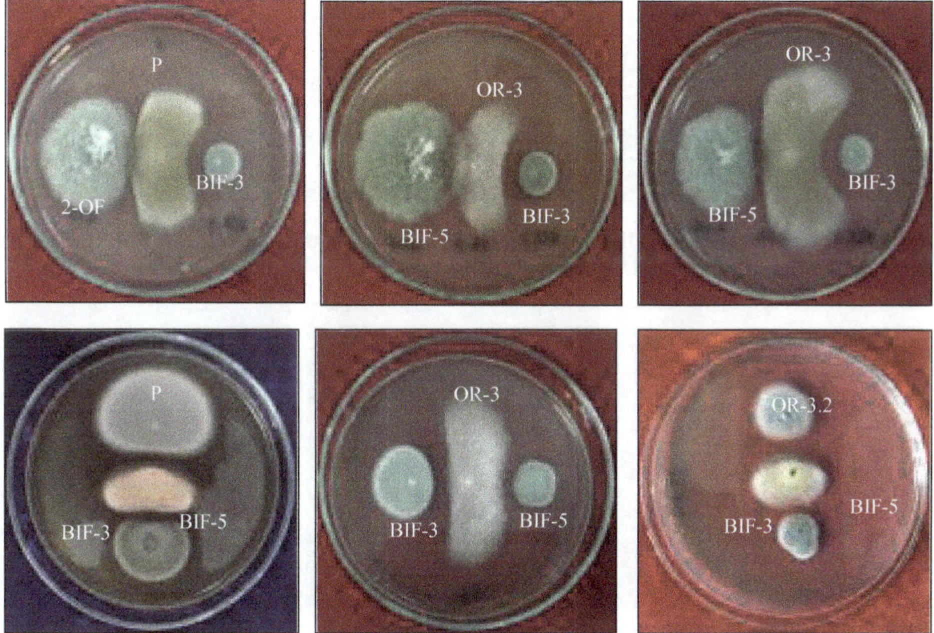


**Figure 11.5: Antifungal Activities of Effective Fungi against Plant Pathogenic Fungi on PDA Media after 2 Weeks Incubation Period.**

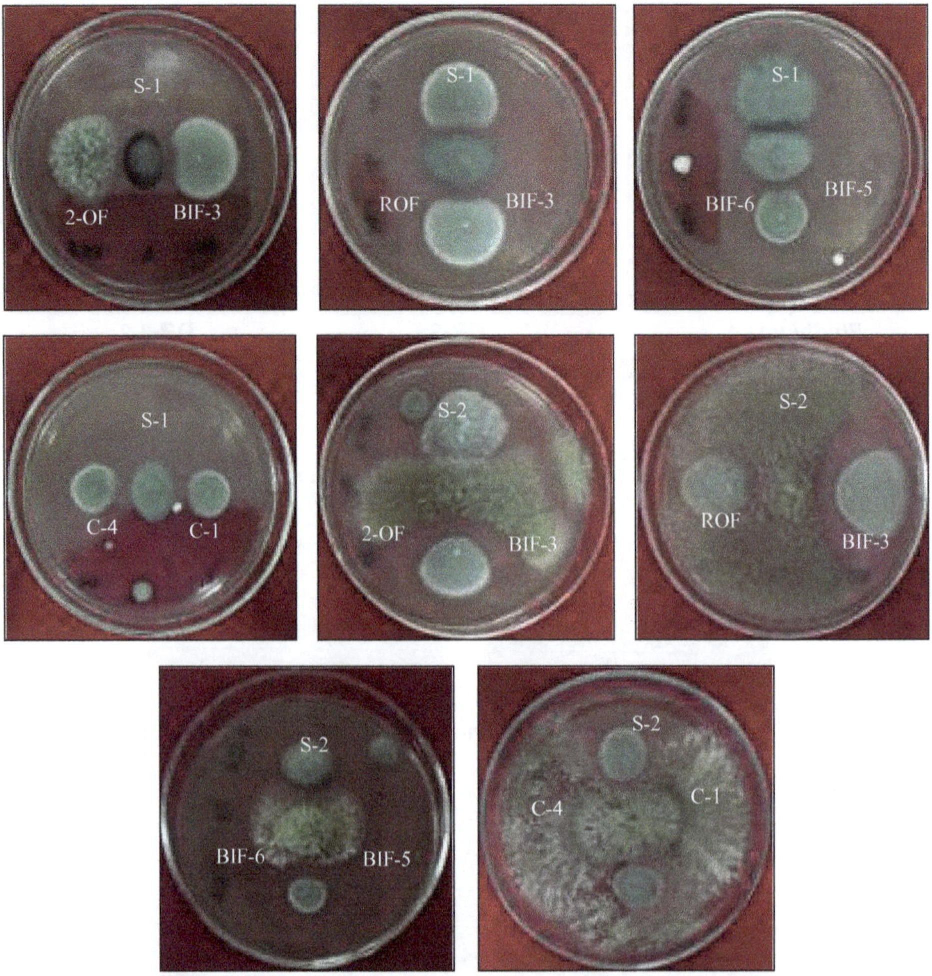

**Figure 11.6: Antifungal Activities of Effective Fungi against Plant Pathogenic Fungi on PDA Media after 2 Weeks Incubation Period.**

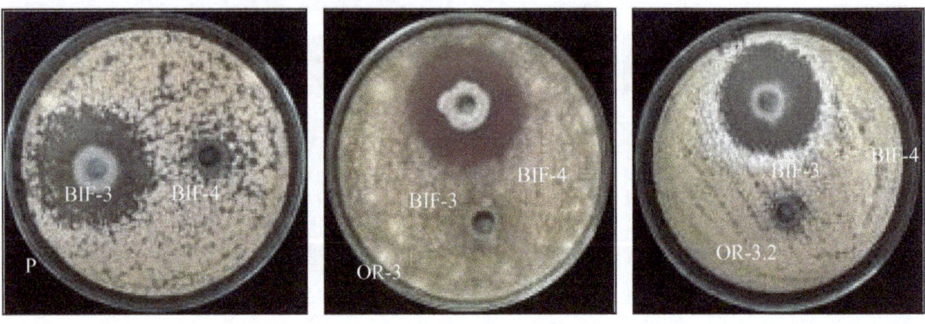


**Figure 11.7: Antifungal Activities of Effective Fungi – *Penicillium* sp. (BIF-3) against Plant Pathogenic Fungi (*Phythium* sp., OR-3 and OR-3.2) on PDA Media after 2 Weeks Incubation Period (100µL/well).**

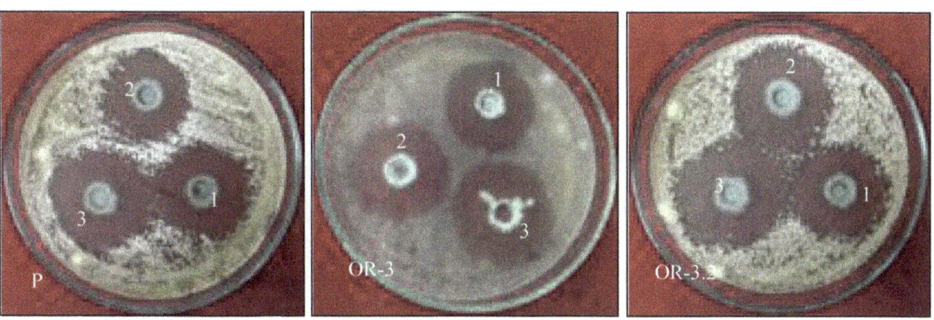


**Figure 11.8: Antifungal Activities of Effective Fungi – *Penicillium* sp. (BIF-3) against Plant Pathogenic Fungi (*Phythium* sp., OR-3 and OR-3.2) on PDA Media after 2 Weeks Incubation Period (100µL/well).**

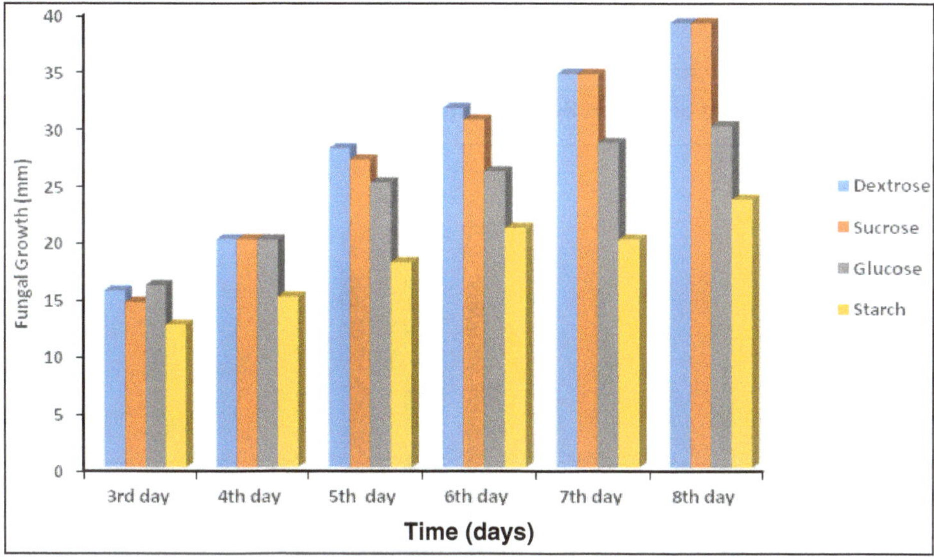


**Figure 11.9: Effects of Carbon Sources on the Growth of BIF-3.**

Antifungal activities of the isolated fungi against various plant pathogenic fungi were tested by dual culture method and well diffusion assay. According to the results, the isolated effective fungi (7 strains) showed the antifungal activities against the common plant pathogenic fungus (*Phythium* sp.) and the isolated plant pathogenic fungi of orange and sesame plants (S-1, S-2, OR-3 and OR-3.2). Among them, the isolated effective fungus (BIF-3) showed the significant antifungal activities on the tested strains.

The cultural conditions of the effective fungi (BIF-3 and 2-OF) were determined in surface and submerged cultures. In carbon Source determination, Dextrose is the best for both strains among four carbon sources tested. In addition, 18g/L and 12g/L

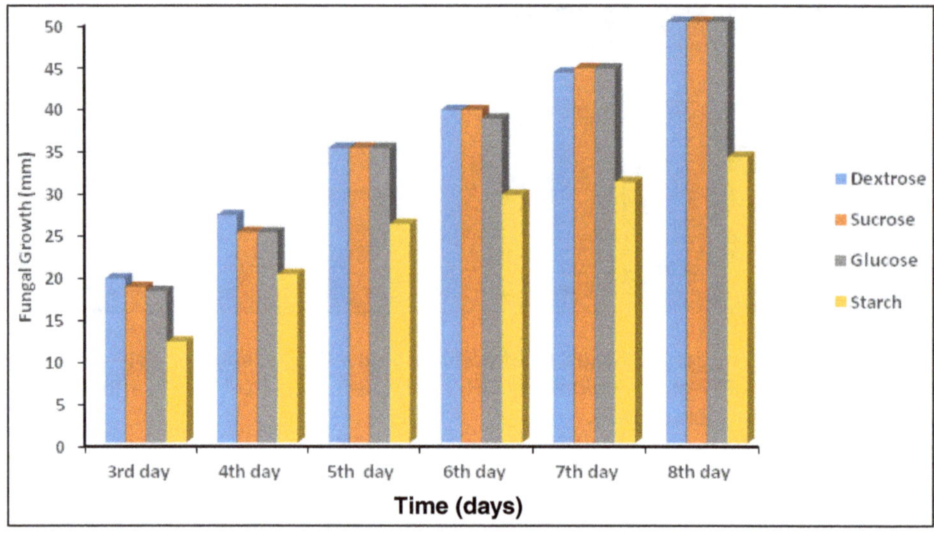


**Figure 11.10: Effects of Carbon Sources on the Growth of 2OF.**

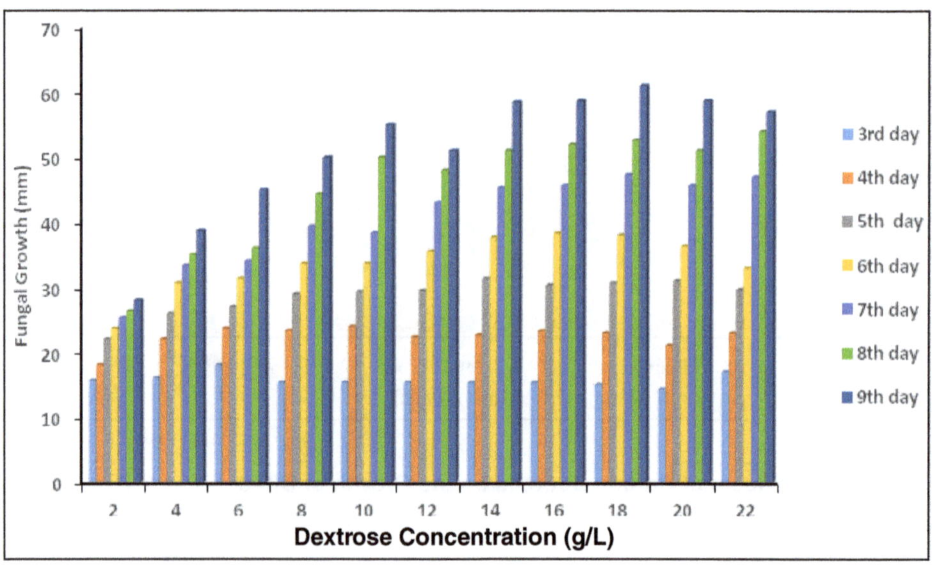


**Figure 11.11: Effects of Dextrose Concentrations on the Growth of BIF-3.**

of Dextrose sugar was the best for the growth of BIF-3 and 2-OF, respectively. The optimum pH for the growth of BIF-3 and 2-OF was pH 5 and pH 3, respectively. However, the maximum antifungal activities showed at pH 9 and pH 10 for BIF-3 and 2-OF during the course of fermentation. It showed that the antifungal metabolites affect the cultural or medium pH.

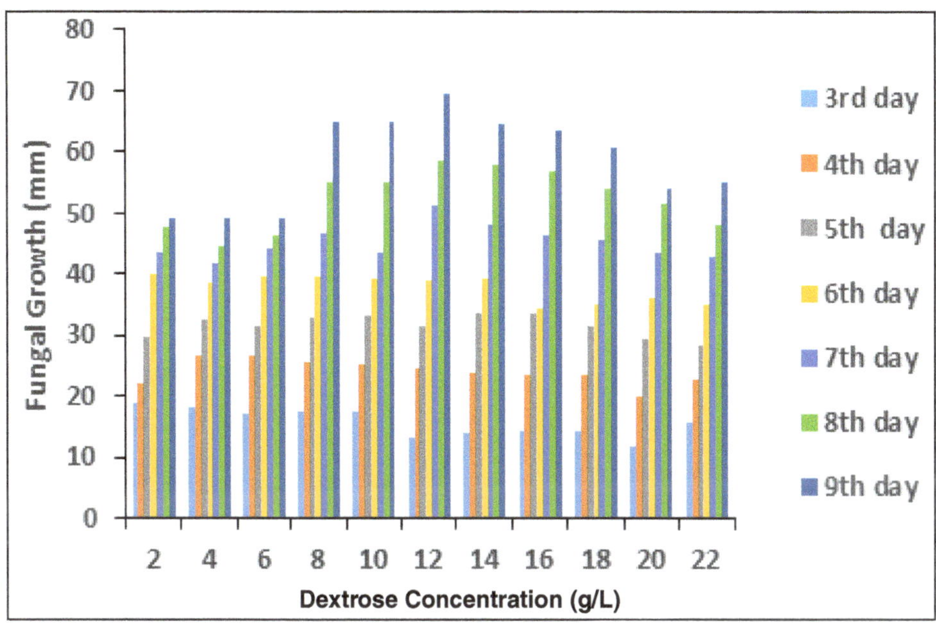


Figure 11.12: Effects of Dextrose Concentrations on the Growth of 2OF.

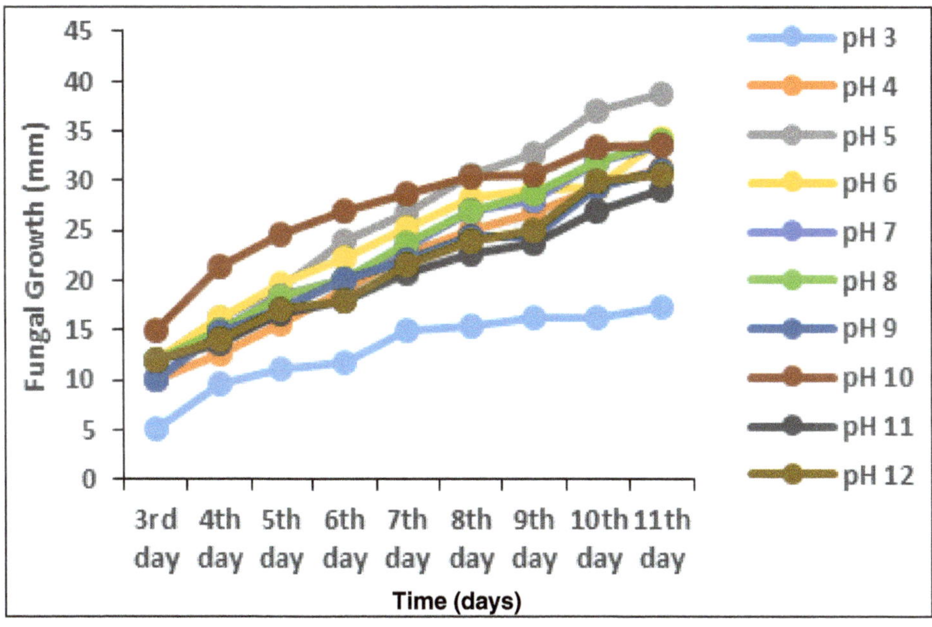


Figure 11.13: Effect of pH on the Growth of BIF-3.

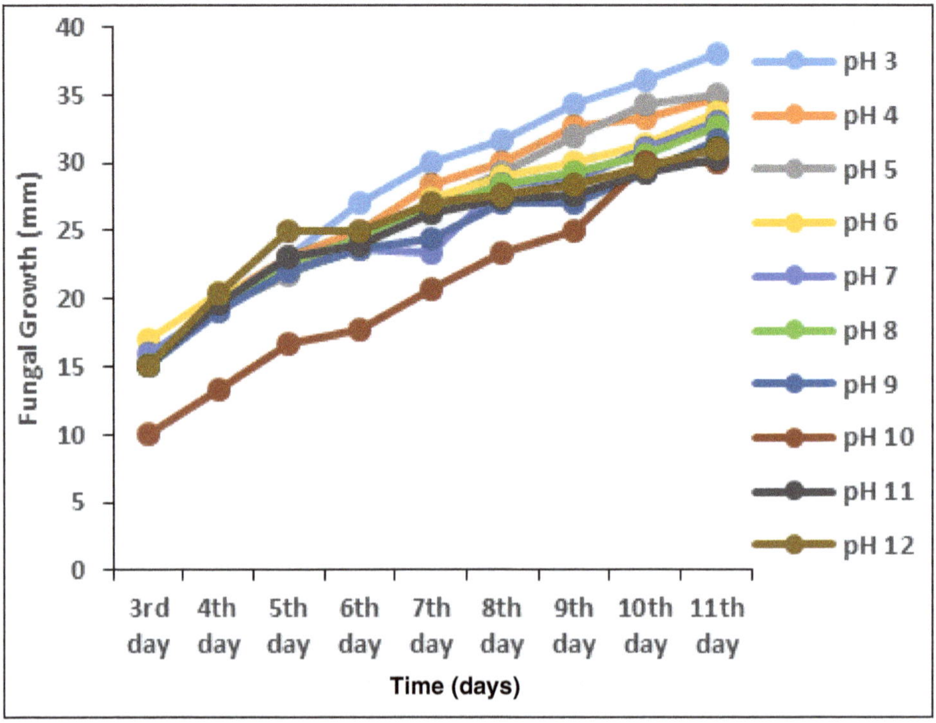

**Figure 11.14: Effect of pH on the Growth of 2OF.**

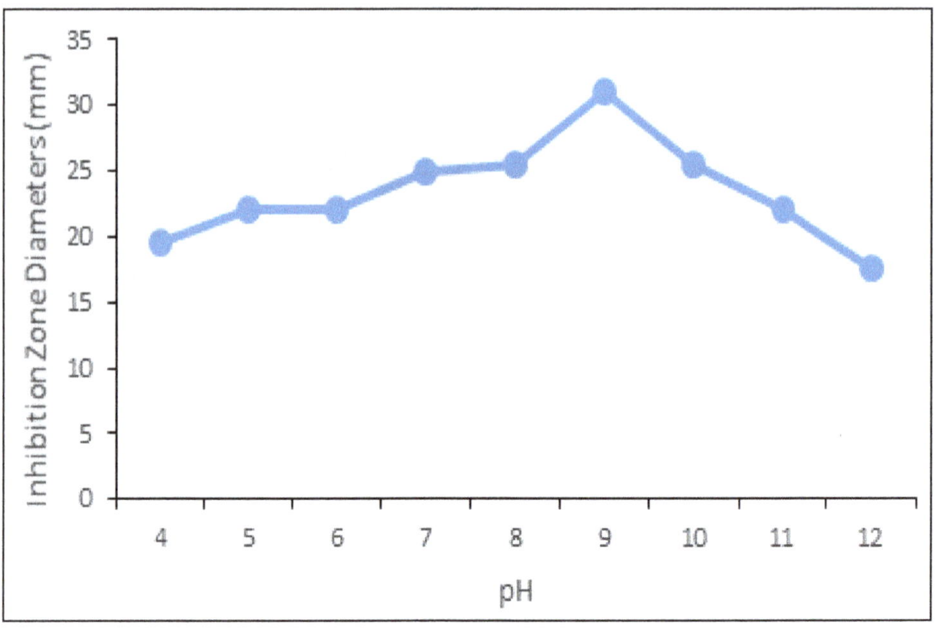


**Figure 11.15: Effect of pH on Antifungal Activities of BIF-3.**

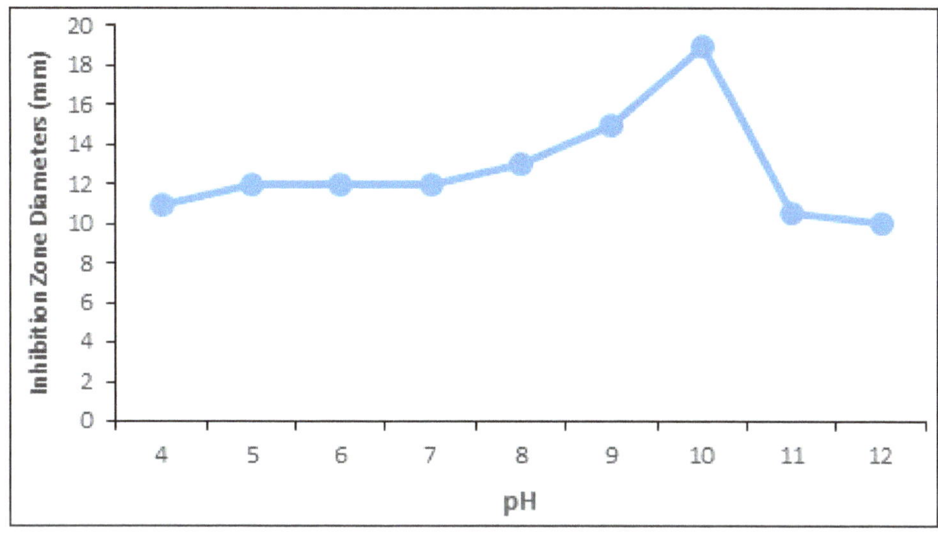


**Figure 11.16: Effect of pH on Antifungal Activities of 2OF.**

## Conclusions

The isolated effective fungi – *Penicillium* spp. (BIF-3 and 2-OF) have a potential role for controlling plant pathogenic fungi. Among them, *Penicillium* sp. (BIF-3) is the best strain for antifungal activities. Dextrose (18g/L and 12g/L) can be used as a carbon source for cultivating BIF-3 and 2-OF, respectively. The optimum pH for the growth of BIF-3 and 2-OF was pH 5 and pH 3, respectively. However, the optimum pH for antifungal activities were pH 9 and pH 10 for BIF-3 and 2-OF, respectively during the course of fermentation.

## Acknowledgement

The author wishes to express his profound gratitude to his Excellency, the Honorable, Dr. Myo Thein Gyi, Minister, Ministry of Education for permission to make this research work. The author wishes to express his gratitude to Dr. Aye Aye Khai, Head of Biotechnology Research Department, Ministry of Education, Kyaukse, Myanmar for permission and valuable advice on this research topic. The author specially wishes to acknowledge his gratitude to Dr. Myo Myint and Dr. Zaw Khaing Oo for their close suggestions, helpful advice and kind understanding for the success of his research work. Finally, the author likes to acknowledge his deep and sincere gratitude to his parents for their financial support and moral encouragement throughout his life and all his teachers from kindergartens to University.

## REFERENCES

1. A Espinel-Ingroff, F Barchiesi, K Hazeen, *et al.* 1998. Standarardization of antifungal susceptibility testing and clinical relevance, *Medical Mycology*, 36: 293-304.

2. A Espinel-Ingroff, D.W Warnock, *et al.* 2000. *In vitro* antifungal susceptibility methods and clinical implications of antifungal resistance *Medical Mycology*, 38: 68-78.
3. Brian Mcneil and Linda M. Harvey 2008. Practical fermentation technology Strathclyde Fermentation Centre, Strathclyde University, UK, ISBN: 978-0-470-01434-9.
4. Brian Steinwand, What are Biopesticides? Communications Officer and Ombudsman, Biopesticides and Pollution Prevention Division, (703) 305-7973.
5. Crueger, W. and Crueger, A 1989. A textbook of Industrial Microbiology 2$^{nd}$ ed, Panima Publishing Corporation, New Delhi.
6. Jarvis, W. R 1992. Managing diseases in greenhouse crops APS Press, Minnesota.
7. Kamal Krishna Pal and Brian Mc Spadden Gardenar 2006. Biological control of plant pathogen The Plant Health Instrucror, pp. 17-22.
8. Kamal Krishna Pal and Brian Mc Spadden Gardenar 2006. Biological control of plant pathogen The Plant Health Instrucror, pp. 17-22.
9. M. B. Ellis 1971. Dematiaceous Hypomycetes Commonwealth Mycological Institute, Kew, Surrey, England.
10. M. B. Ellis 1976. More Dematiaceous Hypomycetes Commonwealth Mycological Institute, Kew, Surrey, England.
11. Pauline Lowrie and Susan Wells 1994. Microbiology and biotechnology Cambridge UniversityPress.
12. S. Irshad, *et al.* 2012). *In vitro* anti-bacterial activities of three medicinal plants using agar welldiffusion method Research Journal of Biology, Vol. 02, Issue 01, pp. 1-8. ISSN 2049 1727.
13. Skidmore, A.M. and Dickinson, C.H 1976. British Mycol.Soc., 66(1): 57-64.
14. Smith, I. M., *et al.* 1988. European handbook of plant diseases Blackwell Scientific Publications, Oxford, UK.

*Chapter 12*

# Commercialization of Bioorganic Fertilizer for Sustainable Agriculture

***Buddhi Ratna Khadge***

*Secretary,*
*Nepal Academy of Science and Technology*
*P.O. Box Lalitpur, NEPAL*
*E-mail: buddhi.khadge@gmail.com*

## ABSTRACT

Nepal is an agricultural country. Thirty five percent of its GDP comes from agriculture sector and 65 per cent of its population depends directly or indirectly on agriculture. So-called modern agriculture depends highly on imported high inputs, like fertilizers and pesticides. Nepal government imported about 17 thousand metric tons of chemical fertilizer worth millions dollar. Use of chemical fertilizer has environmental effect and causes degradation of soil fertility. Now-a-days Integrated Plant Nutrient System (IPNS) is the key word for the supply of plant nutrients required to achieve sustainable agricultural products. One of the main components of IPNS is organic fertilizer, which supplies not only nutrients to plants, but also helps to maintain soil fertility. Traditionally, Nepalese farmers have been using organic manures in their field since time unmemorable. But because of easy availability of chemical fertilizer, farmers started to abandon organic manures. The so-called modern agriculture has become addicted to chemical fertilizer and pesticides. Because of sole use of chemical fertilizer without addition of carbon, the fertility status of the soil is decreasing day by days. The organic matter, which is considered as heart of soil is decreasing together with beneficial microbes in the soil. Other soil related problems like soil-borne plant diseases, acidic soil, and low water holding capacity; soil erosion and others are increasing.

To tackle above-mentioned problems, the local appropriate technology of Bio-organic fertilizer (BOF) was developed. Two strains of *Trichoderma, Trichoderma herzianum* and *Trichoderma viride* were selected after rigorous laboratory and greenhouse experiment works. The strains of *Trichoderma* have biocontrol and biofertilizer properties respectively. The inoculum production technology for bioagent was developed using locally available cheap raw materials like rice husk and rice bran. One local strain of *Azotobacter chroococcum* was selected for nitrogen fixation in the composting process. The use of *Azotobacter* increased the nitrogen contents of the biofertilizer produced.

Composting technology for the production of BOF using locally available raw materials like plant residue, chicken manures or biogas slurry. The product were tested on farmers field using participatory approach on the vegetable crops. The products was packaged and sold to the farmers.

Farmer groups or co-operative of the farmers were trained for the entrepreneurship development skill. The value-added products was branded as "Bhu- Bardan" (Soil Blessing) and commercialized. The problems and difficulties faced during the process of value addition and commercialization of BOF are discussed

***Keywords:*** *Bio-fertilizer, Sustainable agriculture, Trichoderma, Azotobacter, Organic agriculture, Soil fertility.*

## INTRODUCTION

Integrated Plant Nutrient System (IPNS) is the key work for the supply of plant nutrients required to produce different agricultural products. One of the main components of IPNS is organic manure, which supplies not only nutrients to plants but also help to maintain soil fertility. Traditionally, Nepalese farmers have been using organic manures since time unmemorable. But because of easy availability of chemical fertilizers to supply plant nutrients, particularly major nutrients like nitrogen, phosphorus and potash farmers started to abandon organic manure. The modern agriculture has become addicted to chemical fertilizers. Because sole use of chemical fertilizer without addition of carbon, the fertility status of the soil is decreasing day by day (Cook, R.J.,1983). The organic matter, which is considered heart of the soil, is decreasing together with beneficial microbial population of the soil. Other soil related problems like soil-borne plant diseases, acidic pH, low water holding capacity, soil erosion and others are increasing.

Nepalese Government imported about 177 thousand metric ton of chemical fertilizer worth billions rupees in 2012-13. Ministry of Agriculture Development (MOAD) Government of Nepal (GON) is spending billion of rupees to subsidize chemical fertilizers. One of the studies done with NARD fund showed that farmers of Chitwan are using far more chemical fertilizers than recommended dose. The participatory field trial conducted at farmers' fields proved that almost equal yield of vegetable could be taken with the use of well scientifically prepared bio-fortified bio-organic fertilizer using bio-agents like *Trichoderma* spp. and *Azotobater* without using chemical fertilizer (Brozová J. 2004). MOAD has the policy to promote Organic Fertilizer.

The management practice of organic manure is not scientific. Farmers know only to pile the animal waste nearby the animal shade to make organic manure and take to the field without complete decomposition. The partially decomposed organic manure in anaerobic condition could be source of disease inocula and poor in nutrient contents. The quality of the organic manure can be enhanced by following scientific decomposition process like improving aeration, balanced C/N ratio and avoiding nutrient losses at the time of production and using in the crop field.

The main purpose of the project was to develop technology to convert organic manure into very effective bioorganic fertilizer. The farmer would change the way they prepare organic manure in their composting yard. It was expected that in five-year time 50 per cent of the farmers in the area would switch over to the bio-fertilizer technology. The soil fertility status of the area would be improved. There would be reduction in the use of chemical fertilizer in the area. The way the farmer thinks of organic matter as dirty business would be changed. Seventy percent of the agriculture waste of the project area would be converted into bio-fertilizer. Because of easy availability of bio-fertilizer, the production of organic farm would be improved. There would be more organic product available in the market. The organic product would be cheaper and affordable to the consumers.

## Materials and Methods

Selection of *Trichoderma* and *Azotobacter*- Two local isolates of *Trichoderma harzianum* (TH1) and *Trichoderma viride* (TV1) were selected to be used in the bioorganic fertilizer technology (Khadge, B.R., 1994, 2002). Mass production technology of *Trichoderma* using simple substrates, rice husk and rice bran (4:1 volume base) was developed. These isolates were selected after series of laboratory, plastic house, and on-farm experimentation at the Plant Pathology Division, Khumaltar, Lalitpur. Biofertilizer technology was developed using local raw materials like biogas slurry (160 kg), chicken manure, plant residue or bioproduct (330 kg), mustard seed cake (5 kg). Ten packets of *Trichoderma* and ten packets of *Azotobacter* for composting were used in the composting process. Air flow to facilitate composting process was enhanced by inserting plastic pipes, 4in. diameter with 3 cm holes at 5 in. apart inside the compost hips. The compost was turned thoroughly three times (Khadge, 2012). The bio-fertilizer was ready to be used in the field in 35-40 days. The bioorganic fertilizer was analysed for N, P, K, and Trichoderma content.

On-farm testing of bioorganic fertilizer was done with local farmers' participation. There were four treatments, Bioorganic fertilizer (BOF) at the rate of 2 ton per hectare, BOF 2 tons per hectare added to half the dose of recommended chemical fertilizer. Biogas slurry directly was used at the rate of 1.3 ton per hectare. Same rate of biogas slurry was added to half the dose of recommended dose of chemical fertilizer. The treatments were replicated 7 (one farmer's plot as one replication. The bioorganic fertilizer was tested in tomato var. BL 401. The experimental design was the Randomized Complete Block Design (RCBD). Before and after the experiment, soil samples were taken for the soil and microbial analysis. Yield parameters like marketable tomato, height of the plants and biomass were recorded and statistical analysis was done using statistical package.

For commercialization of BOF, two co-operative farmer's groups were selected. Farmers were trained both for production of BOF and entrepreneurship development. The farmers produced about 4 tons of BOF on each site. They developed skills for packing and selling the products. The product was named. They were also taught about the promotion scaling-up of the BOF.

## Results and Discussion

### Mass Production of *Trichoderma*

Different combinations of substrate, rice wheat, millets and their byproducts were tested for the mass production of *Trichoderma*. The combination of rice husk and rice bran was selected because it was easily available and cheap in Nepal. The average production of colony forming units (*c.f.u.*) achieved was $10^7$ per gram of substrate. These living units were good for the production of bioorganic fertilizer. It might not be good to sell *Trichoderma* as sole bioagent. Simple technique using polypropylene bags with cotton plug for aeration was used to mass-produce the bioagent, *Trichoderma* (Saxena, M.C., 1993).

**Table 12.1: Effect of Biofertilizer, Biogas Slurry, Fertilizer and their Combination on Tomato (BL 401) Yield Parameters at Chitwan**

| *No.* | *Treatment* | *Marketable Yield *kg/15 sq. meter* | *Plant Height at Flowering*(cm)* |
|---|---|---|---|
| 1. | Bioorganic fertilizer (BOF), 2 tons/hectare | 7.5 | 71 |
| 2. | BOF 2 ton/h + half chemical fertilizer dose | 6.15 | 67 |
| 3. | Biogas slurry 1.3 ton/hacter | 4.25 | 66 |
| 4. | Biogas slurry 1.3 ton/h+ half dose of fertilizer | 5.65 | 60 |

* Data is average of 10 experiment plots.

**Table 12.2: Effect of Biofertilizer, Biogas Slurry, Fertilizer and their Combination on Tomato (Unsari) Yield Parameters at Pokhara**

| *No.* | *Treatment* | *Marketable Yield kg/plot (50 plants grown in plastic house)* | *Plant Height at Flowering (cm)* |
|---|---|---|---|
| 1. | Bioorganic fertilizer (BOF), 2 tons/hectare | 147.5 | 2.1 |
| 2. | BOF 2 ton/h + half chemical fertilizer dose | 203.0 | 2.2 |
| 3. | Biogas slurry 1.3 ton/hacter | 105.00 | 1.75 |
| 4. | Biogas slurry 1.3 ton/h+ half dose of fertilizer | 115.5 | 1.63 |

From the Table 12.1 data of Chitwan, It was found that Bioorganic fertilizer treatment gave highest tomato yield, 5 ton per hectare which was not significantly different from Biofertilizer treatment with half the dose of recommended fertilizer dose (N:P:K=120:60:40). Use of biogas slurry alone yielded less tomato. The data from showed that the highest yield of tomato was obtained with the application of Bio-organic fertilizer together with half dose of recommended fertilizer dose. The two experimental sites were different as far as soil properties and climate were considered. Chitwan site was in hot zone with soil pH ranging from 4.5 to 5.5. Pokhara site was cold zone in the mid-hill with highly acidic pH ranging from 4-5. Plant height data were not significantly different at both experiment sites. Farmers at Chitwan were convinced that they could grow profitable tomato crops without using chemical fertilizer. In Pokhara, the experimental plots were low fertility with too low pH. The farmers experienced the need to apply both BOF and chemical fertilizer to get better yield of tomato.

Demonstration of BOF technology were done on cauliflower, cabbage, maize and potato. Farmers who conducted the demonstration were convinced that BOF increased yield of from 15-20 per cent. BOF treated crops were more resistant to pest and diseases. BOF treated vegetables were tastier than chemical fertilizer treated vegetable. The vegetable products applied with BOF had longer post-harvest life.

Cooperative organization of one project site, Chitwan was given technical and financial support for the commercial production of BOF. The members of the cooperative were given training for both commercial production and entrepreneurship development. About four tons of bioorganic fertilizer was produced using local inputs. They were able to market some of the products. They branded their product with name "Bhu-wardan". Literally, Bhu-wardan" means gift for soil. They made attractive packaging of 10 and 25 kg. The retail price of the BOF was Rs.15.00 per Kg (about US$ 0.15). The cost of production was Rs. 10.00 per kg. The profit margin was Rs. 5.0 per kg.

Due to commercial productions constraints, the cooperative could not continue with the business of BOF production and marketing once the assistance was stopped from the project. One of the main reasons was inadequate experience on entrepreneurship and commercialization. The members of the cooperative were less educated, below high school graduate. Their BOF product was not big enough to penetrate big market. It was difficult to convince the local farmers and stakeholders the benefits of BOF. The profit margin for the users was not attractive to switch over to BOF from chemical fertilizer.

## Conclusions

From the project work, it could be concluded that farmers could be trained for the production and commercialization of bioorganic fertilizer. BOF increased different types of vegetable crops. Farmers at local rural level needed continue support from the project or government side at least for 5 years to make them sustainable in the production and commercialization of bioorganic fertilizer.

## Acknowledgements

This paper is the product of the project funded by National Agriculture Research and Development Fund (NARDF), Kathmandu, Nepal. The author would like to acknowledge NARDF and its staff for the fund and cooperation to run the project successfully. The project was executed under Innovative Agricultural Initiative (IAI) Pvt. Ltd. The staff and the farmers of the project sites are also acknowledged for their hard work and cooperation.

## REFERENCES

1. Brozová J. 2004. Mycoparasitic fungi *Trichoderma* spp. in plant protection. *Plant Prot. Sci.* 40 (2): 63–74.

2. Cook R.J., Baker K.F. 1983. The Nature and Practice of Biological Control of Plant Pathogens. APS Press, St. Paul, Minnesota, USA, 539 pp.
3. De Castro A.M., Ferreira M.C., Da Cruz J.C., Pedro K.C.N.R., Carvalho D.F., Leite S.G.F., Pereira Jr N. 2010. High-yield endoglucanase production by *Trichoderma harzianum* IOC- 3844 cultivated in pretreated sugarcane mill byproduct. *Enzyme Res.* 1 (1): 1–8.
4. Elad Y. 2000. *Trichoderma harzianum* T39 preparation for bio-control of plant diseases-control of *Botrytis cinerea, Sclerotinia sclerotiorum* and *Cladosporium fulvum. Biocontrol Sci. Technol.*, 10 (4): 499–507.
5. Harman G.E. 2006. Overview of mechanisms and uses of *Trichoderma* spp. *Phytopathology* 96 (2): 190–194.
6. Harman G.E., Howell C.R., Viterbo A., Chet I., Lorito M. 2004. *Trichoderma* species opportunistic, avirulent plant symbionts. *Nat. Rev. Microbiol.*, 2 (1): 43–56.
7. Khadge B.R. 1994. Preliminary screening of *Trichoderma* spp. against white blight disease of mustard. Proceeding, National Winter crops seminar, NARC.
8. Khadge, B.R. 2008. *Trichoderma* for composting chicken manure. Paper presented in SAS conference.
9. Khadge B.R. 2002. *Trichoderma:* a novel fungi for biological control of soil-borne disease. *Proceeding, National Seminar on IPM in Nepal.*
10. Khadge, B.R. 2012. Effect of Bio-organic Fertilizer on Vegetables. *Proceeding SAS Journal.*
11. Saxena M.C. 1993. The challenge of developing biotic and abiotic stress resistance in cool-season food legumes. p. 3-14. In: "Breeding for Stress Tolerance in Cool Season Food Legumes" (K. B. Singh, M. C. Saxena, eds.). Wiley, Chichester, UK, 474 pp.
12. Dawadi, V.R. and B.R. Khadge, 2000. Training Manual on Soil-borne disease and their Management (In Nepali Language). 2000. Published by DEPROSC-Nepal for SSMP, Nepal.

# Chapter 13

# A Review on the Role of Tissue Culture in the Propagation of Planting Materials in Zimbabwe: Sweet Potato

*L.G. Muusha*[1] *and T.O. Nyarumbu*[1] *and C. Moffat*[2]

[1]*Horticulture Research Institute,*
*Box 810, Marondera, ZIMBABWE*
*E-mail: lindagmuusha@gmail.com, nyarumbutrish@gmail.com*
[2]*National Biotechnology Authority of Zimbabwe,*
*22 Princess Drive, Newlands, Harare, ZIMBABWE*
*E-mail: moffatcathrine21@gmail.com*

## ABSTRACT

Tissue culture is an application of agricultural biotechnology which is defined as the *in vitro* techniques used to grow or maintain cells or tissue derived from a living organism in artificial nutrient-specific media.Tissue culture is a biotechnological technique used in the production of disease free planting materials. In Zimbabwe the technique is being used mainly in the production of virus free sweet potato planting material. The use of tissue culture material is still low as many small holder farmers are still relying on recycled material that they circulate amongst themselves. The disadvantage of this is that the material will be infected with pests and diseases that cause yield reductions and lower the quality of the tubers. Currently, in Zimbabwe, most reported tissue culture work has been done on sweet potatoes and Irish potatoes with emerging interests on cassava, bananas and strawberries. In the year 1996, the Horticulture Research Institute (HRI) and the Biotechnology Trust of Zimbabwe (BTZ) collaborated to promote sweet potato production in Zimbabwe through the promotion and provision of clean planting materials. The research work involved trials on collection, selection, cleaning and evaluation of suitable varieties for distribution to commercial, small-scale and communal farmers in Hwedza and Buhera districts. The micro-propagation project helped resource poor communal farmers to access clean material at low prices. Farmers were also trained in sweet potato production and awareness was raised on the importance of using virus free planting material in order to achieve high yields. Today this approach is being encouraged in collaboration with National Biotechnology Authority (NBA) and work was carried out in Murewa, Rusape and Bulawayo.

***Keywords:*** *Tissue culture, Sweet potato, Viral diseases, Micropropagation, Variety.*

## INTRODUCTION

Agriculture is the backbone of the Zimbabwean economy contributing to foreign currency earnings through the export of cash crops such as tobacco and flowers. The sector contributes 11-14 per cent of GDP and approximately 70 per cent of the Zimbabwean population is dependent on the agriculture sector for a livelihood (Ministry of Foreign Affairs, 2015). Zimbabwe, like many African countries is still vulnerable in terms of food security. Farmers are faced with challenges which include climate change leading to unpredictable weather and rainfall patterns, low mechanisation and expensive seed. Five factors have been identified as being key in the improvement of food production on the African continent and these are; use of appropriate agrochemicals, sustainable irrigation, and efficient high yielding (adapted) varieties, crop management and plant biotechnology (Brink *et al.*, 1998). While research in agronomy and breeding has been providing good results and has helped farmers to improve yields, the use of biotechnology is still very low in sub-Saharan Africa. The most advanced country in the use of biotechnology is South Africa.

In Zimbabwe strides are being made in the use of plant biotechnology for the improvement of the agriculture sector. Biotechnology is being applied in both plant and livestock production. 80 per cent of the work is on plants while 20 per cent is on livestock (Parawira *et al.*, 2009). Biotechnology projects that are being conducted in the country range from those using traditional biotechnology to experimental work on genetically modified organisms (Sithole-Niang, 2001).Tissue culture is an application of agricultural biotechnology which is defined as the *in vitro* techniques used to grow or maintain cells or tissue derived from a living organism in artificial nutrient-specific media. Traditional biotechnology techniques are used in Zimbabwe because they require less scientific knowledge, less time, less finance, less risk and are closer to the market. The only institutes using more advanced genetic engineering techniques are the Biotechnology Research Institute (BRI), University of Zimbabwe and Veterinary Research Laboratories (VRL) (Parawira *et al.*, 2009). BRI has been conducting biotechnology research on maize and sweet potato since 1996. VRL has been working on the use of biotechnology in the diagnosis, and prevention of livestock diseases which are of major economic importance since 1989. The Department of Research and Specialist Services has three institutes that apply biotechnology research work. The Horticultural Research Institute uses tissue culture to produce virus free sweet potato planting materials, the Soil Productivity Research Laboratory produces legume inoculants while the Cotton Research Institute works on transgenic cotton (Woodend, 1995; Parawira *et al.*, 2009). The Tobacco Research

Board is another institute using tissue culture techniques on tobacco and researching on transgenic tobacco plants.

Tissue culture is currently being used to produce planting materials for sweet potato, cassava and Irish potato on a commercial scale. These crops are important in small holder agriculture as they contribute towards household food security. Sweet potato and Irish potato were recently upgraded by the Zimbabwean government into the class of staple foods for the nation; therefore, the availability of clean planting materials of these key crops is essential for the achievement of household and national food security. This paper will review the use of biotechnology in the production of sweet potato planting material in Zimbabwe.

Communal farmers play a crucial role in agriculture but they are the least trained and informed in proper food production techniques, post-harvest processing, utilization and marketing. Access to clean, disease free planting materials is a stumbling block for small-scale farmers as they sometimes fail to afford purchasing of the planting material. This leads to reduced yields and the production of poor quality crops that will not fetch good selling prices on the market.

Sweet potato (*Ipomoea batatas* (L.) Lam) is a Native American plant belonging to the Convolvulaceae family, order Polmoniales (Burden, 2005). It is a crop that can adapt to a wide range of environmental conditions and grow on marginal areas with poor soils of limited fertility and inadequate moisture (Bioethics, 2004). The effects of climate change are becoming evident with the increasing temperatures being experienced in the country. It is therefore, prudent for farmers to grow sweet potatoes as they can withstand high temperatures and will be a reliable food source for resource poor communities.

Sweet potatoes are propagated vegetatively using mainly terminal and middle vine cuttings (Kapinga *et al.*, 1995) but also using sprouts from tuberous roots from the previous crop. The majority of small holder farmers across Zimbabwe grow sweet potato for household consumption and as a source of income. The fact that sweet potato can be grown on marginal areas has enabled it to be grown across Zimbabwe. Small holder farmers use volunteer sprouts from the previous crop following the first.

In urban areas, it is estimated that between 1-7 kg of sweet potatoes are consumed per capita while rural households consume between 3-5 kg of sweet potatoes per capita (Zimbabwe National Vulnerability Assessment Committee, 2004). The Midlands province has the largest area under sweet potato cultivation with an area of 7069 ha and an average yield of 6.46t/ha. Manicaland province has the highest average yield of 10.65t/ha on an area of 3693 ha, while Mashonaland East is averaging 9.38t/ha on an area of 4817 ha.

This paper reviews the use of biotechnology to increase sweet potato production, utilisation and marketing through the provision of virus free planting materials to small holder farmers. The project was carried out in Hwedza and Buhera districts of Zimbabwe. It was a collaborative project involving the following institutions: Biotechnology Trust of Zimbabwe, Biotechnology Research Institute,

Tobacco Research Board, Horticulture Research Institute and Agricultural Extension (Biotechnology Trust of Zimbabwe, 2003).

## Materials and Methods

The sweet potato project began in 1996 and was implemented in Hwedza and Buhera districts of Zimbabwe. The project involved collection of sweet potato varieties and virus elimination. The cleaned varieties were then distributed to pilot nurseries in Murambinda and Mawire, where the local farmers would have easy access to the planting materials (Munyulwa, 1999).

The start of the project activities followed a survey of sweet potato varieties that were grown in the area. About 109 sweet potato varieties were collected from Buhera, Hwedza and other districts and these were taken for virus cleaning at BRI and TRB. In 1998, 25 varieties which included new varieties from HRI, traditional varieties collected from the project area and commercial check cultivars were taken back to Buhera and Hwedza for inclusion in demonstration trials. The commercial check cultivars used were Brondal, Cordner, Magutse and Pamhai. Twenty three varieties were planted under irrigation at Murambinda Irrigation scheme on 21 December 1998. Xushu, Japon, Germany II, Imby, Kori and Matebeleland South Mhlope were introduced from HRI. Chigogo (BTZ98/H001), Kerotsi, Botswana, Madhura and Chi Zambia were farmers varieties collected from Hwedza district whereas Mai farai A, Mai farai B, Sibhamu Zijena, Chigogo (BTZ98/B111), Kanyimo, Chena and Mupedzanzara were from Buhera district.

Another 25 varieties were planted under rainfed conditions at Mombeyarara (Ward 31), Nerutanga (Ward 4), and Gosho (Ward 1) in Buhera 0n 22 – 24 February 1999 and compared to the four commercial check varieties. Varieties from HRI were Xushu, Japon, Germany II, Imby, Kori, Matebeleland South Mhlope and Matabeleland South Bomvu. Varieties from Hwedza were Chigogo (BTZ98/H001), Kerotsi, Madhura, Chizambia, Mukadziusaende, and Tumbe while from Buhera there was Madhuve, Kanyimo, SibhamuZijena, Mupedzanzara, Muuyu, Chigogo (BTZ98/B111), Chena, Kanyembamudiki, Chikaranga (BTZ98/B115), Chikaranga (BTZ98/B100) and Chivise.

Three rainfed trials were planted at Mabaye (Zviyambe East), Musvinu (Goneso ward) and Mukondwa (Mashaya Ward) in Hwedza district on 2-3 February 1999. Twenty-three varieties were planted at each site and compared to the four commercial check varieties. Seven varieties from HRI were used:Xushu, Imby, Japon, Kori, Matebeleland South Mhlope, Matebeleland South Bomvu and Germany II. Chigogo (BTZ98/H001), Tumbe, Mdhura, Dhubhe, Botswana, Mukadziusaende, ChiZambia, Kerotsi, Bhanabhasi and ex-Waddilove were from Hwedza while Kanyimo, Madhuve, Sibhamu, Zijena, Muuyu, Mupedzanzara and Chena were from Buhera.

At each site 40m$^2$ plots were arranged in a randomised complete block design with three replications. Forty-centimetre sweet potato vine cuttings were planted using a spacing of 30cm along the ridge with the ridges being 1m apart (33,333 plants/ha). Compound D fertiliser (8:14:7 $N, P_2O_5, K_2O$) was applied at a rate of 40kg/ha during preparation of the ridges. The crops were top dressed with 50kg/

ha ammonium nitrate (34.5 per cent N) and 30kg/ha muriate of potash (60 per cent $K_2O$) a one and five weeks after planting. There were five nursery farmers who managed the crop at Murambinda Irrigation Scheme. Sweet potato trials at each of the rainfed sites were managed by a group of between 12 and 18 farmers who met once every month to continuously assess the performance of the varieties. Sweet potatoes were harvested approximately four months after planting on 27 April at Murambinda, 14 June at Mabaye, 16 June at Musvinu and 21 June at Mukondwa. Sweet potatoes failed at each of the three rainfed sites in Buhera because no rains fell after planting (Nzima *et al.*, 1999).

Parameters that were evaluated at these demonstration trials were adaptability, yield potential, agronomic characteristics and organoleptic tests. The best ten varieties that were identified from this evaluation were adopted for further trials in three research areas. The three trials were: a re-infection trial; performance of virus cleaned and uncleaned planting materials and a fertiliser management trial (Nzima *et al.*, 1999).

## Results and Discussion

Total yield of tuberous roots at Murambinda Irrigation Scheme was good and ranged between 6.90 to 29.12t/ha with a trial mean of 14.43 (6.802t/ha). In contrast yields of marketable tuberous roots were between 5.32 and 25.18t/ha with a trial mean of 10.16 (6.526t/ha). Weevil damage was severe on some varieties accounting for over 50 per cent of the unmarketable tuberous roots.

Tuberous root yield at Hwedza were comparatively low averaging 6.65t/ha at Goneso ward and 5.81t/ha at Zviyambe East and 1.590t/ha at Mashaya ward. Weevil damage was very severe at some sites shown bya large differences between total and marketable yields. The poor yields were attributed to the short growing season and low rainfall (300mm) that fell after the late planting in early February 1999. The sweet potato yields obtained were greater than yields that could have been produced by maize planted at the same time. The commercial checks Magutse, Brondal and Pamhai were among the top 10 heavy yielders which included the introduced, improved variety Sibhamu Zijena from Buhera which was yielding up to 11.18t/ha.

On organoleptic tests, the tastes of farmers traditional sweet potato varieties were most preferred. Pamhai was the only improved variety that was in the preferred top ten varieties by the participants at all the sites. In contrast, improved varieties were regarded highly with respect to yield.

Work done by Mutandwa in 2008, in Hwedza district showed that 93 per cent of the farmers that he interviewed were still using disease free, tissue cultured materials. 32 per cent of the farmers purchased their materials from BTZ while 21.8 per cent obtained their materials from the nursery sites established in the 1999/2000 season (Mutandwa, 2008). However, at Mawire irrigation scheme only 9 out of the 27 varieties were still available due to the unavailability of a reliable irrigation system. The yields noted by Mutandwa showed that tissue cultured sweet potatoes were yielding 1.8t/ha while non-tissue cultured material was yielding 0.5t/ha. These yields are lower than expected but this could be due to the fact that the farmers grew their crop on marginal land with no fertiliser. Work done in other parts of the world, including Peru have shown that tissue cultured sweet potatoes produce higher yields than non-tissue cultured materials (Fonseca *et al.*, 2003). The higher yields gave a higher net economic return for tissue cultured material of US$91.58 while non-tissue cultured material gave a return of US$36.05 (Mutandwa, 2008). In Peru, the use of tissue cultured materials lowered production costs by US$500 to US$700/ha (Zuger, 2003).

## Conclusions

The work done on the use of tissue culture to improve sweet potato yields produced positive results. It can be noted that from project inception in 1996, small holder farmers have increased awareness on the importance of using virus free planting materials in order to achieve high yields. This is evidenced by the increase in the number of farmers who come to HRI to purchase tissue cultured planting material and requesting for training in sweet potato propagation. There is also an increase in the number of requests for orange fleshed sweet potato varieties which have high vitamin A content. The next step is to increase production of the tissue cultured materials and to establish more satellite nurseries across the country.

## Acknowledgements

I would like to acknowledge the work done by Dr. M. Nzima and the BTZ team on the sweet potato micropropagation project. I would also like to thank the HRI team and National Biotechnology Trust staff who have continued with the work.

## Abbreviations

BRI: Biotechnology Research Institute
GDP: Gross Domestic product
HRI: Horticultural Research Institute
TRB: Tobacco Research Board
VRL: Veterinary Research Laboratories
t/ha: tonnes per hectare
ha: hectare

## References

1. Bioethics Nuffield council 2004.The Use of GM Crops in Developing Countries. Case study 5: Improved resistance to viruses in sweet potato.
2. Biotechnology Trust of Zimbabwe 2003. Biological Nitrogen Fixation, Mushroom and Sweet potato projects: A socio-economic evaluation. Harare: Biotechnology Trust of Zimbabwe.
3. Brink, J.A., Woodward, B.R., and DaSilva, E.J. (1998). Plant biotechnology: A Tool for development in Africa. *Electronic Journal of Biotechnology*, 1(3), 1-12.
4. Burden D (2005). Sweet Potato Profile, Agricultural Marketing and Resource Centre (AgMRC) A National Information Resource for Valueadded Agriculture. Iowa State University Publishers.

5. Fonseca, C., Zuger, R., Walker, T., and Molina, J 2003. Impact study of the adoption of new varieties of sweet potatoes released by INIA in Peru: Case of the Canete valley. Lima, Peru: CIP
6. Kapinga R.E., P.T. Ewell, S.C Jeremiah and R. Kilo 1995. Sweet potato in Tanzania Farming and Food Systems: Implications for Research. International Potato Centre (CIP), Nairobi, Kenya; Ministry of Agriculture, Dar-es-Salaam. Tanzania.
7. Mnyulwa D 1999. Highlights of the year.Biotechnology Newsletter. Volume 4 No. 5. August 1999-January 2000
8. Ministry of Foreign Affairs 2015. Agriculture. Accessed on 31 August 2017.
9. Mutandwa E 2008. Performance of Tissue cultured sweet potatoes among smallholder farmers in Zimbabwe. *AgBioForum*, 11(1): 48-57
10. Nzima, M.D.S, H.H. Dhliwayo, K. Mazivazvose, P.R. Mazaiwana, B.A Mundeiri, P. Dhliwayo, A. Matibiri, T. Chirara, F. Gatsinzi, J.M Gopo and V. Mandishona 1999. Preliminary results of participatory evaluation of introduced sweet potato varieties in Hwedza and Buhera districts. Biotechnology Newsletter.Volume 4 No. 5. August 1999-January 2000
11. Parawira W and Khosa Mpandi E 2009. Biotechnology research, development, applications and management in Zimbabwe: Review. Scientific Research and Essay Vol.4 (9), pp. 825-841.
12. Sithole-Niang 1 2001. Future of plant science in Zimbabwe. Trends in Plant Science 6(10): 493-494.
13. Woodend J.J 1995. Technical Paper No. 109, "Biotechnology and Sustainable Crop Production in Zimbabwe".Produced as part of the research programme on Sustainable Develoment: Environment, Resource Use, Technology and Trade.
14. Zuger, R 2003. Impact study of the adoption of new varieties of sweet potatoes released by INIA in Peru: Case of the Canete valley. Lima, Peru: CIP
15. Zimbabwe National Vulnerability Assessment Committee 2004. February. Zimbabwe urban areas food security and vulnerability assessment report: September 2003 (Urban Report No. 1). Harare, Zimbabwe: UNDP Publications

# Specific Biotechnology Efforts — *Industrial*

# *Chapter 14*

# Engineering Fatty Acid Biosynthesis Pathway in Microbes for Production of Long Chain Polyunsaturated Fatty Acids

*Narendra Kadoo*, Smrati Sanghi, Tejas Chirmade, Ashwini Rajwade and Vidya Gupta*

*Biochemical Sciences Division,*
*CSIR-National Chemical Laboratory,*
*Dr. Homi Bhabha Road, Pashan, Pune – 411 008, INDIA*
*Email: ny.kadoo@ncl.res.in, s.sanghi@ncl.res.in,*
*tp.chirmade@ncl.res.in, a.rajwade@ncl.res.in, vs.gupta@ncl.res.in*

## ABSTRACT

The long chain polyunsaturated fatty acids (LCPUFAs) are of great importance from the nutritional point of view. Omega 3 fatty acids (ω-3 FAs), especially the eicosapentaenoic acid (EPA) and docosahexaenoic acid (DHA), play crucial roles in human brain development and are an integral part of biological membranes. They not only serve as the precursors for biosynthesis of a variety of eicosanoids, growth regulators and hormones, maintain membrane fluidity and cell permeability, but also reduce the risk of several ailments like cardiovascular disease, obesity, rheumatoid arthritis and cancer. The commercial sources of ω-3 FAs are fishes and sea foods, whereas the primary producers of ω-3 FAs are algae, some fungi, bacteria and lower plants. Fishes feed on these primary sources and accumulate large amounts of LCPUFAs in them. However, there are certain concerns regarding the consumption of fishes for this purpose, such as depletion of fish stock from water bodies due to overfishing, accumulation of heavy met als *etc.* An alternative source is therefore required which fulfills the basic need of LCPUFAs on a large-scale. Therefore, microbes are considered as the best option for producing LCPUFAs at commercial scale.

Several diatoms produce good amount of EPA and DHA. However, their very slow growth and low biomass are the major limitations for their use in commercial production of LCPUFAs. Therefore, we are isolating the desired genes from the selected diatoms and plan to transfer them into a suitable fungus/yeast, which are the good producers of the precursors of EPA, like linoleic acid (LA) and alpha linoleic acid (ALA). Hence, we isolated few desaturase and elongase genes from diatoms as well as *Linum usitatissimum* for transformation in the fungus *Rhizopus meihei* (NCIM 1306), which was identified as the candidate for commercial production of EPA. The transformants will be evaluated for production of EPA and those producing the highest amount of EPA will be evaluated for their suitability for commercial production of EPA.

***Keywords:*** *Omega-3 fatty acids, Long chain polyunsaturated fatty acids, LCPUFAs, Desaturase, elongase, Gas chromatography.*

## INTRODUCTION

The long chain polyunsaturated fatty acids (LCPUFAs) are the fatty acids, which contain 20 or more carbon atoms with more than one methylene-interrupted *cis* double bond (Abbadi *et al.*, 2004). Omega 3 (ω-3) LCPUFAs such as eicosapentaenoic acid (EPA) and docosahexaenoic acid (DHA) are essential for proper fet al development, including neuronal and retinal development as well as immune function. ω-3 LCPUFAs play magnificent roles in maintaining the cell membrane integrity (Wallis *et al.*, 2002) and brain development (Qi *et al.*, 2004). They not only play significant roles in synthesis of eicosanoids (Sayanova and Napier, 2004), but also minimize the risks of several ailments like cardiovascular disease and cancer (Li and Hu, 2009), inflammatory, thrombotic and autoimmune disease (Calder, 2006; Li and Hu, 2009), hypertension (Appel *et al.*, 1993), type 2 diabetes (Graham *et al.*, 2004), Crohn's disease (Belluzzi *et al.*, 1996) and arthritis (Kremer *et al.*, 1989). For humans, fishes are the main sources of ω-3 LCPUFAs (Abedi and Sahari, 2014); however, microalgae, some fungi and lower plants are the primary producers of these fatty acids. Fishes feed on these primary producers and accumulate LCPUFAs (Napier, 2007). However, several major constraints are associated with the use of fish oils such as undesirable odors, contamination of heavy met als, carcinogens and mutagens, overfishing leading to depletion of fishes from water bodies, and non-preference from vegetarians (Sidhu, 2003; Foran *et al.*, 2005; Abedi and Sahari, 2014). Considering these issues, the microbes, being the primary producers of ω-3 LCPUFAs, are the best alternative sources for large-scale production of ω-3 LCPUFAs.

In several microbes, the conventional ω-3 LCPUFAs biosynthesis pathway is present (Figure 14.1) (Chirmade *et al.*, 2016). Linoleic acid (LA) and alpha linolenic acid (ALA) are the precursors for LCPUFA biosynthesis. Various desaturase and elongase enzymes are involved in the biosynthesis of LCPUFAs. For EPA synthesis from ALA, three enzymes are required: Δ6 desaturase, Δ6 elongase and Δ5 desaturase; while for DHA synthesis, two additional enzymes *viz.* Δ5 elongase and Δ4 desaturase are essential (Wu *et al.*, 2005). However, most of these microbes produce EPA and DHA in very small amounts; hence they cannot be directly used for commercial production of the LCPUFAs. In view of these constraints, either these or other microbes could be genetically engineered to produce high amounts of the LCPUFAs, so that they could be used for industrial production of the fatty acids.

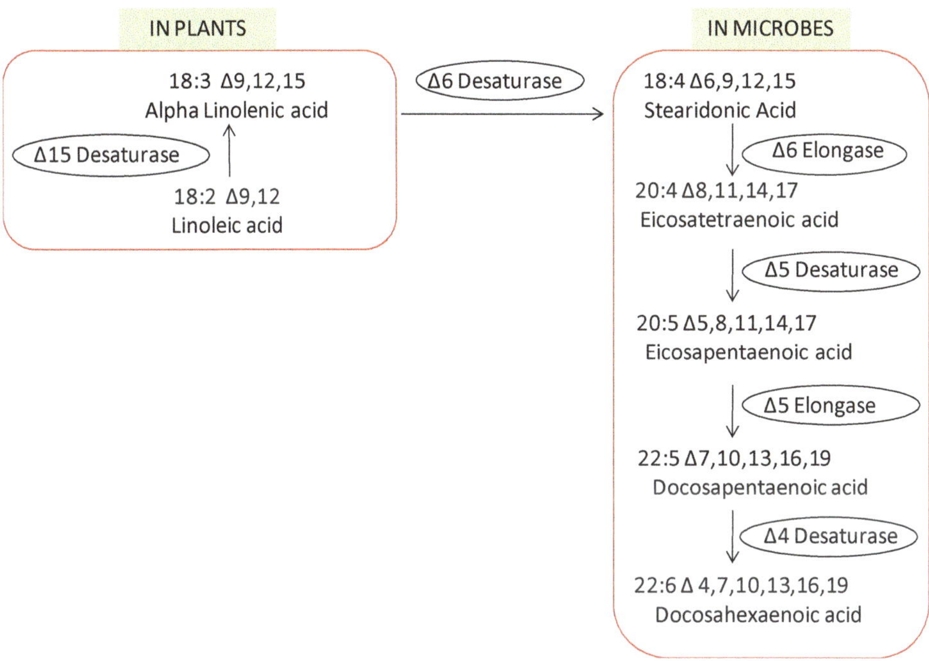


**Figure 14.1: Steps Involved in EPA and DHA Biosynthesis (Modified from Chirmade *et al.*, 2016).**

Engineering microbes for the large-scale production of ω-3 LCPUFAs is a process involving five major steps. The first step is to evaluate the oleaginous microbes producing EPA and DHA and select the desired microbes. The second step is to select and isolate the genes necessary for EPA/DHA biosynthesis from one or more of these microbes. The third step is selection of a suitable microbial host for transformation, which should be rich in LA/ALA and can produce high biomass in short-time. Transformation of the genes from the source microbes into the microbial host is the fourth step; while the fifth and the last step is the selection of transformants producing high amounts of the desired ω-3 LCPUFAs.

Diatoms are good sources of ω-3 LCPUFAs like EPA and DHA (Tonon *et al.*, 2002). However, they are photoautotrophic and utilize huge amount of light energy to proliferate and synthesize fatty acids (Sevilla *et al.*, 2004). Therefore, diatoms cannot be used for commercial production of ω-3 LCPUFAs because of the high costs required for providing sufficient illumination for the optimal growth of diatoms in large-scale (Kroth, 2007). Moreover, even after providing the optimal growth conditions, diatoms produce much less biomass compared to many other microbes. Hence, for commercial production of the ω-3 LCPUFAs, it would be better to isolate the desired genes from diatoms and transfer them into other fermentation friendly microbes like yeast or fungi, which can produce very high biomass. With this objective, we isolated diatoms from a saline and soda lake in Maharashtra, India, which produce high proportion of EPA. We identified desaturase and elongase genes from them and currently isolating full-length genes from them. Similarly, we also screened several fungi and yeasts as the possible hosts/recipients to transform the desired genes from the diatoms to develop genetically modified microbe producing high EPA.

## Materials and Methods

### Screening Fungi and Yeasts as Possible Hosts of the Diatom Genes

Ten microbial cultures were screened as possible hosts for the diatom genes, *viz. Mucor hiemalis* (NCIM 873), *Mucor* spp. (NCIM 881), *Mucor hiemalis* (NCIM 984), *Penicillium notatum* (NCIM 1206), *Rhizopus oligosporous* (NCIM 1215), *Beauveria tenella* (NCIM 1216), *Rhizopus meihei* (NCIM 1306), *Rhizopus* Jk., Yeast (NCIM 3623) and *Yarrowia lipolitica* (NCIM 3229).All the cultures except *Rhizopus* Jk.(RJK) were obtained from the National Collection of Industrial Microorganisms (NCIM), CSIR-National Chemical Laboratory(CSIR-NCL), Pune, India; while *Rhizopus* Jk. was provided by Dr. Asmita Prabhune, CSIR-National Chemical Laboratory, Pune, India.

### Growth Conditions of Fungi and Yeasts

Potato dextrose broth (24g/l) (HiMedia, India) was used for growing the fungal cultures, whereas MGYP media (HiMedia, India) was used for growing the yeasts. In both cases, 50ml media was inoculated with 10 per cent inoculum and allowed to grow at 28°C in a shaker at 160 rpm.

### Lipid Analysis

#### Sample Preparation for Gas Chromatography (GC)

The cultures were harvested after four days of growth and washed twice with sterile distilled water. The tissue was finely crushed in liquid nitrogen and used for preparing fatty acid methyl esters (FAMES). For this, about 100 mg tissue was suspended in 5 ml 0.6 N methanolic-HCl for esterification and the fatty acids were extracted in 4 ml hexane. Before the gas chromatography (GC) run, hexane was evaporated using centrivap (Labconco, USA) and the samples were reconstituted in 100 µl of chloroform (Deshpande *et al.*, 2016).

#### Fatty Acid Analysis

Agilent 7890B GC system was used for GC-FID analysis. The Supelco SP™-2560 capillary GC column and the following parameters, temperature gradient (130°C hold for 5 min; raised up to 230°C by 20°C/min; final hold at 230°C for 20 min), inlet temperature (250°C), carrier gas (helium, flow rate 1 ml/min), 1/10 split ratio and 1 µl sample (injection volume) were used for lipid profiling. For authentication, 14-24 carbon containing fatty acid methyl esters (Sigma-Aldrich, USA) were used as standards. Three biological samples with two technical replicates each were analyzed and all the values for determination were the mean of six replicates.

## Results and Discussion

### Fatty Acid Profiling of Fungi and Yeasts

Fatty acid profiling of two yeast and eight fungal samples (Figure 14.2) was performed, which showed that the yeasts were rich inoleic acid (OA), a monounsaturated fatty acid; whereas the fungi were rich in the polyunsaturated fatty acid, linoleic acid (LA). Maximum production of LA was seen in *Rhizopus meihei* (NCIM 1306) (57.75±0.55 per cent). In addition, these fungi also produced small amounts of gamma linolenic acid (GLA), alpha linolenic acid (ALA) and arachidonic acid (AA). Therefore, *Rhizopus meihei* (NCIM 1306) having high LA content was selected as a suitable potential host for engineering the ω-3 LCPUFAs biosynthesis pathway using the genes isolated from diatoms as well as *Linum usitatissimum*.

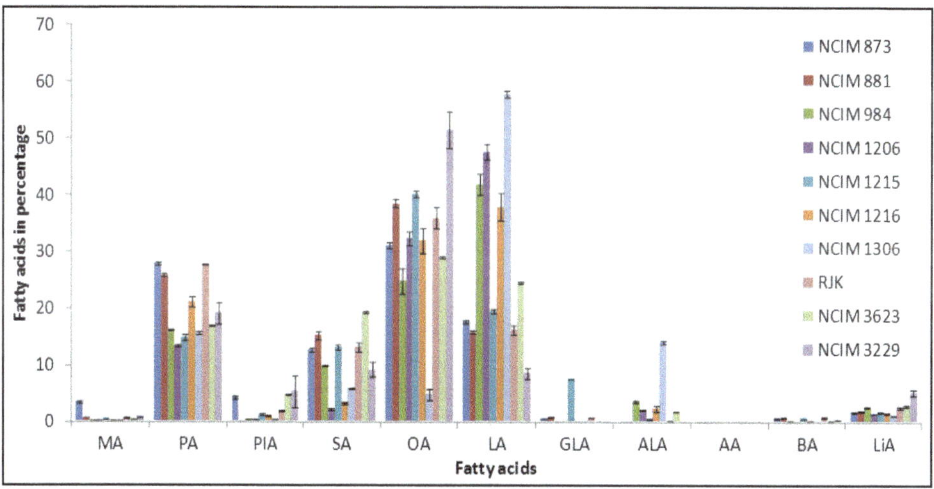


**Figure 14.2: Fatty Acid Profiles of the Fungal and Yeast Samples; Vertical bars at each data point represent standard errors calculated for all biological and technical replicates considered for the study.**

### Engineering the ω-3 LCPUFAs Biosynthesis Pathway in *Rhizopus meihei* (NCIM 1306)

To produce EPA from LA in the fungus *Rhizopus meihei* (NCIM 1306), four additional enzymes, *viz.* Δ15 desaturase, Δ6 desaturase, Δ6 elongase and Δ5 desaturase are required. We have already isolated Δ15 desaturase from *Linum usitatissimum*, an oilseed crop known for its high ALA content (Rajwade *et al.*, 2014). The gene will be used to convert LA to ALA in this fungus. Further, Δ6 desaturase, Δ6 elongase and Δ5 desaturase genes from the diatoms will be used for carrying out ALA to SDA, SDA to ETA and ETA to EPA reactions. Partial sequences of Δ6 desaturase and Δ5 desaturase genes have been obtained and isolation of full-length genes is underway. We have also developed an *Agrobacterium tumefaciens* LBA4404 strain containing a modified pCAMBIA 1302 vector, which will be used for transformation of these genes in *Rhizopus meihei* (NCIM 1306) under the control of *citA* promoter (Upasani *et al.*, 2016). The fungus transformed with these genes can then serve as a potential source for commercial production of EPA.

## Conclusions

Omega-3 LCPUFAs play several vital roles in development and functioning of the human body. Compared to the historical human diets, current diets severely lack in omega-3 LCPUFAs. The sources of omega-3 LCPUFAs are depleting due to several reasons; hence to fulfill their daily demand, alternative sources are required. There have been several attempts of development of transgenic crops to produce EPA and DHA, but these have not been very successful. Hence, commercial production of the omega-3 LCPUFAs using transgenic plants could be a long-term goal; and microbial production of these fatty acids could be a more feasible alternative. Hence, in this study we identified diatoms as the promising sources of EPA and are isolating full-length Δ6 desaturase, Δ6 elongase and Δ5 desaturase genes from them. In addition, full-length Δ15 desaturase gene has also been obtained from *Linum usitatissimum*. The fungus *Rhizopus meihei* (NCIM 1306), producing high biomass and high LA content, was identified as the possible host for engineering the fatty acid biosynthesis pathway. The transformants producing the highest amount of EPA could be used for commercial production.

## Acknowledgements

The authors acknowledge the Department of Science and Technology (DST), India for the INSPIRE fellowship to SS and the University Grants Commission (UGC), India for junior and senior research fellowships to TC. Financial support in the form of CSIR (Council of Scientific and Industrial Research, India) (CSC 0112) and ICAR (Indian Council of Agricultural Research, India) (GAP 311926) to NYK and DBT Bio-CARe grant (GAP 308426) to AVR are gratefully acknowledged. We thank Dr. Asmita Prabhune, CSIR-NCL, Pune, India for providing the microbial strain *Rhizopus* Jk and Dr. Ashish Deshpande, CSIR-NCL, Pune, India for his help in our initial GC studies.

## Abbreviations

AA: Arachidonic acid
ALA: Alpha linolenic acid
BA: Behenic acid
DHA: Docosahexaenoic acid
EPA: Eicosapentaenoic acid
GLA: Gamma Linoleic acid
LA: Linoleic acid
LCPUFAs: Long chain polyunsaturated fatty acids
LiA: Lignoceric acid
MA: Myristic acid

MTCC: Microbial Type Culture Collection
NCIM: National Collection of Industrial Microorganisms
OA: Oleic acid
PA: Palmitic acid
PIA: Palmitoleic acid
RJK: *Rhizopus* Jk.
SA: Stearic acid

## REFERENCES


1. Abbadi A, Domergue F, Bauer J *et al.* 2004. Biosynthesis of very-long-chain polyunsaturated fatty acids in transgenic oilseeds: constraints on their accumulation. *The Plant Cell,* 16(10): 2734-2748.
2. Abedi E, Sahari MA 2014. Long-chain polyunsaturated fatty acid sources and evaluation of their nutritional and functional properties. *Food Science and Nutrition,* 2 (5): 443-463.
3. Appel LJ, Miller ER, Seidler AJ, Whelton PK 1993. Does supplementation of diet with 'fish oil' reduce blood pressure?: A meta-analysis of controlled clinical trials. *Archives of Internal Medicine,* 153 (12): 1429-1438.
4. Belluzzi A, Brignola C, Campieri M *et al.* 1996. Effect of an enteric-coated fish-oil preparation on relapses in Crohn's disease. *New England Journal of Medicine,* 334 (24): 1557-1560.
5. Calder PC 2006. n-3 polyunsaturated fatty acids, inflammation, and inflammatory diseases. *The American Journal of Clinical Nutrition,* 83 (6): S1505-1519S.
6. Chirmade TP, Sanghi S, Rajwade AV, Gupta VS, Kadoo NY 2016. Balancing ω-6: ω-3 Ratios in Oilseeds. In: ω-3 Fatty Acids. Springer, pp 203-220.
7. Deshpande AB, Chidley HG, Oak PS *et al.* 2016. Data on changes in the fatty acid composition during fruit development and ripening of three mango cultivars (Alphonso, Pairi and Kent) varying in lactone content. *Data in Brief* 9: 480-491.
8. Foran JA, Good DH, Carpenter DO *et al.* 2005. Quantitative analysis of the benefits and risks of consuming farmed and wild salmon. *The Journal of Nutrition,* 135 (11): 2639-2643.
9. Graham I, Cirpus P, Rein D, Napier J 2004. The use of very long chain polyunsaturated fatty acids to ameliorate metabolic syndrome: transgenic plants as an alternative sustainable source to fish oils. *Nutrition Bulletin,* 29 (3): 228-233.
10. Kremer JM, Lawrence DA, Jubiz W 1989. Different doses of fish-oil fatty acid ingestion active rheumatoid arthritis: a prospective study of clinical and immunological parameters. In: Dietary ω3 and ω6 fatty acids. Springer, pp 343-350.

11. Kroth P 2007. Molecular biology and the biotechnological potential of diatoms. In: Transgenic Microalgae as Green Cell Factories. pp 23-33.
12. Li D, Hu X-J 2009. Fish and its multiple human health effects in times of threat to sustainability and affordability: are there alternatives? *Asia Pacific Journal of Clinical Nutrition,* 18 (4): 553-563.
13. Napier JA 2007. The production of unusual fatty acids in transgenic plants. *Annu. Rev. Plant Biol.,* 58: 295-319.
14. Qi B, Fraser T, Mugford S *et al.* 2004. Production of very long chain polyunsaturated ω-3 and ω-6 fatty acids in plants. *Nature Biotechnology,* 22(6): 739.
15. Rajwade AV, Kadoo NY, Borikar SP *et al.* 2014. Differential transcriptional activity of SAD, FAD2 and FAD3 desaturase genes in developing seeds of linseed contributes to varietal variation in α-linolenic acid content. *Phytochemistry,* 98: 41-53.
16. Sayanova OV, Napier JA 2004. Eicosapentaenoic acid: biosynthetic routes and the potential for synthesis in transgenic plants. *Phytochemistry,* 65(2): 147-158.
17. Sevilla J, García C, Sánchez Mirón A *et al.* 2004. Pilot plant scale outdoor mixotrophic cultures of *Phaeodactylum tricornutum* using glycerol in vertical bubble column and airlift photobioreactors: studies in fedbatch mode. *Biotechnology Progress,* 20(3): 728-736.
18. Sidhu KS (2003) Health benefits and potential risks related to consumption of fish or fish oil. *Regulatory Toxicology and Pharmacology,* 38(3): 336-344.
19. Tonon T, Harvey D, Larson TR, Graham IA 2002. Long chain polyunsaturated fatty acid production and partitioning to triacylglycerols in four microalgae. *Phytochemistry,* 61(1): 15-24.
20. Upasani ML, Gurjar GS, Kadoo NY, Gupta VS 2016. Dynamics of colonization and expression of pathogenicity related genes in *Fusarium oxysporum* f. sp. *ciceri* during chickpea vascular wilt disease progression. *PloS One,* 11(5): e0156490.
21. Wallis JG, Watts JL, Browse J 2002. Polyunsaturated fatty acid synthesis: what will they think of next? *Trends in Biochemical Sciences,* 27(9): 467-473.
22. Wu G, Truksa M, Datla N *et al.* 2005. Stepwise engineering to produce high yields of very long-chain polyunsaturated fatty acids in plants. *Nature Biotechnology,* 23(8): 1013.

*Chapter 15*

# Lipase Production Potential of a Locally Isolated Extreme Halotolerant *Aspergillus* sp. FIMT2 Strain using Agro-industrial Wastes as Substrate

*Farizul Hafiz Kasim*[1], *Haliru Musa*[1], *Ahmad Anas Bin Nagoor Gunny*[2] and *Mohammad Azmier Ahmad*[3]

[1]*Centre of Excellence for Biomass Utilization, School of Bioprocess Engineering, Universiti Malaysia Perlis, Kompleks Pusat Pengajian Jejawi 3, 02600 Arau, Perlis, MALAYSIA*
*E-mail: farizul@unimap.edu.my, hallyruh@gmail.com*
[2]*Department of Chemical Engineering Technology, Faculty of Engineering Technology, Universiti Malaysia Perlis, Kampus Uni CITI Alam, Sungai Chuchuh, 02100 Padang Besar, Perlis, MALAYSIA*
*E-mail: ahmadanas@unimap.edu.my*
[3]*School of Chemical Engineering, Engineering Campus, UniversitiSains Malaysia, Seri Ampangan, 14300 NibongTebal, Pulau Pinang, MALAYSIA*
*E-mail: chazmier@eng.usm.my*

## ABSTRACT

Lipase production by halophilic and halotolerant strains has been relatively understudied, especially when utilizing agro-industrial residues as substrates for fermentation. This study is aimed at screening various agro-industrial wastes as the substrate for lipase production by an extreme halotolerant strain *Aspergillus* sp. FIMT2. This strain was locally isolated from a salted sardine fish (*Sardina pilchardus*) and screened for lipolytic activity on tributyrin and Tween 80-containing agar. No activity was detected during the primary screening on tributyrin and Tween 80 solid agar, hence the strain was further subjected to secondary screening by submerged fermentation using olive oil as lipase inducer. Lipase production of 0.100 U/μL was observed under static condition of fermentation while 0.142 U/μL production was recorded for the strain under agitation condition. Morphological and physiological studies of the strain were conducted. The strain was outsourced for molecular characterization. It was identified as *Aspergillus* sp. FIMT2 and has been deposited in the gene bank with the accession number JN585932.1. The strain's potential for halotolerant lipase production was further determined by solid state fermentation using various agro-industrial residues such as coconut fibre, rice husk, banana peels, oil palm empty fruit bunch, sugarcane bagasse, coconut oil cake, and palm kernel cake. Among the substrates studied, palm kernel cake supported the best lipase production of 0.211 U/g by *Aspergillus* sp. FIMT2 under static condition and 0.154 U/g under agitation condition. Coconut oil cake was also found to support good lipase production (0.107 U/g) by the strain, although, in this case under agitation condition. It can be concluded that palm kernel cake and coconut oil cake best supported lipase production by the extremely halotolerant strain, *Aspergillus* sp. FIMT2. The implication of the study is that these agro-industrial residues (palm kernel cake and coconut oil cake) can be utilized as inexpensive substrates for considerable halotolerant lipase production.

***Keywords:*** *Halophilic, Halotolerant, Aspergillus sp. FIMT2, Sardina pilchardus, Lipase production, Solid state fermentation, Agro-industrial residues.*

## INTRODUCTION

Halotolerant enzymes are enzymes that are active and stable in high salt concentration (Sana, 2015). These enzymes are isolated from organisms dwelling in saline or hypersaline environment and possess diverse applications and functions that will efficiently accelerate bioprocess technology. Halotolerant lipases may perform the same function as their non-halophilic counterparts; however, they surpass mesophilic enzymes in their ability to carry out reaction under high salt condition. These enzymes display a phenomenon known as polyextremophilicity, which is activity and stability in more than one extreme condition *e.g.* high salt concentrations, alkaline pH, long periods in high temperature, and non-aqueous medium (Delgado-García *et al.*, 2012; Karan *et al.*, 2012; Munawar and Engel, 2013). These characteristics are being exploited for some industrial and environmental applications such as biofuel, textiles, pharmaceuticals, oleochemicals, wastewater treatment, and bioremediation (Sana, 2015).

Filamentous fungi are regarded as an interesting source of lipases because of their ability to produce extracellular enzymes in high quantity (Quintanilla *et al.*, 2015; Ramos-Sánchez *et al.*, 2015). Although most industrial enzymes are currently produced by submerged fermentation (SMF), solid state fermentation (SSF) seems to be a more promising technology because of the several advantages it offers, such as high enzyme yield (Gopalan and Nampoothirir, 2016), low cost of production, higher oxygen distribution, simpler equipment and control system, fewer operational problems (Ramos-Sánchez *et al.*, 2015), and environmentally-friendly approach (Kumar and Kanawar, 2012). SSF is the preferred method for the production of various enzymes from agro-industrial residues, especially when the residues are water insoluble.

The accumulation of vast quantities of agro-industrial residues as a result of agro-industrial practices necessitate the need to utilize them as fermentation substrate for bio-conversion into value-added products such as enzymes, feed, biofuel, and a variety of chemicals. Several agro-industrial substrates such as palm kernel cake (Anusha *et al.*, 2017), coconut oil cake (Venkatesagowda *et al.*, 2015), wheat bran (de Almeida *et al.*, 2016), sugar cane bagasse, mustard seed oil cake (Salihu*et al.*, 2013), olive cake, *Jatropha curcas* seed cake, shea nut cake (Salihu*et al.*, 2016),babassu oil cake, groundnut oil cake, gingelly oil cake, and canola seed oil cake (Amin *et al.*, 2014) have been successfully used for lipase production. Amongst these substrates, oil cake has been reported to show tremendous potential for lipase production due to the nutritional and residual lipid contents that induce the production of lipase (Anusha *et al.*, 2017).

The approach of utilizing agro-industrial residues as fermentation substrate in SSF by an extremely halotolerant *Aspergillus* sp. FIMT2 for lipase production is a novel approach that requires further exploration through medium optimization and enzyme concentration studies. Furthermore, the industrial demand for new sources of lipases with unique catalytic properties such as hyperthermostability, halostability, organic solvent, and pH tolerance that can adapt to extreme harsh reaction conditions is on the increase. Hence, this report presents a study on lipase production potential of an extremely halotolerant *Aspergillus* sp. FIMT2 using various agro-industrial residues as substrate under SSF.

## Materials and Methods

### Strain Isolation

*Aspergillus* sp. FIMT2 was isolated from salted sardine fish collected from a local fish market in Kuala Perlis, Perlis, Malaysia. The salted fish sample was crushed into smaller pieces and about 1g of the sample was inoculated into 50 mL of halophilic nutrient medium contained in a 250 mL Erlenmeyer flask. The halophilic medium is composed of (per cent w/w): Yeast extract: 1.0; glucose: 6.0; malt extract: 1.0; $FeSO_4{\cdot}7H_2O$: 0.01; $MgSO_4{\cdot}7H_2O$: 0.5; $K_2HPO_4$: 0.5; peptone: 2.0; and NaCl: 3-7 (for moderate halotolerants) and 15-30 (for extreme halotolerants) (Annapurna *et al.*, 2012). The medium was adjusted to pH 7.0 using 1M NaOH solution. The flask was then incubated on a rotary shaker with a speed of 150 rpm at 27°C for 4 to 5 days. The obtained turbid culture was spread on the above halophilic medium with the inclusion of 2 per cent w/w agar and then incubated for 6 to 7 days. The fungal colonies obtained were checked for cultural and morphological characteristics. The pure fungal colony obtained thereof was maintained on the halophilic medium and stored in the cold room at 4°C until further use.

### Cultural, Micromorphological and Physiological Characterization of Halotolerant Fungal Strains

The cultural characteristics of the fungal strains were carried out by visual observation of the matured distinct colony on halophilic agar plate. Micromorphological characterization of the strains was done by slide culture technique following the method of Nazareth and Gonsalves (2014). A 3 to 5-day old fungal plug was placed on a clean grease-free microscopic slide already stained with a few drops of lactophenol cotton blue dye, covered with sterile cover slip and examined microscopically using ×40 objectives. The morphological aspect of the fungal colony was analyzed. The physiological studies of the strains in terms of testing salinity tolerance, tolerance for pH and incubation temperature of the fungal colony were determined by cultivating the strains under different NaCl concentrations (0 per cent, 5 per cent, 10 per cent, 15 per cent, 20 per cent, and 25 per cent), pH (6.0, 6.5, 7.0, 7.5, 8.0, and 8.5) and temperature (30°C, 35°C, 40°C, 45°C, 50°C, 55°C, and 60°C). This was done according to the modified method described by Batista-Garciá*et al.* (2014). The colony diameter of the fungal strains was measured on the 7$^{th}$ and 14$^{th}$ day of incubation for those strains showing delayed growth.

## Primary Screening of Fungal Strains for Lipase Production on Solid Agar

The preliminary screening of fungal strains with lipolytic potential was carried out in petri plates using halophilic medium (described above) supplemented with 1 per cent v/v triglyceride substrates, tributyrin, and Tween 80. The prepared petri plates were inoculated with pure fungal colonies and incubated at 27°C for 3-5 days. Lipolytic activity was determined by the zone of hydrolysis around the fungal growth.

## Secondary Screening of Fungal Strains for Lipase Production using Submerged Fermentation (SMF) and Solid-State Fermentation (SSF) Techniques

### Submerged Fermentation

Fungal inoculum preparation was carried out following the method of Rai *et al.* (2014). Spore suspension was prepared by adding 10 mL of sterile distilled water to fungal culture plates and the spores were gently scrapped with an inoculation needle. The aqueous spore suspension obtained thereof was counted on a haemocytometer chamber as the number of spores per mL of suspension. The fungal spore suspension was then transferred into sterile empty McCartney bottles (25 µL) and was ready to be inoculated into the fermentation vessel.

The fungal strains were cultivated in halophilic production medium containing 1 per cent v/v olive oil as the source of natural triglyceride and inducer. About 2 mL ($1.0 \times 10^{-6}$ spores/µL) of spore suspension was inoculated into 50 mL halophilic production medium (supplemented with 1 per cent v/v olive oil) contained in 250 mL Erlenmeyer flask. The flasks were incubated at 27°C for 5 days under static condition, as well as on a rotary shaker maintained at 150 rpm. Experiments were conducted in duplicate. The fermentation broth was filtered with a sterile muslin cloth and the clear filtrate was used as the source of crude lipase. The wet fungal biomass retained on the muslin cloth was gently scraped on Whatman No. 1 filter paper (110 mm diameter) and dried to constant weight in an oven at 80°C for 48 h. The dry weight of the fungal biomass was calculated using the Equation 1:

Fungal dry weight (g/L) = (Weight of dry filter paper with dried fungal biomass – Weight of dry filter paper) [1]

## Solid State Fermentation

The culture medium used for SSF was based on agro-industrial wastes (such as banana peels, coconut fibre, coconut oil cake, palm kernel cake, oil palm empty fruit bunch, sugarcane bagasse, and rice husk) that were obtained from local markets in Perlis, Malaysia. These substrates were ground in the laboratory with a grinder and separated in a sieve shaker AS 200 (Retsch) to obtain particles between 0.125 and 0.80 mm. The ground substrates were then washed twice with sterile distilled water and dried in the oven at 80°C for 48 h.

About 5 g of the substrates were transferred into a series of 250 mL Erlenmeyer flasks, moistened with the halophilic production medium containing 1 per cent v/v olive oil inducer to give 70 per cent moisture content, and then sterilized in the autoclave at 120°C for 20 min. The flasks were allowed to cool to room temperature and then inoculated with 2 mL ($1.0 \times 10^{-6}$ spores/µL) spore suspension. At this point, the inoculated substrates were stirred with a sterile glass rod for even distribution of inoculum suspension. The flasks were cotton plugged and incubated at 27°C for 5 days under static condition and also on a rotary shaker at the speed of 150 rpm. All experiments were performed in duplicate.

## Lipase Extraction

At the end of the fermentation, crude lipase was extracted by mixing the fermented substrates with 50 mL of 0.1 M phosphate buffer (pH 7.0) containing 0.1 per cent v/v Tween 80. The mixture was shaken on a rotary shaker (150 rpm) at 28°C for 1 h. The extract was collected and filtered through muslin cloth, and the resultant filtrate was centrifuged at 10,000 rpm for 15 min at 4°C in a refrigerated centrifuge (Sigma 3-18k, Sartorius) (Dayanandan *et al.*, 2013; Rehman *et al.*, 2011). The obtained supernatants were used for enzyme assay.

## Lipase Assay

Lipase activity was determined by the method described by Gutarra *et al.* (2009) with slight modification. Lipase activity was determined by the addition of 0.05 mL of the crude enzyme to a solution of 2.2 mL of 25 µM phosphate buffer (pH 7.0) and 0.25 mL of 2.5 µMpNPL. The hydrolysis reaction was carried out at 60°C for 10 min, after which 0.25 mL of 0.1M $Na_2CO_3$ was added to terminate the reaction and the activity was determined at 412 nm wavelength. One unit of lipase activity is defined as the amount of enzyme which releases 1 mol of p-nitrophenol per minute from pNPL in 10 min under the assay conditions. Lipase activity was expressed as units per gram of the dry agro-industrial residues or as units per millilitre as in the case of SMF.

## Molecular Identification and Phylogenetic Analysis of the Selected Halotolerant Fungal Strain

The fungal strain with the highest lipase producing potential under SSF condition was outsourced for molecular identification by determination of the ITS region sequencing that was provided by Macrogen, Seoul, Republic of Korea. The ITS region sequencing was performed by sequencing of the ITS1 region from the amplified DNA templates using highly specific universal primers ITS1 5' (TCC GTA GGT GAA CCT GCG G) 3' and ITS4 5' (TCC TCC GCT TAT TGA TAT GC) 3'. The obtained sequences were annotated and integrated into the database using the automatic alignment tool. The sequences were analyzed and DNA similarity searches were performed using the BLASTn program and the information contained in the GenBank of the National Centre for Biotechnology Information (NCBI) website (www.ncbi.nih.gov). The phylogenetic analyses and molecular evolutionary analyses for 18S rRNA gene sequences were conducted for sequence alignments using the computer programs ClustalW and MEGA5 software. The phylogenetic tree was constructed using the maximum likelihood algorithm method and the tree topology was evaluated by means of bootstrap analysis.

## Results and Discussion

### Strain Isolation

Diverse halotolerant fungal strains flourish in natural hypersaline environment and thus are consistently isolated from such environment with high salt concentration. Salt tolerant fungi have been found to inhabit diverse hypersaline ecosystem such as freshwater, seawater; water with saturated solution of NaCl salt, and are also known as associated contaminants of salted food products (Gunde-Cimerman and Zalar, 2014; Karan *et al.*, 2012). In this study, 3 fungal strains (FIMT1, FIMT2 and FIMT4) were isolated from a salted local sardine fish, *Sardina pilchardus* on halophilic medium agar plates. Youssef *et al.* (2003) earlier isolated several genera and species of halotolerant fungi from a local salted fish 'Moloha', amongst which *Aspergillus* and *Penicillium* were the predominant genera encountered. The main groups of fungi inhabiting hypersaline environments include the filamentous genera *Wallemia, Scopulariopsis* and *Alternaria,* as well as different species of anamorphic genera *Aspergillus* and *Penicillium*, and some of the teleomorphic genera *Eurotium* and *Emericella* (Gunde-Cimerman and Zalar, 2014).

### Cultural, Micromorphological and Physiological Characterization of Halotolerant Fungal Strains

The cultural and morphology characterizations of the isolated halotolerant fungal strains (FIMT1, FIMT2 and FIMT4) are presented in Table 15.1. Presumptive identification of the strains was based on colony surface colour, hyphal structure, and spore type. Figure 15.1(A) shows that the surface colony colour for strain FIMT1 is brown while Figure 15.1(B) shows that the surface colour of strain FIMT2 is brownish-white. The growth rate in the two strains (FIMT1 and FIMT2) was fairly rapid, and the texture of the colonies varies from downy to powdery. Based on the morphology and growth pattern, the three strains were identified as fungi. Microscopic appearance as depicted in Figure 15.2(A) shows the micromorphology of FIMT2, where the strain has a conidiophore (stipe), conidia and vesicle. Numerous conidiogenous cells appeared synchronically on the vesicle to form a structure known as phialides. The phialides are formed by short branches known as metulae.

A biseriate conidial head is the result of bilayer arrangement of phialides and metulae on the vesicle. These are the characteristic features of *Aspergillus* sp. and have been explained by Guarro *et al.* (2009). Figure 15.2(B) shows the scanning electron micrograph (SEM) of FIMT2 conidia, which further suggests that the organism could be *Aspergillus* sp.

**Table 15.1: Cultural and Morphological Characterization of Halotolerant Fungal Isolates**

| *Sl.No.* | *Strain Code* | *Colony Morphology* | *Reverse Mycelium Colour* |
|---|---|---|---|
| 1. | FIMT1 | Brown, powdery aerial mycelium. Fast growing -full growth attained within 5 days. | White |
| 2. | FIMT2 | Brownish-white mycelium forming concentric rings. Scanty growth at early stage. Turns brown when matured. | Brown |
| 3. | FIMT4 | White, woolly mycelium. Forming distinct ring pattern. | White |

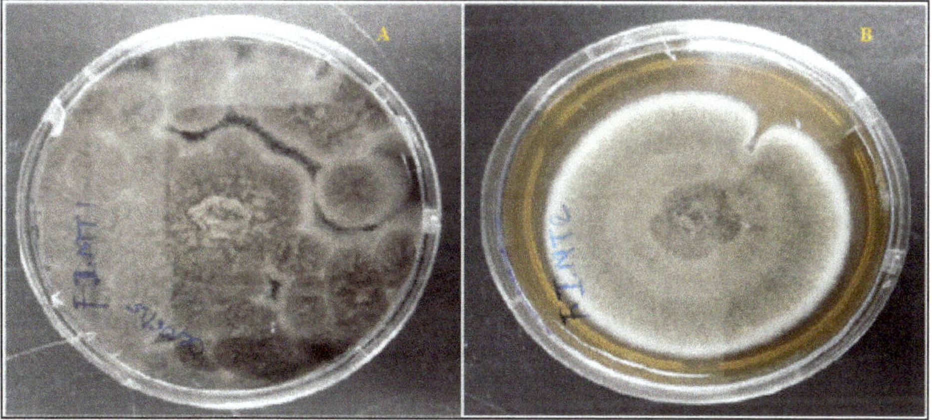


**Figure 15.1: Pure Culture Plate of (A) FIMT1 and (B) FIMT2.**

The physiological characterization of the isolated strains involved halotolerance test, growth temperature tolerance test, and pH tolerance test. Halotolerance of the fungal strains was determined by measuring their colony diameter (growth) on agar plate with different salt concentration range (Figure 15.3). On the 7$^{th}$ day of incubation, FIMT1 and FIMT2 grew at a salinity range of 0-25 per cent and the maximum growth obtained at 0-15 per cent NaCl. As the NaCl concentration increased from 15-25 per cent, a decrease in growth was observed for all the strains in which FIMT4 showed no visible growth at 20-25 per cent NaCl concentrations. The strain had its optimal growth at 0-5 per cent NaCl concentration. Similar growth pattern was observed for all strains on the 14$^{th}$ day of incubation except that in this case, they had close to full growth at low (0-5 per cent) and moderate (5-10 per cent) salinity. These results show that none of these strains are halophilic in nature since they were all capable of growth at 0 per cent NaCl concentration, indicating they do not require NaCl for growth. Hence, they can be regarded as halotolerant

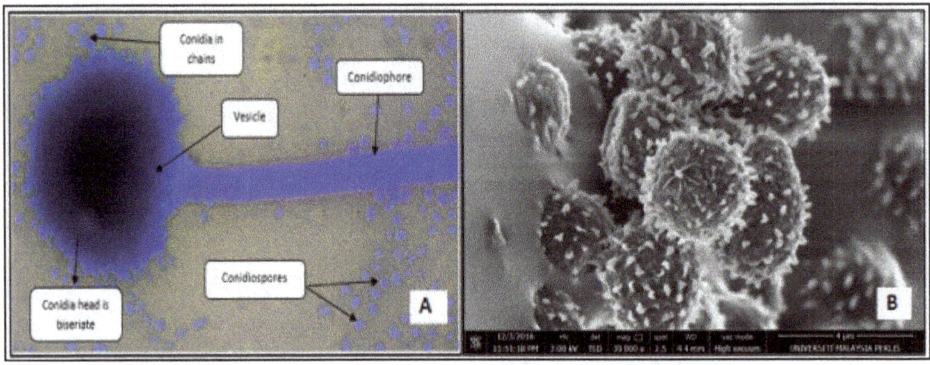


**Figure 15.2: (A) Micromorphology of FIMT2 and (B) Scanning Electron Micrograph (SEM) of FIMT2 Conidia.**

fungi with strains FIMT1 and FIMT4 being categorized as moderately halotolerant and FIMT2 being categorized as extremely halotolerant due to the considerable growth noticed on the 14$^{th}$ day of incubation at 15-25 per cent NaCl concentrations. Halotolerant microorganisms can grow in various high concentrations of salt and at the same time survive in the absence of high salt; those halotolerants that are capable of growth at approximately 15 per cent or 2.5M NaCl and above are considered as extremely halotolerant (Margesin and Schinner, 2001)

Although there are different definitions given for halotolerance and halophilia in microorganisms, the most widely used definition is that of Kushner (1978) where he categorized organisms as moderate, extreme, and borderline extreme. Further still, it could be observed that FIMT2 in Figure 3 exhibits improved growth (55mm colony diameter) at elevated (25 per cent) NaCl concentrations on the 14$^{th}$ day of incubation. The probable explanation for this escalated growth may be due to strain adaptation as a result of prolonged exposure to high salinity. Salt tolerant organisms possess adaptive mechanisms that ensure their survival in harsh environmental conditions (Gunde-Cimerman *et al.*, 2009). All the strains in this study were euryhaline in nature; they were able to adapt to a wide range of salt concentrations. Nazareth *et al.* (2012) and Nazareth and Gonsalves (2014) earlier reported some

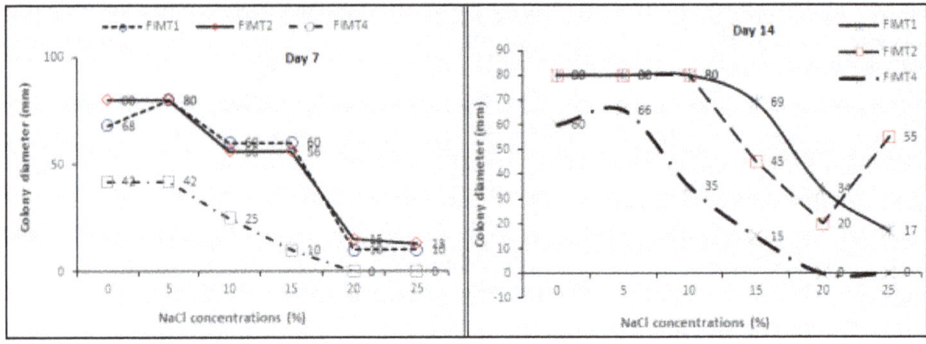


**Figure 15.3: Salinity Tolerance of Fungal Isolates.**

*Aspergillus* sp. and other fungal isolates that are extremely halotolerant in nature and exhibited broad salinity tolerance.

The fungal strains tolerance to growth temperature is depicted in Figure 15.4. The growth of the three strains was restricted to mesophilic temperature range of 30-40°C even until the 14th day of incubation. It could be observed that FIMT1 and FIMT2 showed increased growth at the temperature range of 30-35°C but less growth at 40°C. However, FIMT4 showed lesser growth at 30-35°C and refused to grow at 40°C even though it was isolated from the same source with the other strains. Environmental tolerances differ among varying microbial strains and even more so amongst strains that are phylogenetically related (Evans *et al.*, 2013). Martinelli *et al.* (2017) have similarly reported halotolerant *Aspergillus* strains with colony growth restricted to mesophilic temperature range of 25-37°C. Mesophilic organisms grow at the temperature range of 25-40°C.

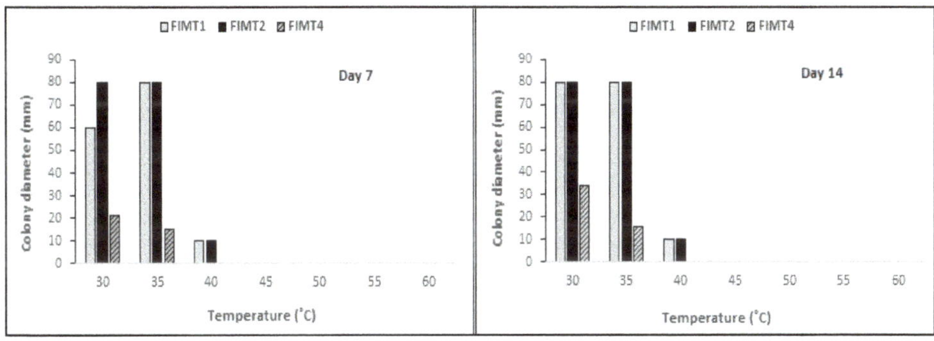


**Figure 15.4: Temperature Tolerance of Fungal Strains.**

pH tolerance of the isolated fungal strains was broad (Figure 15.5). All the strains grew across the pH range of 6.0-8.5. On the 7th day of incubation, FIMT1 had the best growth over the entire pH range while FIMT2 and FIMT4 grew best at the pH range of 6.5-7.5. However, all the strains showed very good growth across the entire pH range (6.0-8.5) on day 14 of incubation except FIMT4 that grew less at the extremes of the pH (6.0 and 8.5). These results show that the fungal strains have optimum growth pH close to neutral (pH 7.0).

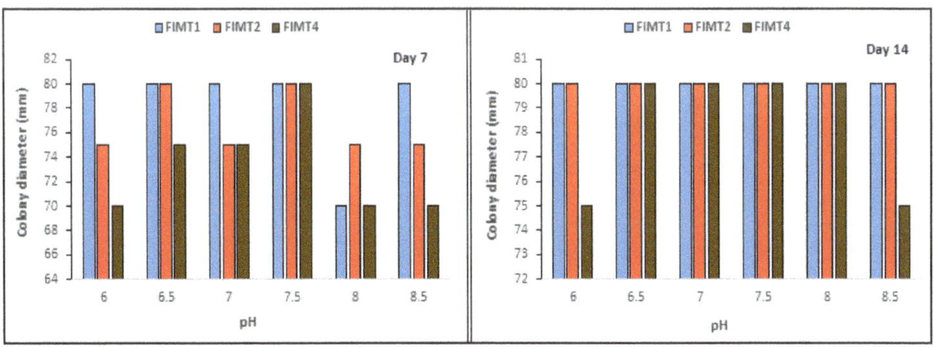


**Figure 15.5: pH Tolerance of Fungal Strains.**

## Primary Screening of Fungal Strains for Lipase Production on Solid Agar

The isolated fungal strains were screened for lipase production on tributyrin (1 per cent v/v) and Tween 80-containing halophilic medium on agar plate. No lipolytic activity was detected in the strains tested, hence they were further subjected to secondary screening for lipase production in a SMF medium containing longer chain fatty acids, that is, olive oil (1 per cent v/v) as lipidic inducer. The inability to detect lipolytic activity on the agar plate using tributyrin and Tween 80 lipidic inducer might be because the lipase produced by these organisms is true lipase, and as such repressed in the presence of short-chain fatty esters (tributyrin). Another possibility for lack of lipase activity could be as a result of catabolite repression than normally occurs when a medium contains a soluble carbon source alongside a fatty acid inducer. In such a case, biomass production can be higher and no increase in lipolytic activity is observed (Zarevúcka, 2012).

## Secondary Screening of Fungal Strains for Lipase Production using Submerged Fermentation Technique

All the strains initially screened on agar plate were further screened in submerged culture under static and agitation conditions using olive oil as lipidic inducer. It could be seen from Figure 15.6A-B that the best lipase production (0.142 U/µL) was achieved under agitation condition by FIMT2 followed in order by FIMT1 (0.124 U/µL) and FIMT4 (0.088 U/µL), respectively. The maximum lipase production (0.115 U/µL) under static condition was produced by FIMT1. On the other hand, the largest dry fungal biomass (2.7039 g/L) was produced under agitation condition by FIMT2 followed in order by FIMT1 (2.5796 g/L) and FIMT4 (0.1001 g/L), respectively. It could be seen from this study that the maximum lipase production was achieved at the maximum mycelial biomass. This suggests that lipase production by these strains is directly associated with growth. It could be assumed that the fungal strains were able to effectively utilize olive oil both for biosynthesis of lipase and biomass production. Lipase production was induced by the presence of lipid substrate (olive oil). Lipidic carbon sources are very

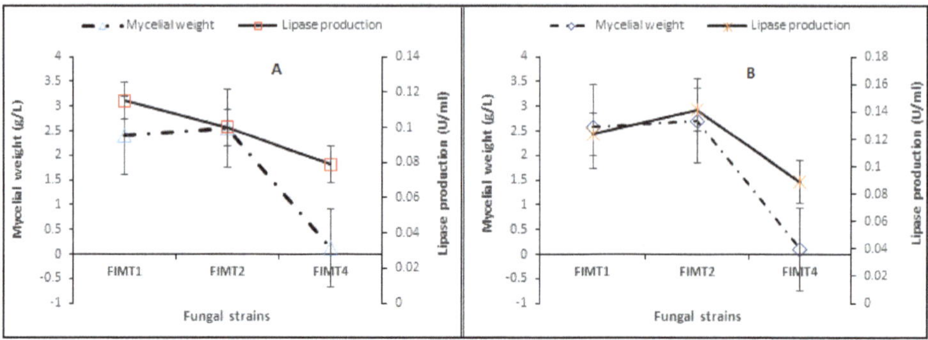


**Figure 15.6: Secondary Screening of Fungal Strains for Lipase Production in Submerged Culture Under (A) Static and (B) Agitation Conditions.**

essential for stimulating high amount of lipase; consequently, lipases are normally produced when the medium is supplemented with lipid such as triacylglycerols, hydrolysable esters, fatty acids, and bile salts (Sharma *et al.*, 2016). In order to attain optimal biomass and enzyme production, it is important to reach a good mix of the fermentation broth since agitation not only produces the dispersion of air in the culture medium but also homogenizes the temperature and pH, as well as improves nutrient transference rate. However, high agitation speed causes stress condition that may negatively affect cell growth and enzyme stability (Ducros *et al.*, 2009).

## Screening Fungal Strains for Lipolytic Potential and Agro-industrial Substrates as Support for Lipase Production using Solid State Fermentation Technique

The three (3) halotolerant fungal strains (FIMT1, 2 and 4) were screened on various agro-industrial substrates such as banana peels, coconut fibre, coconut oil cake, palm kernel cake, oil palm empty fruit bunch, sugarcane bagasse, and rice husk for lipase production potential. The importance of this study is that it has allowed us to determine lipase producing potential of the halotolerant strains and at the same time allowed screening of the various agroresidues as substrate/support for lipase production. The results in Figure 15.7A-B showed that FIMT2 gave the best lipase production (0.211 U/g) under static fermentation condition and this was accomplished when palm kernel cake was used as the substrate. Lipase production yield in SSF vary according to the strain, solid support (substrate), culture medium, and cultivation conditions such as pH, temperature, and moisture content. The main important lipases from filamentous fungi produced in SSF belong to the genus *Aspergillus*, *Rhizopus* and *Penicillium*(Ramos-Sánchez *et al.*, 2015; Sivaramakrishnan and Gangadharan, 2009). Similarly, a lipase production of 0.202 U/g was recorded for FIMT1 under agitation condition when palm kernel cake was also used as the fermentation substrate. The result in Figure 15.7A-B further revealed that coconut oil cake also supported good lipase production of 0.150 U/g by FIMT1 under static condition and lipase production of 0.107 U/g by FIMT2 under agitation fermentation condition using the same substrate. Substantial lipase production of 0.124 U/g by FIMT2 and 0.108 U/g by FIMT4 respectively under agitation condition was attained

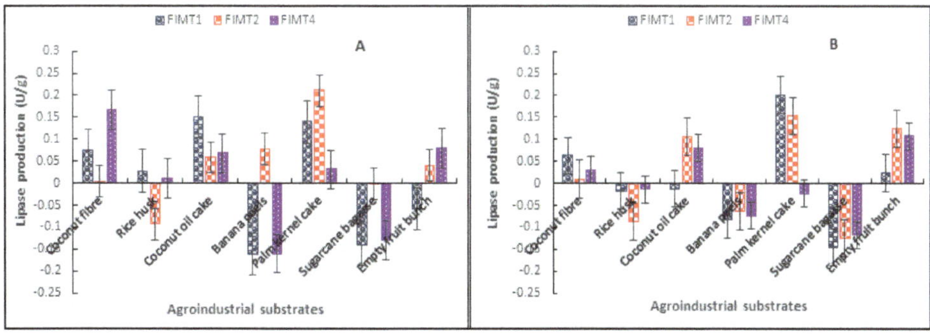


**Figure 15.7: Screening of Fungal Strains on Agro-industrial Substrates for Lipase Production Potential using SSF Technique under (A) Static and (B) Agitation Condition.**

when palm oil empty fruit bunch was used as the fermentation substrate. However, FIMT4 had its best lipase production (0.167 U/g) under static condition when coconut fibre was used as the substrate for fermentation. The remaining substrates; rice husk, banana peels and sugarcane bagasse inhibited lipase production and as such they are not good substrates for lipase fermentation by the 3 strains used in this study. It is therefore fair to say that palm kernel cake, coconut oil cake, oil palm empty fruit bunch, and coconut fibre induced good lipase production by the strains but palm kernel cake and coconut oil cake are the best substrates for lipase production by the halotolerant strains FIMT1 and FIMT2. It appears that the residual oil in the coconut oil cake and palm kernel cake acted as the inducer and additional nutrient source for lipase production as well as for fungal growth. Oil cakes are used either as a single substrate or mixed with other substrates in different combination for SSF (Sivaramakrishnan and Gangadharan, 2009). Different oil cakes have been extensively studied and utilized as suitable substrate for lipase production using fungal species by SSF because they provide carbon and nitrogen sources of nutrients (Ramachandran *et al.*, 2007). Moreover, several studies dealing with fungal lipase production have previously reported the superiority of coconut oil cake and palm kernel cake when used as the solid support or fermentation substrate for lipase production (Anusha *et al.*, 2017; Balaji and Ebenezer, 2008; Venkatesagowda *et al.*, 2015). Benjamin and Pandey (1997) earlier evaluated the potential of coconut oil cake as the substrate for lipase production by *Candida rugosa* where they achieved 88 U/g activities. Lipase production was also studied by Alam *et al.* (2013) where they used palm kernel cake as a cost-effective substrate for the production of lipase by *Candida cylindracea*. A 4-fold lipase production corresponding to 400 U/gds was obtained under optimized fermentation condition.

A brief comparison of the lipase production performance under SMF (0.142 U/µL) and SSF (0.211 U/g) by strain FIMT2 in this study shows that lipase production using SSF was favourable, where it was about 1.5-fold higher in enzyme titre. This result is in conformity with the study recently conducted by Anusha *et al.* (2017). They investigated lipase production by fungal strains using both SMF and SSF; with palm kernel cake as the substrate. All the *Aspergillus* strains used in the study showed higher lipase production in SSF when compared with SMF. Previous studies that dealt with fungal lipase production have reported the advantages of using SSF culture techniques (Barrios-Gonzalez and Tarragó-Castellanos, 2016; Kumar and Kanwar, 2012; Ramos-Sánchez *et al.*, 2015).

## Molecular Identification and Phylogenetic Analysis of the Selected Halotolerant Fungal Strain

Strain FIMT2 with the best lipase production potential on palm kernel cake medium in SSF culture technique was chosen for molecular identification based on ITS region sequence analysis. The phylogenetic analysis obtained from the alignment of ITS region of rDNA of *Aspergillus* species is shown in Figure 15.8. Based on sequence homology and phylogenetic tree analysis, the 18S rDNA sequence of strain FIMT2 showed a nucleotide identity of 94 per cent with that of *Aspergillus* sp. (JN585932.1). Thus, strain FIMT2 was classified into the genus *Aspergillus*. The

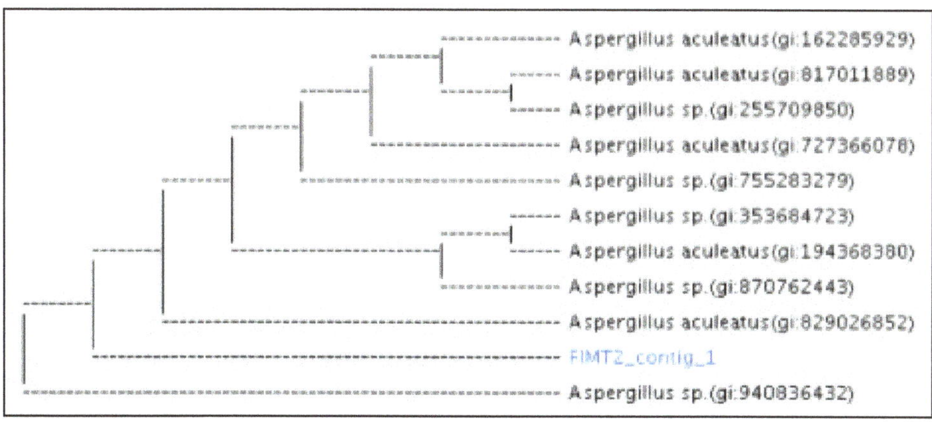


**Figure 15.8: Phylogenetic Tree Obtained from the Alignment of ITS Region of rDNA of *Aspergillus* Species. The sequence accession numbers are given at the end of each species name.**

gene sequence has been deposited in the NCBI GenBank and assigned accession number JN585932.1.

## Conclusions

The present investigation demonstrated that the fungal strains tested produced substantial amount of lipase but extreme halotolerant *Aspergillus* sp. FIMT2 produced the maximum lipase concentration of 0.211 U/g under static condition using palm kernel cake as the substrate for SSF. The oil cakes; palm kernel cake and coconut oil cake, as well as oil palm empty fruit bunch supported good lipase production which could be as a result of the residual lipid content present in them. These agro-industrial residues especially palm kernel cake and coconut oil cake could be used as low-cost substrates for the production of salt tolerant lipase by halotolerant fungal strains. Further optimization and concentration studies via SSF are required in order to maximize the potential of this extreme halotolerant strain.

## Acknowledgements

The work was supported by the Research Acculturation Collaborative Effort (RACE) Grant Scheme (Grant number: 9017-00007), the Ministry of Higher Education (MOHE), Malaysia.

## REFERENCES

1. Alam, M. Z., Elgharbawy, A. A. and Salleh, H. M., 2013. Optimization and characterization of *Candida cylindracea* lipase produced from palm kernel cake by solid-state bioconversion. In: AIChE Annual Meeting. San Fransisco, USA. Conference Proceedings: Food, Pharmaceutical and Bioengineering Division: Biocatalysis and Biosynthesis III: Applications.

2. Amin, M., Bhatti, H. N., Zuber, M., Bhatti, I. A. and Asgher, M., 2014. Potential use of agricultural wastes for the production of lipase by *Aspergillus melleus* under solid state fermentation. *Journal of Animal and Plant Sciences*, 23, 1430–1437.
3. Annapurna, S. A., Singh, A., Garg, S., Kumar, A. and Kumar, H., 2012. Screening, isolation and characterisation of protease producing moderately halophilic microorganisms. *Asian Journal of Microbiology, Biotechnology and Environmental Sciences*, 14(4): 603-612.
4. Anusha, N. C., Hirzun, M. Y., Umikalsom, M. S. and Ling, T. C. A. A., 2017. Comparative study on lipase production using solid state and submerged fermentation systems by several fungal strains and the predicted molecular characteristics. *Minerva Biotecnologica*, 29(2): 53–61.
5. Balaji, V. and Ebenezer, P., 2008. Optimization of extracellular lipase production in *Colletotrichum gloeosporioides* by solid state fermentation. *Indian Journal of Science and Technology*, 1(7): 1–8.
6. Barrios-González, J. and Tarragó-Castellanos, M. R., 2016. Solid-State Fermentation: Special Physiology of Fungi. *Fungal Metabolites*, 1–29.
7. Batista-García, R. A., Balcázar-López, E., Miranda-Miranda, E., Sánchez-Reyes, A., Cuervo-Soto, L., Aceves-Zamudio, D. and Folch-Mallol, J., 2014. Characterization of Lignocellulolytic Activities from a Moderate Halophile Strain of *Aspergillus caesiellus* Isolated from a Sugarcane Bagasse Fermentation. *PloS One*, 9(8): e105893.
8. Benjamin, S. and Pandey, A., 1997. Coconut cake–a potent substrate for the production of lipase by *Candida rugosa* in solidstate fermentation. *Acta Biotechnologica*, 17(3): 241–251.
9. Dayanandan, A., Rani, S., Shanmugavel, M., Gnanamani, A. and Rajakumar, G. S., 2013. Enhanced production of *Aspergillus tamarii* lipase for recovery of fat from tannery fleshings. *Brazilian Journal of Microbiology*, 44(4): 1089–1095.
10. de Almeida, A. F., Dias, K. B., da Silva, A. C. C., Terrasan, C. R. F., Tauk-Tornisielo, S. M. and Carmona, E. C., 2016. Agroindustrial wastes as alternative for lipase production by *Candida viswanathii* under solid-state cultivation: purification, biochemical properties, and its potential for poultry fat hydrolysis. *Enzyme Research*, 1-15.
11. DelgadoGarcía, M., ValdiviaUrdiales, B., AguilarGonzález, C. N., ContrerasEsquivel, J. C. and RodríguezHerrera, R., 2012. Halophilic hydrolases as a new tool for the biotechnological industries. *Journal of the Science of Food and Agriculture*, 92(13): 2575–2580.
12. Ducros, E., Ferrari, M., Pellegrino, M., Raspanti, C. and Bogni, C., 2009. Effect of aeration and agitation on the protease production by *Staphylococcus aureus* mutant RC128 in a stirred tank bioreactor. *Bioprocess and Biosystems Engineering*, 32(1): 143–148.

13. Evans, S., Hansen, R. W., Stone, H. M. and Schneegurt, M. A., 2013. Isolation and characterization of halotolerant soil fungi from the Great Salt Plains of Oklahoma (USA). *Cryptogamie, Mycologie*, 34(4): 329–341.

14. Gopalan, N. and Nampoothiri, K. M., 2016. Biotechnological Production of Enzymes Using Agro-Industrial Wastes: Economic Considerations, Commercialization Potential, and Future Prospects. In: Agro-Industrial Wastes as Feedstock for Enzyme Production: Apply and Exploit the Emerging and Valuable Use Options of Waste Biomass. 313-330.

15. Guarro, J., Xavier, M. O. and Severo, L. C., 2009. Differences and similarities amongst pathogenic *Aspergillus* species. ***In*** *Aspergillosis: From Diagnosis to Prevention*, Springer. pp. 7–32.

16. Gunde-Cimerman, N. and Zalar, P., 2014. "Extremely halotolerant and halophilic fungi inhabit brine in solar salterns around the globe. *Food Technology and Biotechnology*, 52(2): 170.

17. Gunde-Cimerman, N., Ramos, J. and Plemenitaš, A., 2009. Halotolerant and halophilic fungi. *Mycological Research*, 113(11): 1231–1241.

18. Gutarra, M. L. E., Godoy, M. G., Maugeri, F., Rodrigues, M. I., Freire, D. M. G. and Castilho, L. R., 2009. Production of an acidic and thermostable lipase of the mesophilic fungus *Penicillium simplicissimum* by solid-state fermentation. *Bioresource Technology*, 100(21): 5249–5254.

19. Karan, R., Kumar, S., Sinha, R. and Khare, S. K., 2012. Halophilic microorganisms as sources of novel enzymes. ***In***: Microorganisms in Sustainable Agriculture and Biotechnology, Springer, pp. 555–579.

20. Kumar, A. and Kanwar, S. S., 2012. Lipase production in solid-state fermentation (SSF): recent developments and biotechnological applications. *Dynamic Biochemistry, Process Biotechnology and Molecular Biology*, 6(1): 13–27.

21. Kushner, D. J., 1978. Life in high salt and solute concentrations: halophilic bacteria. *Microbial Life in Extreme Environments*, 317–368.

22. Margesin, R.and Schinner, F., 2001. Potential of halotolerant and halophilic microorganisms for biotechnology. *Extremophiles*, 5(2): 73–83.

23. Martinelli, L., Zalar, P., Gunde-Cimerman, N., Azua-Bustos, A., Sterflinger, K. and Piñar, G., 2017. *Aspergillus atacamensis* and *A. salisburgensis*: two new halophilic species from hypersaline/arid habitats with a phialosimplex-like morphology. *Extremophiles*, 21(4): 755–773.

24. Munawar, N. and Engel, P. C., 2013. Halophilic enzymes: characteristics, structural adaptation and potential applications for biocatalysis. *Current Biotechnology*, 2(4): 334–344.

25. Nazareth, S., Gonsalves, V. and Nayak, S., 2012. A first record of obligate halophilic *Aspergilli* from the Dead Sea. *Indian Journal of Microbiology*, 52(1): 22–27.

26. Nazareth, S. W. and Gonsalves, V., 2014. Halophilic *Aspergillus penicillioides* from athalassohaline, thalassohaline, and polyhaline environments. *Frontiers in Microbiology*, 5, 412.

27. Quintanilla, D., Hagemann, T., Hansen, K. and Gernaey, K. V., 2015. Fungal Morphology in Industrial Enzyme Production–Modelling and Monitoring. ***In***: *Filaments in Bioprocesses*, Springer, pp. 29–54.

28. Rai, B., Shrestha, A., Sharma, S. and Joshi, J., 2014. Screening, Optimization and Process Scale up for Pilot Scale Production of Lipase by *Aspergillus niger*. *Biomedicine and Biotechnology*, 2(3): 54–59.

29. Ramachandran, S., Singh, S. K., Larroche, C., Soccol, C. R. and Pandey, A., 2007. Oil cakes and their biotechnological applications–A review. *Bioresource Technology*, 98(10): 2000–2009.

30. Ramos-Sánchez, L. B., Cujilema-Quitio, M. C., Julian-Ricardo, M. C., Cordova, J. and Fickers, P., 2015. Fungal lipase production by solid-state fermentation. *Journal of Bioprocessing and Biotechniques*, 5, 203–212.

31. Rehman, S., Bhatti, H. N., Bhatti, I. A. and Asgher, M., 2011. Optimization of process parameters for enhanced production of lipase by *Penicillium notatum* using agricultural wastes. *African Journal of Biotechnology*, 10(84): 19580.

32. Salihu, A., Bala, M. and Alam, M. Z., 2016. Lipase production by *Aspergillus niger* using sheanut cake: An optimization study. *Journal of Taibah University for Science*, 10(6): 850–859.

33. Sana, B., 2015. Marine microbial enzymes: current status and future prospects. In: *Springer Handbook of Marine Biotechnology*, Springer.905–917.

34. Sethi, B. K., Rout, J. R., Das, R., Nanda, P. K. and Sahoo, S. L., 2013. Lipase production by *Aspergillus terreus* using mustard seed oil cake as a carbon source. *Annals of Microbiology*, 63(1): 241–252.

35. Sharma, A. K., Sharma, V. and Saxena, J., 2016. A review on optimization of growth parameters for enhanced fungal lipase production. Indo American *Journal of Pharmaceutical Sciences*, 3(10): 1196–1202.

36. Sivaramakrishnan, S. and Gangadharan, D., 2009. Edible Oil Cakes. In: P. nee' Nigam and A. Pandey (Eds.), Biotechnology for Agro-Industrial Residues Utilisation: Utilisation of Agro-Residues,Dordrecht: Springer Netherlands. 253–271.

37. Venkatesagowda, B., Ponugupaty, E., Barbosa, A. M. and Dekker, R. F. H., 2015. Solid-state fermentation of coconut kernel-cake as substrate for the production of lipases by the coconut kernel-associated fungus *Lasiodiplodia theobromae* VBE-1. *Annals of Microbiology*,65(1): 129–142.

38. Youssef, M. S., Abo-Dahab, N. F. and Farghaly, R. M., 2003. Studies on Mycological Status of Salted Fish. *Mycobiology*, 31(3): 166–172.

39. Zarevúcka, M., 2012. Olive oil as inductor of microbial lipase. In: Olive Oil-Constituents, Quality, Health Properties and Bioconversions. InTech. www.intechopen.com.

*Chapter 16*

# Sri Lankan Finger Millet (*Elucine coracana*) Variety 'Raavana' as Potential Probiotic Source

*D.M.W.D. Divisekera*[1], *J.K.R.R. Samarasekera*[1], *J. Goonerathne*[1], *C. Hettiarachchi*[2] *and S. Gopalakrishnan*[3]

[1]*Food Technology Section, Industrial Technology Institute, 363, Bauddhaloka Mawatha, Colombo, 00700 SRI LANKA*
*E-mail: mb.wasu@gmail.com*
[2]*Faculty of Science, University of Colombo, SRI LANKA*
[3]*International Crops Research Institute for the Semi-Arid Tropic, Telangana, INDIA*

## ABSTRACT

This study aims to isolate and identify probiotic potential lactic acid bacteria from fermented Sri Lankan finger millet variety *"Raavana"* and to investigate the probiotic characteristics, *in vitro* safety and efficacy. A bacterial isolate with typical lactic acid bacterial phenotypic and biochemical characteristics was isolated and identified. Partial sequence of the 16S rRNA gene of the Sri Lankan strain was deposited in the NCBI gene bank as *Lactococcus lactis* subsp. *lactis* FM_19LAB and the accession number MF480428 was obtained. It did not demonstrate hemolysis, DNase, gelatine hydrolysis activity as well as did not acquire complete resistance to any of the antibiotics tested hence indicating the safety. *Lactococcus lactis* subsp. *lactis* FM_19LAB had the capacity to tolerate different concentrations of acid, bile, phenol, salt, simulated gastric juices and range of temperatures. Further it exhibited anti-microbial, anticancer and anti-oxidant activities. Further, *Lactococcus lactis* subsp. *lactis* FM_19LAB assimilated cholesterol and produced lactic acid during the fermentation.

***Keywords:*** *Sri Lankan finger millet, Lactococcus lactis* subsp. *lactis FM_19LAB, Probiotics, Prebiotics.*

## INTRODUCTION

Probiotics are defined as "live microorganisms, which when administrated in adequate amounts confer a health benefit on the host" by the Food and Agriculture Organization/World Health Organization (FAO/WHO 2006). Lactic Acid Bacteria (LAB) are widely recognized among probiotic bacteria that are gram positive, non-spore forming and catalase negative organisms. The beneficial effects include promoting gastrointestinal and genitourinary health improving the immune system, managing irritable bowel syndrome and inflammatory bowel diseases, reducing *H. pylori* associated gastric ulcers, and improving constipation (Bergonzelli *et al.*, 2006; D'Souza *et al.*, 2002; Whelan *et al.*, 2013; Koebnick *et al.*, 2003). Lactic acid bacteria (LAB), if functional as a probiotic it should exhibit resistance to acid, bile and gastric juices, adhere and colonize in-gastric mucosa (Kos *et al.*, 2003), exhibit co-aggregation preventing colonization by pathogens (Collado *et al.*, 2008) and efficacy to host which support their use as alternative therapy. Therefore, probiotic LABs are increasingly recognized in food industrial applications. As a result, novel bacterial strains with probiotic properties are been introduced in to food and pharmaceutical market particularly in dairy products (Penna *et al.*, 2007). Currently consumer demand exists for non-dairy probiotic products in beverages, supplements, capsules and freeze-dried preparations (Schrezenmeir and de Vrese, 2001). Therefore, cereals rich in prebiotics play a major role as substrate for many non-dairy probiotic products. Finger millet (*Eleusine coracana*) is known since ancient times and rich in carbohydrates, dietary fibre, minerals, and sulfur containing amino acids when compared with rice, the current major staple in south Asia (Sripriya *et al.*, 1994). Fermentation of finger millet using different starter cultures to develop functional foods has been extensively reported in Africa and Asia (Charalampopoulos *et al.*, 2002). Due to the presence of water-soluble fibres, oligosaccharides and resistant starch, it fulfils the prebiotic effects and therefore can stimulate the growth of probiotic bacteria. Though, plenty of research available on prebiotic and probiotic potential of finger millet varieties grown on different regions in the world, there is a paucity of data on Sri Lankan scenario. Furthermore, due to the increasing interest in the application of probiotics and their metabolites as an alternative strategy for treatment and prevention of infections, antimicrobial activity against human pathogens is an important property of a potential probiotic candidate. In addition, antimicrobial metabolites of probiotic LAB in preventing food spoilage, extending the shelf life stability of food and enriching the food with bioactive properties are the challenges facing food industry today. The objective of the research was to isolate probiotic potential organisms associated with Sri Lankan finger millet variety *'Raavana'* and to explore its' probiotic potential through series of experiments at the industrial technology institute of Sri Lanka.

## Materials and Methods

### Collection and Processing of Finger Millet Samples

Sri Lankan finger millet (*Elucine coracana*) variety namely *Raavana* was selected for the present study. Seeds of the variety represented the six different provinces of the island including North, North Central, Eastern, Southern, Sabaragamuva and Uva, were obtained from the germplasm of the Field Crop Research and Development Institute (FCRDI), Mahailluppallama. The seeds were transported to the Microbiology Laboratory, Industrial Technology Institute (ITI) within 3 h by maintaining the temperature at 20 ± 2 °C. Samples were washed with sterilized distilled water inside a Biological safety cabinet (Thermoforma,USA) and dried at 35 ± 2 °C in an oven (Memmert Universal Oven U, Germany) till the moisture content reduced to 10 per cent. The moisture content of the samples was measured by drying the samples at 105 ± 2 °C in an oven (Memmert drying oven UF, Germany) for 5 h and calculated the water loss. Each dried sample was ground in a variable Speed Rotar Mill (Fritsch PULVERISETTE 14, Germany) and passed through a 0.5 mm sieve attached to the mill. The milled and sieved samples were packed separately in air tight containers and stored in cold room (Viessmann Tecto compact 80, Finland) at 12 ± 2 °C till use.

## Fermentation of Finger Millet Samples

Six samples (n=6) containing 25 g of each was measured and transferred in to pre-sterilized glass beakers covered with aluminium foils. The flour samples were mixed with sterilized tap water in 1:3 (w/v) ratios to prepare the batter. The batters were allowed to ferment inside a biological safety cabinet at room temperature (24 ± 3 °C) for 18 h.

## Isolation of Probiotic Potential Lactic Acid Bacteria from Fermented Finger Millet

Each fermented sample was serially diluted up $10^6$ in sterilized physiological saline (0.9 per cent NaCl w/v). Isolation was carried out by following both spread plate and pour plate technique in duplicates. Both pour and spread plates were incubated at 37 ± 1 °C for 24 h.

## Phenotypic Characterization of Lactic Acid Bacteria

Colonies appeared on MRS agar plates were picked carefully and streaked on fresh MRS agar plates. The plates were incubated at 37 ± 1 °C for 24 h. After incubation, colony morphology of isolates such as form, size, shape, surface, texture, color, elevation and margin were recorded. Gram staining, endospore staining and motility test was performed to differentiate the isolates based on their phenotypic characteristics (Aswathy *et al.*, 2008).

## Biochemical Characterization of Isolates

Biochemical tests including indole, methyl red, vogeus prosker, citrate utilization, gelatin liquefaction, $H_2S$ production, starch hydrolysis, urease and catalase were performed to characterize isolates. Sugar fermentation pattern of potential LAB isolates were investigated in triplicate (n=3) for sixteen different sugars; glucose, fructose, maltose, lactose, galactose, melezitose, melibiose, arabinose, ribose, sucrose, salicinsorbitol, mannitol, cellulose, cellobiose and dextrose.

## *In vitro* Safety Attributes of the Newly Isolated Probiotic Isolates

### Bile Salt Hydrolysis (BSH) Test

Bile Salt Hydrolysis screening medium was prepared by supplementing MRS agar with (0.5 per cent porcine bile w/v, 0.5 per cent sodium tauroglycocholate w/v, 0.5 per cent taurodeoxycholic acid sodium Salt w/v and 0.37 $CaCl_2$ g/l. The media was sterilized for 121 ± 1°C for 15 min and poured in to sterile Petri plates in triplicates and allowed to solidify. Cell density of each test bacterial isolate was adjusted to $10^5$cfu/ml. From each culture, 10 µl were spotted on BSH screening media plates. Plates were incubated at 37 ± 1°C for 72 h. BSH activity was determined by observing and measuring the precipitation zones.

### Hemolysis Test

Blood agar base (Himedia, India) was prepared and sterilized at 121 ± 2 °C for 15 min. The sterilized media was cooled up to 50 ± 1°C and supplemented with 5 per cent sheep blood (v/v) aseptically followed by mixing; the media was poured in to sterile petri plates and allowed to solidify. Six colonies (n=6) from each test bacterial isolate was inoculated in to blood agar plates followed by streaking. The plates were incubated at 37 ± 1 °C for 72 h. After incubation, the plates were observed for presence of hemolysis zones (β-hemolysis- clear zone of hydrolysis of blood cells around the colonies, α-hemolysis- green zone around the colonies, γ-hemolysis- no clear or no green zone around the colonies). Haemolysing strain *Streptococcus pyogene* ATCC 19615 was used as the positive control.

### DNase Test

DNase agar was prepared and sterilized at 121 ± 2 °C for 15 min. Six colonies (n=6) from each bacterial isolate was spotted on the surface of the DNase agar plates. The plates were incubated at 37 ± 1 °C for 18 h and observed for thick plaque of growth around the colonies. Pathogenic strain *Serratia marcescens* ATCC 13880 was used as the positive control.

### Gelatin Hydrolysis

TND agar containing 1.7 per cent tryptone (w/v), 0.3 per cent peptone (w/v), 0.25 per cent dextrose (w/v), 0.5 per cent NaCl (w/v), 0.25 per cent $K_2HPO_4$ (w/v), 1.5 per cent agar (w/v) and 0.4 per cent gelatine bacteriological (w/v) was prepared and sterilized for 121 ± 1 °C for 15 min. Sterilized media was poured in to sterile plates and allowed to solidify. Cell density of each test probiotics was adjusted to $10^5$cfu/ml. From each culture, 10µl were spotted on TND agar plates in triplicates. Plates were incubated at 37 ± 1 °C for 72 h. After incubation, the plates were treated with saturated solution of ammonium sulphate and observed for the clear zones around the inoculated spot against the opaque background. Gelatine hydrolysing strain *Serratia marcescens* ATCC 13880 was used as the positive control.

## Evaluation of the *In vitro* Probiotic Attributes of Newly Isolated Potential LAB

The newly isolated LAB were further investigated for its' ability to grow in the presence of acid, bile, salt, phenol, temperature and gastric juice (Aswathy *et al.*, 2008). Isolates were inoculated into sterile MRS broth tubes and incubated at 37 ± 1 °C for 18 h. After incubation, the tubes were centrifuged at 10,000 × *g* at 4 ± 1 °C for 15 min. Subsequently the pellet was washed with sterile saline solution and centrifuged at 10,000 × *g* at 4 ± 1 °C for 15 min. Finally, the pellets were dissolved in 10 ml of MRS broth and adjusted to 0.5 Macfarl and turbidity standards to use in the tolerance tests.

For acid tolerance assay, MRS broth tubes were sterilized and pH was adjusted to 2, 3, and 4 using 1 M HCl. The pH adjusted broths were inoculated with 100 µl of each test bacteria (n=3). For bile tolerance assay, MRS broth tubes were adjusted with 0.2 per cent, 0.5 per cent, 1.0 per cent, 1.5 per cent and 2.0 per cent porcine Bile (w/v). The media were sterilized by filtering through 0.45 µm diameter syringe filters. Sterilized media were inoculated with 100 µl of each test bacteria (n=3). For simulated gastric juice tolerance assay, simulated gastric juice was formulated using 3.5 g/l glucose, 2.05 g/l NaCl, 0.60 g/l $KH_2PO_4$, 0.11 g/l $CaCl_2$, 0.37 g/l KCl. The pH of the mixture was adjusted to 2 by 1M HCl (Corcoran *et al.*, 2005). The mixture was sterilized for 121 ± 1 °C at 15 min. Prior to analysis 0.05 g/l porcine bile, 0.10 g/l lysozyme, and 0.10 g/l pepsin, were added to stock solution. The simulated gastric juice solution was sterilized by filtering through 0.45 µm diameter syringe filters. Subsequently 100 µl of each test bacteria were inoculated in to the tubes containing sterile simulated gastric juice (n=3). For salt tolerance assay (Menconi *et al.*, 2014) MRS broth tubes were prepared and adjusted to 4 per cent, 5 per cent, 8 per cent and 12 per cent (w/v) with NaCl. The media was sterilized at 121 ± 1 °C for 15 min. Aseptically 100 µl of each test bacteria were inoculated in to the MRS broth tubes and adjusted to different salt concentrations (n=3). For phenol tolerance assay MRS broth were prepared and adjusted to 0.1 per cent, 0.2 per cent, 0.3 per cent, 0.4 per cent and 0.5 per cent phenol (v/v) separately (Aswathy *et al.*, 2008). The media were sterilized for 121 ± 1 °C at 15 min. Inoculated 100 µl of each test bacteria in to the MRS broth tubes adjusted in to different phenol concentrations (n=3). All the assay tubes were mixed for 30 sec. Under aseptic condition, 200 µl of each test sample was loaded into 9 wells of the microplate and initial cell density was measured spectrophotometrically at 620 nm and the cell densities of the experimental wells were measured hourly at 1, 2, 3, 4, 5 and 6 h intervals.

For temperature tolerance assay, MRS broth was dispensed equally in to tubes and sterilized. The tubes were inoculated with 100 µl of each test bacteria (n=3). Under aseptic condition, 200 µl of each test sample was loaded into 3 sterile micro plates where in each plate 9 wells were loaded from same inoculums (n=9). Initial cell density was measured spectrophotometrically at 620 nm and the three plates were incubated at three different temperature 30 ± 1 °C (Memmert INC 153, G), 37±1°C (Gemmyco IN-010, France) and 42 ± 1 °C (MemmertINplus, Germany), respectively for 6 h. Cell density was measured hourly at 1, 2, 3, 4, 5 and 6 h intervals.

Among the isolates, an isolate with superior probiotic attributes was selected for molecular identification.

## Molecular Characterization of Potential Lactic Acid Bacteria Isolates

### Extraction of Genomic DNA

Test isolate was inoculated in to sterilized MRS broth tubes and incubated at 37 ± 1 °C for 24 h. after incubation; 2 ml of the inoculums was transferred in to 2.5 ml micro centrifuge tubes and centrifuged at 14000 × *g* at 4 ± 1 °C for 2 min. The supernatant was separated without disturbing the pellets and 200 µl of Tris EDTA buffer was added to pellet followed by centrifugation at 14000 × *g* at 4 ± 1 °C for 2 min. Supernatant was discarded and the pellet was re-suspended in 200 µl Tris EDTA buffer and added 10 µl of 100 µg/µl (w/v) Proteinase K enzyme. Subsequently 10 µl of 10 per cent Sodium Dodecyl Sulfate was added and mixed thoroughly. The reaction tube was incubated in a water bath at 50 ± 1 °C for 1 h. After incubation, 110 µl of phenol and 110 µl of chloroform were added and centrifuged at 14000 × *g* at 4 ± 1 °C for 2 min. Aqueous layer (approximately 150 µl) was separated without disturbing the organic layers. To the organic layer, 30 µl of ≥99.8 ethanol (v/v) and 15 µl of 3 M sodium acetate were added. The tube was mixed by vortexing and incubated in ice for 1 h. After incubation, the tube was centrifuged at 14000 × *g* at 4 ± 1 °C for 5 min. Supernatant was discarded and 1 ml of 70 per cent ethanol (v/v) was added to the tubes and mixed by inverting several times followed by centrifugation at 14000 × *g* at 4 ± 1 °C for 5 min. Supernatant was discarded and ethanol was evaporated and the pellet was dissolved in 40 µl of PCR water and stored at -20 ± 2 °C (Shahriar *et al.*, 2011 modified). The extracted genomic DNA was quantified using gel documentation system (Gel Doc™ XR+ BIO RAD, USA).

### Polymerase Chain Reaction (PCR)

Bacterial DNA was amplified by Dr. MAX DNA Polymerase using DNA Engine Tetrad 2 Peltier Thermal Cycler (BIO-RAD, UK) at MACROGEN, South Korea (www.macrogen.com). Universal primers 27F (5c-AGAGTTTGATCCTGGCTCAG -3c) and 1492R (5c-GGTTACCTTGTTACGACTT -3c) were used as forward and reverse primers, respectively. The PCR was performed under the following thermocycler program; Initial denaturation at 95 ± 1 °C for 5 min followed by denaturing step conducted in 35 cycles at 95 ± 1 °C for 30 sec. Annealing of the primers to the single stranded DNA template was done at 55 ± 1 °C for 30 sec. Elongation was conducted at 72 ± 1 °C for 1 min; the final elongation was carried out at 72 ± 1°C for 10 min. The PCR products were purified using multiscreen filter plate (Millipore Corp, UK).

### Sequencing of 16S rRNA Region

Sequencing of 16S rRNA region was performed using 96 capillary type ABI PRISM 3730XL Analyzer (UK). Forward primer 5′ TGTCGTGAGATGTTGGGTTAAGTC 3′ and Reverse primer 5′ CGGTATTAGCATCTGTTTCC 3′ were used. Purified PCR product was sequenced at MACROGEN, South Korea in a thermocycler program consisting of initial denaturation at 96 ± 1 °C for 1 min followed by 25 cycles at 96 ± 1 °C for 10 sec. Annealing was done at 50 ± 1 °C for 4 sec followed by elongation at 60 ± 1 °C for 4 min; and hold at 4 ± 1 °C. DNA sequences were obtained as FASTA format were compared with those from GenBank (http://www.ncbi.nlm.nih.gov) using the Basic Local Alignment Tool (http://www.ncbi.nlm.gov/BLAST/).

Sequence with a percentage of identity of 98 per cent or higher to those in databases were allocated to the same species. The sequence was aligned using the Clustal W multiple sequence alignment program (Thompson *et al.*, 1997). The 16S rRNA gene sequences of potential probiotic isolate was submitted to NCBI (http://www.ncbi.nlm.nih.gov) and GenBank accession number was obtained.

## Investigating Antibiotic Susceptibility of Potential Probiotic by Alamar Blue Cell Viability Assay

Newly isolated probiotic strain was investigated for their susceptibility to 24 different antibiotics including netilmicin, amikacin, gentamycin, ofloxacin, cefoxitin, doxycycline, sulbactam, neomycin, ampicillin, vancomycin, oxacillin, streptomycin, penicillin, nitrofurantoin, sulfamethoxazole, chloramphenicol, trimethoprim and clindamycin. Antibiotic solutions were prepared at a concentration of 100 µg/ml (w/v) by dissolving the above antibiotics in sterilized distilled water followed by filtering through 0.22 µm syringe filters. Potential probiotic isolate was adjusted to 0.5 McFarland turbidity standards and stored at 4±1 °C until use. Antibiotic susceptibility was measured spectrophotometrically by performing Alamar blue assay. Each test antibiotic solution in a volume of 20 µl was aseptically added to the wells (n=9) of the sterile 96 well plate. Subsequently 173 µl of sterile MRS broth was added to all the wells followed by test probiotics (each 7 µl). Micro plates were sealed with parafilm and incubated at 37 ± 1 °C for 20 h. After incubation, 20 µl of Alamar blue cell viability reagent® was added to all the wells in dark environment. The plates were covered with aluminum foils and incubated in a shaker (CPS-350, Korea) at 30 ± 1 °C for 2 h at 100 × g. After incubation, the wells were sealed and absorbance were measured (Spectra Max plus, USA) at both λ=570 nm and λ=600 nm. Negative control was performed omitting antibiotics and replacing the volume with 193 µl of MRS broth.

Percentage inhibition of test probiotics by antibiotics was calculated by following formula.

$$\text{Per cent inhibition} = \frac{(\varepsilon ox)\lambda 2 A\lambda 1 - (\varepsilon ox)\lambda 1 A\lambda 2}{(\varepsilon red)\lambda 1 A\lambda 2 - (\varepsilon red)\lambda 2 A\lambda 1} x100$$

*where,*

$(e_{ox})$ = molar extinction coefficient of Alamar blue oxidized form (blue)

$(e_{red})$ = molar extinction coefficient of Alamar blue reduced form (pink)

A = absorbance of test wells

A2 = absorbance of negative control well

$\lambda_1$ = 570 nm, and $\lambda_2$ = 600 nm.

## Investigating *In vitro* Anti-microbial Activity by Well Diffusion Assay

Ten strains of drug sensitive and five strains of Multi Drug Resistant (MDR) pathogens were obtained from Microbial Bank of PCMD, ICCBS University of Karachi, Pakistan. These strains were *Escherichia coli* ATCC 2592, *Escherichia coli* ATCC 35218 (MDR), *Staphylococcus aureus* ATCC 6571, *Staphylococcus aureus* EMRSA

17 COCR (MDR), *Staphylococcus aureus* EMRSA 16 NCTC 13143 (MDR), *Klebsiella pneumonia* ATCC 35594, *Klebsiella pneumonia* ATCC 700603 (MDR), *Enterococcus faecalis* ATCC 49532, *Enterococcus faecalis* ATCC 700802 (MDR), *Streptococcus mutans* ATCC 25175, *Streptococcus pyogenes* ATCC 700294, *Streptococcus sanguinis* ATCC 10556, *Streptococcus salvarius* ATCC 13419, *Salmonella enterica* ATCC 700408 (MDR), *Acinetobacter baumannii* ATCC 17978 and *Shigella flexneri* ATCC 12022. The well diffusion assay was conducted according to Naderi *et al.*, 2013 with modifications. Probiotic isolate was adjusted to 0.5 McFarland turbidity standards. Soft agar was melted and at 45 ± 2 °C, 100 µl of each pathogenic culture was added to separate soft agar tubes in triplicates and poured on to the solidified agar plates (n=3). Plates were rotated to evenly distribute the culture and allowed to solidify. By using sterile 6 mm diameter borer, wells were made on the solidified plates; wells were clearly marked and 100 µl of probiotic inoculums was added to the well (n=9). The plates were sealed and incubated at 37 ± 1 °C for 24 h. Disc of 10 µg concentration of imipenem was used as the control. After incubation, the inhibition zones were measured using a calibrated scale. Antimicrobial activity was expressed as the diameter of the inhibition zones in mm around the wells.

## Investigating *In vitro* Anticancer Activity by MTT Assay

Anticancer activity of potential probiotic was evaluated against two Colon cancer cell lines namely HCT 116 and HT 29.

To prepare the Cell free extract (CFE), isolate was inoculated in to sterile MRS broth followed by incubation at 37 ± 1 °C for 18 h. After incubation, the tubes were centrifuged at 11,000 × *g* for 30 min at 4 ± 1 °C. The supernatants were sterilized by passing through 0.22 µm syringe filter. The CFE was stored at 4 ± 1 °C until use. To prepare Cell Free Lyophilate (CFL), the CFS of test probiotic was freeze dried (Lablyo HSL 4, UK) by storing the CFE at -20 ± 1 ° C for 10 h initially and transferred to freeze drier for 45 h with 10 min initial freezing followed by 40 h of primary (when internal pressure reduced to -100 torr) and 5 h of secondary freezing at -80 ± 2 °C. The resulted CFL was stored at -20 ± 1 °C until use.

Dulbecco's Modified Eagle's Medium (DMEM) was used to maintain the cell lines. DMEM was prepared by supplementing DMEM F-12 with 10 per cent Fet al Bovine Serum (v/v), 1 per cent l-glutamine (v/v), 1 per cent penicillin-streptomycin solution (v/v) and 7.5 per cent $NaHCO_3$. The medium was sterilized by filtration and stored at 4 ± 1 °C until use.

The cryo vials containing two different cell lines were reviewed in DMEM flasks and incubated (Nuaire NU-8700E, USA) at 37 ± 1 °C with 5 per cent $CO_2$ for 24 h. The flasks were observed through microscope for the 80 per cent confluence. Cell viability was determined by MTT assay. HT 29 and HCT 116 cell lines were inoculated separately in to wells (n=9) of 96 well plate at a concentration of 15 × $10^3$ cells/well. Probiotic CFE (5, 25, 50, 250 and 500 µl/ml) and CFL (750 µg/ml, 1250 µg/ml, 2500 µg/ml, 3750 µg/ml, 5000 µg/ml and 7500 µg/ml) at different concentrations were investigated for their anti-cancer assay. Plates were incubated at 37 ± 1 °C for 24 h with 5 per cent $CO_2$. After incubation, the media were discarded and 100 µl of MTT solution (3-[4, 5-dimethylthiazol-2-yl]-2, 5- diphenyl tetrazolium bromide thiazolyl blue; 5 mg/ml in sterile PBS) was added to all the wells. The plates were incubated for 2 h at 37 ± 1 ºC with 5 per cent $CO_2$. After incubation, 100 µl of Dimethyl sulfoxide was added and the plates were shaked to dissolve the blue crystals. The absorbance of plates was measured at λ=570 nm.

The percentage anticancer activity (per cent) was calculated using following formula,

$$\text{Percentage anticancer activity (per cent)} = \frac{MeanODtreatment}{MeanODcontrol} \times 100$$

The cell viability of controls were calculated using following formula,

$$\text{Percentage cell viability of controls} = \frac{MeanODcontrol}{MeanODcontrol} \times 100$$

Where,

Mean OD treatment = Mean value of the OD of treatment well at λ=570 nm

Mean OD control = Mean value of the OD of control well at λ=570 nm

Cetuximab was used as the positive control with CFE experiment (Lancet, 2011). The half maximum inhibitory concentration ($IC_{50}$) of both CFE and CFL of 8 probiotics were calculated by drawing individual scatter plots with linear regression.

## Investigating *In vitro* Antioxidant Activity by DPPH Radical Scavenging Assay

The 2, 2-diphenyl-1-picrylhydrazyl (DPPH) radical scavenging activity was measured by mixing 140 µl of each CFE with 60 µl of freshly prepared DPPH solution (7 mg/100 ml methanol). Each probiotic was tested for series of concentrations including 5, 25, 50, 250 and 500 µl/ml CFE in PBS. Immediately the absorbance was measured at λ= 517 nm. The reaction mixture was allowed to stand for 30 min. Trolox was used as positive control. The scavenged DPPH was evaluated by measuring the reduction in absorbance at 517 nm.

Similarly, probiotic CFL was dissolved in 25 per cent acetone to prepare the concentrations of 10,000 µg/ml, 20,000 µg/ml and 50,000 µg/ml. Immediately the absorbance was measured at λ= 517 nm. The reaction mixture was allowed to stand for 1 hr. Trolox was used as positive control. The scavenged DPPH was evaluated by measuring the reduction in absorbance at 517 nm.

The scavenging ability was calculated by following formula:

$$\text{Per cent inhibition} = 1 - \frac{A517\ (sample)}{A517\ (blank)} \times 100\%$$

*where,*

A517 (sample) = Absorbance of sample at 517 λ

A517 (blank) = Absorbance of blank at 517 λ

## Investigating the *In vitro* Cholesterol Assimilation

The cells of probiotic culture were adjusted to $OD_{660}$ ($10^{10}$cfu/ml). Modified MRS broth was prepared by mixing 0.3 per cent (w/v) porcine bile and 0.1 g/l cholesterol-water soluble in to MRS broth and adjusted the final concentration of cholesterol in the media in to 100 mg/l. 1 ml ($10^{10}$cfu) of the probiotic culture was transferred in to tubes containing 5 ml of modified MRS broth (n=3). Tubes were incubated at 37 ± 1 °C for 24 h. After incubation, the tubes were centrifuged at 4500 × *g* at 4 ± 1 °C for 5 min. Supernatants (test) and un inoculated Modified MRS broth (control) were assayed for cholesterol.

Each supernatant of 1 ml volume was mixed with 3 ml 95 per cent ethanol and 2 ml of 50 per cent (w/v) potassium hydroxide. The mixture was heated at 60 ± 1 °C for 10 min in water. After cooling, 5 ml of hexane was added in to each tube and mixed thoroughly. Subsequently, 1 ml of distilled water was added to all the tubes followed by mixing and allowed to stand for 10 min to permit phase separation. A 3 ml aliquot of hexane layer from each tube was transferred in to clean tubes. Evaporation of hexane was done under the flow of nitrogen gas. *O*-phtalaldehyde (0.5 mg/ml of acetic acid) solution was freshly prepared and 4 ml was added to each tube. The tubes were allowed to stand for 10 min. Subsequently, 2 ml of concentrated $H_2SO_4$ was added to each tube and allowed to stand for another 10 min. The absorbance of reaction mixture was measured at 550 nm. A standard curve of absorbance verses cholesterol concentrations was generated using the cholesterol concentrations; 0, 2.91, 7.81, 15.63, 31.25, 62.5, 125, 250 and 500µg/mL cholesterol in MRS ($R^2$=0.99). The cholesterol assimilated by test probiotic was calculated using following formula;

Cholesterol assimilated (µg/mL) = $[\text{Cholesterol } (\mu g/mL)]_{oh}$-$[\text{Cholesterol } (\mu g/mL)]_{24h}$

Cholesterol assimilated by each test probiotic strain was also calculated in terms of percentage cholesterol assimilation;

$$\text{Per cent cholesterol assimilation} = \frac{[\text{Cholesterol assimilated cholesterol } (\mu g/mL)]}{\text{Cholesterol } (\mu g/mL)]_{oh}} \times 100 \text{ per cent}$$

## Determination of Lactic Acid Production

Cells of probiotic culture were adjusted to $OD_{660}$ ($10^{10}$cfu/ml).Flasks containing 10 ml of sterile MRS broth were inoculated with test probiotic cells at concentration of $10^{10}$cfu/ml. The fermentations of flasks were carried out in a shaking incubator at 37 ± 1°C for 6 h with shaking speed of 150*g*. Aliquots of 5 ml were withdrawn from each fermentation flasks (in triplicates) at every 30 min intervals till 4.5 h. The aliquots were thermally treated at 95 ± 1 °C for 20 min in a water bath. The thermally treated samples were sealed well with parafilm and stored at 4 ± 1 °C. The samples were analysed for lactic acid using HPLC (Agilent technologies, 1260 Infinity, USA) equipped with a UV-VIS detector HPLC column, PhenomenexRezex™ ROA-Organic Acid H+ (8 per cent). The column was 50 mm x 7.8 mm with a length of

300 mm, 7.8 mm diameter and 8 µm particle sizes. The mobile phase was 0.005 M $H_2SO_4$ with an isocratic elution of a flow rate of 0.6 ml/min. the lactic acid content was quantified by measuring the wave length at 210 nm from the peak area at specific retention time for lactic acid and by considering the regression curve factor.

### Statistical Analysis

All the experiments mentioned in this paper were repeated twice. The mean and the standard error of the data obtained from three parallel experiments were calculated using MINITAB 14.

## Results and Discussion

### Phenotypic Characterization

Four different bacterial strains isolated from fermented finger millet *"raavana"* variety. Among them, gram positive, cocci shaped that grow on MRS agar with typical LAB colony characteristics such as punctiform, glistening colony with entire margins and raised elevation was selected for further studies. Further, the isolate observed to be non-spore forming and non-motile.

### Biochemical Characterization

The isolate demonstrates negative reactions to the biochemical tests including catalase, starch hydrolysis, Indole, Voges Proskeur, Methyl Red and citrate utilization thus exhibited typical LAB biochemical characteristics. Among the tested sugars, it ferments glucose, fructose, maltose, lactose, galactose, sucrose, salicinsorbitol, mannitol, cellulose, cellobiose and dextrose. However do not ferment melezitose, melibiose, arabinose and ribose.

### Genotypic Characterization

The isolate was genotypically identified as *Lactococcus lactis* subsp. *lactis*. Partial sequence of the 16S rRNAgene of the Sri Lankan strain was deposited in the NCBI gene bank as *Lactococcus lactis* subsp. *lac*tis FM_19LAB and the accession number MF480428 was obtained.

### *In vitro* Safety Attributes

*Lactococcus lactis* subsp. *lactis* FM_19LAB did not demonstrate hemolysis, DNAse and gelatin hydrolysis thus indicating its' safety to use as potential probiotic.

### *In vitro* Probiotic Attributes

*Lactococcus lactis* subsp. *lactis* FM_19LAB could tolerate pH 3 and 4 not 2. Further, except 2 per cent, the strain could tolerate all the other bile concentrations tested. Moreover, it tolerate salt only up to 5 per cent. *Lactococcus lactis* subsp. *lactis* FM_19LAB could tolerate simulated gastric juice up to pH 4,wheras it did not survive in gastric juice containing pH 2 and 3. The isolate tolerate phenol up to 0.2 per cent and grow luxuriously in all the tested temperatures (Table 16.1).

**Table 16.1: Probiotic Attributes of *Lactococcus lactis* subsp. *lactis* FM_19LAB**

| *Acid (pH)* | | *Bile (per cent)* | | | | | *Salt (per cent)* | | | | *G.J(pH)* | | | *Phenol (per cent)* | | | | | *Temp (ºC)* | | |
|---|---|---|---|---|---|---|---|---|---|---|---|---|---|---|---|---|---|---|---|---|---|
| *3* | *4* | *0.2* | *0.5* | *1.0* | *1.5* | *2.0* | *4* | *5* | *8* | *12* | *2* | *3* | *4* | *0.1* | *0.2* | *0.3* | *0.4* | *0.5* | *30* | *37* | *42* |
| - + | + | + | + | + | + | - | + | + | - | - | - | - | + | + | + | - | - | - | + | + | + |

+: Tolerate; -: Do not tolerate; G.J: Gastric Juice.

## Investigating Antibiotic Susceptibility of Potential Probiotic by Alamar Blue Cell Viability Assay

Antibiotic sensitivity/resistance pattern of *Lactococcus lactis* subsp. *lac*tis FM_19LAB is illustrated in the Table 16.2.

**Table 16.2: Antibiotic Sensitivity/Resistance Pattern of *Lactococcus lactis* subsp. *lactis* FM_19LAB**

| *Test Antibiotics (100 µg/ml)* | *Percentage Inhibition (Per cent) of Lactococcus lactis subsp. lactis FM_19LAB Cells by the Antibiotic* |
|---|---|
| Netilmycin | 47.56 ± 1.39 |
| Amikacin | 26.97 ±0.34 |
| Gentamycin | 14.71 ± 0.81 |
| Ofloxacin | 14.63 ± 0.55 |
| Cefoxitin | 19.29 ± 0.41 |
| Doxycycline | 12.55 ± 0.68 |
| Sulbactum | 23.66 ± 0.56 |
| Neomycin | 37.15 ± 0.37 |
| Ampicillin | 22.57 ± 0.67 |
| Vancomycin | 31.31 ± 0.42 |
| Oxycillin | 31.81 ± 0.78 |
| Streptomycin | 42.34 ± 0.15 |
| Penicillin | 72.83 ± 1.99 |
| Nitrofurantoin | 55.36 ± 0.42 |
| Sulfamethoxazole | 67.25 ±0.30 |
| Cholramphenicol | 19.05 ±0.17 |
| Trimethoprin | 22.10 ± 0.44 |
| Clindamycin | 0.04 ± 0.01 |
| Ciprofloxacin | 25.85 ± 0.78 |
| Coistin | 35.05 ± 0.84 |
| Ceftazidime | 47.09 ±1.13 |
| Nystatin | 59.42 ± 2.07 |
| Imipanum | 95.70 ±0.35 |
| Tetracycline | 24.21 ± 0.66 |

Data is expresses as mean ± SEM, n=9.

Results of the antibiotic susceptibility pattern of *Lactococcus lactis* subsp. *lac*tis FM_19LAB obtained from the Alamar blue assay revealed that, imipanum have the highest inhibitory activity followed by penicillin and sulfamethoxazole. Furthermore, when the inhibition of test antibiotics observed to be <10 per cent,it was considered as the strain is potentially resistant to particular antibiotic. Such scenario was only observed in clindamycin that exhibit poorest inhibition of the probiotic strain.

## *In vitro* Antimicrobial Activity of *L. lactis* subspp. *lactis* FM_19LAB

**Table 16.3: Antimicrobial Activity of *Lactococcus lactis* subsp. *lactis* FM_19LAB against Sensitive and Multi Drug Resistant Pathogens**

| *Test Pathogen* | *Antimicrobial Activity of Probiotic Strains Diameter of the Zone of Inhibition (in mm)* |
|---|---|
| **Drug sensitive organisms** | |
| *E. coli* ATCC 2592 | 15.33 ± 0.33 |
| *K. pneumonia* ATCC 35594 | 15.00 ± 0.00 |
| *S. aureus* ATCC 6571 | 12.66 ± 0.33 |
| *S. sanguinis* ATCC 10556 | 0.00 ± 0.00 |
| *S. salvarius* ATCC 13419 | 16.00 ± 0.00 |
| *S. flexenari* ATCC 12022 | 16.00 ±0.00 |
| *E. faecilis* ATCC49532 | 0.00 ±0.00 |
| *A. baumani* ATCC 17978 | 11.33 ± 0.33 |
| *S. mutans* ATCC 25175 | 0.00 ± 0.00 |
| *S. pyogenes* ATCC 700294 | 12.33 ± 0.33 |
| **Multi Drug Resistant Organisms (MDR)** | |
| *E. coli* ATCC 35218 | 18.33 ± 0.33 |
| *S.aureus* 17EMRSA COCR | 14.66 ± 0.33 |
| *S.aureus* 16 EMRSA NCTC 13143 | 17.66 ± 0.66 |
| *K.pneumonia* ATCC 700603 | 0.00 ± 0.00 |
| *E.faecilis* ATCC 700802 | 0.00 ± 0.00 |
| *S.enterica* ATCC 700408 | 9.66 ± 0.88 |

Data is expresses as mean ± SEM, n=9.

Among the drug sensitive pathogens, *Lactococcus lactis* subsp. *lac*tis FM_19LAB demonstrated highest inhibition in *S. salvarius* ATCC 13419 and*S. flexenari* ATCC 12022.Whereas, it did not inhibit *S. mutans*ATCC 25175. Among the MDR pathogens, *Lactococcus lactis subsp. lac*tis FM_19LAB demonstrated highestinhibition in *E. coli*ATCC 35218 followed by *S.aureus* 16 EMRSA NCTC 13143. Whereas, it did not inhibit *K.pneumonia* ATCC 700603 and *E.faecilis* ATCC 700802.

As reported by many authors, the antimicrobial activity is one of the most important selection criteria for probiotics. Where, probiotics compete with other infectious bacteria for nutrients and cell surface (Quwehand and Vesterlund, 2004, Cakýr, 2003; Rodriguez *et al.*, 2003).Therefore, the results of the antimicrobial activity of the *Lactococcus lactis* subsp. *lac*tis FM_19LAB revealed its'ability to inhibit both drug sensitive and multi drug resistant human pathogens that are causing infections in the gastrointestinal track, respiratory track as well as in the skin. Thus, provide information regarding it's' potentiality to use them in novel therapeutic food developments. Furthermore, the stranded drug imipeum used as the control with every experiment and it demonstrated highest antimicrobial activity against every tested pathogen.

## In vitro Anti-cancer Activity of *L. lactis* subspp. *lactis* FM_19LAB

The anticancer activity of *L. lactis* subsp. *plactis* FM_19LAB observed to increase with increasing the concentration of CFE and CFL. Further, both CFE and CFL of *lactis sub spplactis* FM_19LAB inhibit HT 29 cell line than HCT 116 (Table 16.4).

**Table 16.4: Results of the Anticancer Activity of different Concentrations of *Lactococcus lactis* subsp. *lactis* FM_19LABCFE and CFL Values against HT 29 and HCT 116 Cell Line**

| Percentage inhibition (per cent) of HT 29 cell line by test probiotic CFE at different concentrations | | | | | |
|---|---|---|---|---|---|
| 5 µl/ml | 25 µl/ml | 50 µl/ml | 250 µl/ml | 500 µl/ml | $IC_{50}$ |
| 6.23 ± 1.62 | 16.20 ± 3.78 | 51.55 ± 3.66 | 65.97 ±1.13 | 80.11 ± 0.58 | 247.12 ± 4.68 |
| **Percentage inhibition (per cent) of HT 29 cell line by test probiotic CFL at different concentrations** | | | | | |
| 1250 µg/ml | 2500 µg/ml | 3750 µg/ml | 5000 µg/ml | 7500 µg/ml | $IC_{50}$ |
| 31.37 ± 1.73 | 39.89 ± 3.08 | 50.23 ± 0.46 | 76.46 ± 1.64 | 95.99 ± 0.49 | 3267.6 ± 76.2 |
| **Percentage inhibition (per cent) of HCT 116 cell line by test probiotic CFE at different concentrations** | | | | | |
| 5 µl/ml | 25 µl/ml | 50 µl/ml | 250 µl/ml | 500 µl/ml | $IC_{50}$ |
| 0.00 ± 0.00 | 13.80 ± 1.80 | 20.87 ± 0.77 | 63.19 ± 2.26 | 73.16 ± 0.60 | 319.43 ± 3.74 |
| **Percentage inhibition (per cent) of HCT 116 cell line by test probiotic CFL at different concentrations** | | | | | |
| 1250 µg/ml | 2500 µg/ml | 3750 µg/ml | 5000 µg/ml | 7500 µg/ml | $IC_{50}$ |
| 10.15 ± 0.45 | 21.15 ± 0.45 | 52.46 ± 1.98 | 73.16 ± 0.60 | 87.15 ± 0.71 | 4174.0 ± 3.03 |

Data is expresses as mean ± SEM, n=9.

## DPPH Radical Scavenging Activity of *L. lactis* subspp. *lactis* FM_19LAB

It was observed that the DPPH radical scavenging activity of *L. lactis* subsp. *plactis* FM_19LAB increased with the increment of both CFE and CFL (Figures 16.1 and 16.2).

## In vitro Cholesterol of *L. lactis* subspp. *lactis* FM_19LAB

*Lactococcus lactis* subsp. *lactis* FM_19LAB observed to be weak cholesterol assimilator that assimilated 4.42 per cent of cholesterol in the growth medium. As reported by many authors, the cholesterol lowering effect is one of the most important selection criteria for probiotics thus can accept as an alternative therapy for treating hyperlipidemia (Homayouni *et al.*, 2012). Although test probiotic do

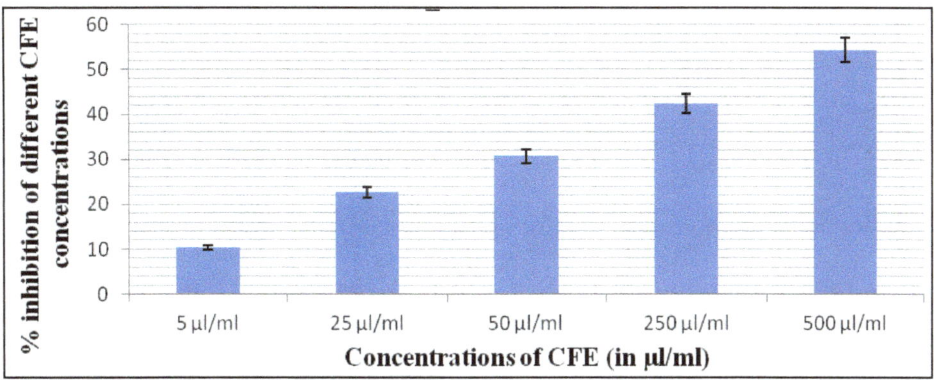


**Figure 16.1: DPPH Radical Scavenging Activity of *Lactococcus lactis* subsp. *lactis* FM_19LAB CFE (Data is expresses as mean ± SEM, n=9).**

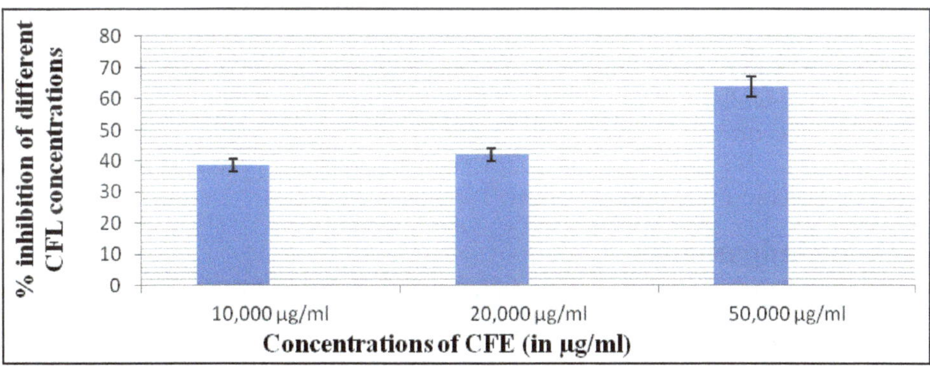


**Figure 16.2: DPPH Radical Scavenging Activity of *Lactococcus lactis* subsp. *lactis* FM_19LAB CFL (Data is expresses as mean ± SEM, n=9).**

not effective in removing cholesterol as a standard drug; however the results of the cholesterol assimilation of the test probiotic used in this study revealed its' ability to assimilate cholesterol at $10^{10}$cfu/ml concentration. Thus, provide information regarding its' potentiality to use them in novel therapeutic food developments.

## *In vitro* Lactic Acid Production by *L. lactis* subspp. *lactis* FM_19LAB

Lactic acid is a commercially important organic acids produced by LAB. Furthermore, lactic acid contributes food preservation as well as exerts antagonistic effect against human pathogenic microorganisms (Asmahan Ali, 2010). Therefore, ability to produce lactic acid is one of the important criteria of probiotics to become commercially successful starter cultures. It was observed that, at the end of the fermentation period, *Lactococcus lactis* subsp. *lactis* FM_19LAB produced 4.62± 0.07 mg/ml lactic acid. Further, it was observed that, the lactic acid synthesis was increased with the time (Figure 16.3).

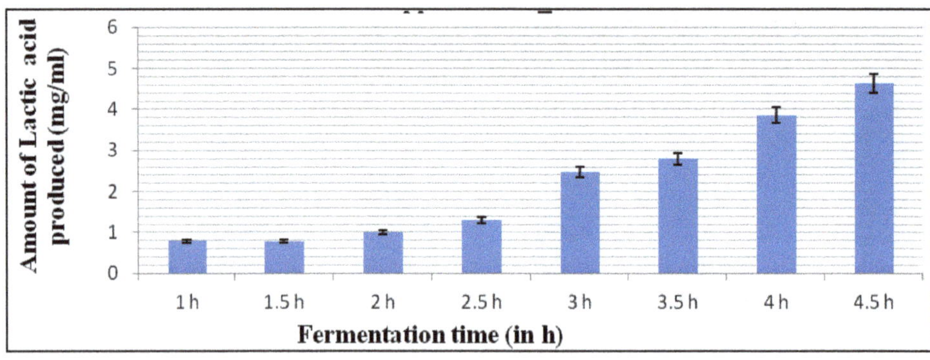


**Figure 16.3: Lactic Acid Production by *L. lactis* subspp. *lactis* FM_19LAB (Data is expresses as mean ± SEM, n=9).**

## Conclusion

This study concludes that *Lactococcus lactis* subsp. *lactis* FM_19LAB isolated from Sri Lankan grown finger millet var. *Raavana* has probiotic attributes, *in vitro* safety properties as well as *in vitro* efficacy. However, the strain needs to be investigated for its' *in-vivo* oral and geno toxicity prior to commercial applications. This is the first report on isolation and characterisation of probiotic potential *Lactococcusspp* from Sri Lankan finger millet variety *'Raavana'*.

## Acknowledgements

Authors like to acknowledge the financial assistance by the Indian - Sri Lankan Inter Governmental Science and Technology Cooperation Program, Government of Sri Lanka and India.

## REFERENCES

1. Aswathy, R.G., Ismail, B., John, R.P., and Nampoothiri, K.M 2008. Evaluation of the probiotic characteristics of newly isolated lactic acid bacteria. *J. Applied Biochemistry and Biotechnology*, 151: 244-255.

2. Bergonzelli G.E., Granato, D., Pridmore, R.D., Marvin-Guy,L.F., Donnicola,D., Corthesy-Theulaz., I.E 2006. GroEL of *Lactobacillus johnsonii* La1 (NCC 533) is cell surface associated: potential role in interactions with the host and the gastric pathogen *Helicobacter pylori. American Society for Microbiology*, 74: 425-434.

3. Charalampopoulos, D., Wang, R., Pandiella, S.S., Webb, C 2002. Application of cereals and cereal components in functional foods: A review. *Int. J. Food Microbiol.*, 79: 131–141.

4. Collado, M., Meriluoto, J., and Salminen, S 2008. Adhesion and aggregation properties of probiotic and pathogen strains. *Eur. Food Res. Technol.*, 226: 1065–1073.

5. D'Souza, A.L., Rajkumar, C., Cooke, J., Bulpitt, C.J 2002. Probiotics in prevention of antibiotic associated diarrhoea: meta-analysis. *British Medical Journal*, 324: 1-6.

6. De Vuyst L., Leroy F 2007. Bacteriocins from lactic acid bacteria: production, purification, and food applications. *J. Mol. Microbiol. Biotechnol.*, 13: 194–199.

7. C. Koebnick, C., Wagner, I., Leitzmann, P., Stern, U and Zunft, H.J 2003. Probiotic beverage containing Lactobacillus casei Shirota improves gastrointestinal symptoms in patients with chronic constipation. *J Gastroenterol.*, 17(11): 655-659.

8. Kos, B., Suskovi, J., Vukovi, S., Simpraga, M., Frece, J and Matosi, S 2005. Adhesion and Aggregation ability of probiotic strain *Lactobacillus acidophilus* M92. *J. Appl. Microbiol.*, 94: 981–987.

9. Laroia, S and Martin, J.H 1991. Effect of pH on survival of *Bifidobacterium bifidum* and *Lactobacillus acidophilusin* frozen fermented dairy desserts". *Cultured Dairy Products Journal*, 26: 13-21.

10. Naderi N.J., Niakan M., Kharazi Fard M.J., Zardi S 2011. Antibacterial activity of Iranian green and black tea on streptococcus mutants: an *in vitro* study. *J Dent.*, 8: 55-9.

11. Penna, A.L.B., Rao-gurram, S. and Barbosa-canovas, G.V 2007. Effect of milk treatment on acidification, physico-chemical characteristics, and probiotic cell counts in low fat yogurt. *Milchwissenschaft*, 62: 48-52.

12. Report of a Joint FAO/WHO Working Group on Drafting Guidelines for the Evaluation of Probiotics in Food, 2002.

13. Schrezenmeir, J and De vrese, M 2001. Probiotics, prebiotics, and symbiotics - approaching a definition. *American Journal of Clinical Nutrition*, 77: 361-364.

14. Sripriya, G., Antony, U., and Chandra, T.S 1994. Changes in carbohydrate, free amino acids, organic acids, phytate and HCl extractability of minerals during germination and fermentation of finger millet (*Eleusinecoracana*). *Food Chem.*, 58(4): 345–350.

15. Whelan, K. and Quigley, E.M 2013. Probiotics in the management of irritable bowel syndrome and inflammatory bowel disease. *Current Opinion Gastroenterol.*, 29: 184-189.

*Chapter 17*

# Isolation, Characterization and Molecular Identification of New Sudanese *Streptomyces* spp. Producing Bioactive Secondary Metabolites

*Abdelhalim Abdullahi Hamza Ahmed*[1], *Benjamin R. Clark*[2], *Cormac D. Murphy*[2] *and Elsheik A. Elobiedc*[3]

[1]*Associate Professor of Microbial Biotechnology, Ministry of High Education and Scientific Research, National Center for Research Commission for Biotechnology and Genetic Engineering, Department Microbial Biotechnology PO Box: 2404, SUDAN E-mail: aahamzaa@yahoo.com*

[2]*School of Biomolecular and Biomedical Science, Centre for Synthesis and Chemical Biology, Ardmore House, University College Dublin, Dublin 4, IRELAND*

[3]*Ahfad University for Women, College of Pharmacology, Khartoum, SUDAN*

## ABSTRACT

300 actinomycete isolates were isolated from 50 soil samples collected from different geographical areas in Sudan. All these isolates were purified and screened for their antimicrobial activity against pathogenic microbes. Out of these, 60 (20 per cent) of the isolates strongly inhibit the growth of Gram positive, Gram negative bacteria and fungi. Three promising strains, with strong antimicrobial activity against pathogenic microbes designated as AH47, AH11.4 and AH4.4 were selected for further studies to be characterized and identified. These isolates were taxonomically characterized on the basis of morphological and physiological characteristics, phylogenetic analysis and genotypic data. These Streptomyces

strains were deposited at the Industrial Microbiology Department (IMD) University College of Dublin (UCD). The 16S rRNA sequences of these strains were submitted to Gene Bank (accession numbers GU013556, GU013557 and GU013558).

The pure active antibiotics were isolated from the culture supernatant and from the biomass using reverse phase HPLC-DAD. Spectroscopical analysis was carried out employing Mass, $^{1}H$ and $^{13}C$ NMR spectra data. Two newly identified *Streptomyces* isolates (AH47 and AH11.4) produced the same antibiotic actinomycin-D; These two new Streptomyces strains (AH47 and AH11.4) were able to produce a large amount of actinomycin-D (44 mg/l and 52 mg/l respectively) and serves as a promising source of this antibiotic. Additionally Strain AH47 yielded two minor compounds, in the UV absorbance maxima comparable to actinomycin D (220, 242 nm and 443 nm). On the basis of their mass fragmentation data we suggested them to be actinomycin $X_2$ (*m/z* 1269) and $X_B$ (*m/z* 1271). The Streptomyces isolate (AH4.4) produced compound was chemically characterized as Cyclo-(Proline—Phenylalnine). Actinomycin-D and cyclo (pro-phe), produced by these identified Streptomyces strains showed significant anticancer effect against human cervical carcinoma cells and Glioma UG-87 cells using MTT assay. The two antibiotics at different concentrations (1µg $ml^{-1}$, 10µg $ml^{-1}$, 20µg, 30µg $ml^{-1}$ and 40µg $ml^{-1}$) for 48 hour incubation caused death of 90 per cent of cancer cells in comparison to the control cells.

***Keywords:*** *Streptomyces sp., Actinomycin-D, Cyclo-(Proline-Phenylalnine), Anticancer activity.*

## INTRODUCTION

Antibiotics play an important role in the medical field; they treat many microbial diseases that affect humans and animals. A large percentage of these antibiotics are naturally produced by medicinal plant, bacteria and fungi. The emergence of antibiotic resistance among pathogenic bacteria has become a serious problem worldwide. Currently, actinomycetes bacteria is considered as one of the most attractive sources of antibiotics and other biologically active substances of high commercial value and they are attracting considerable interest from bacteriologists, biotechnologists, geneticists and ecologists. Streptomycetes are the source of several useful antibiotics that are used not only in the treatment of various human and animal diseases but also as biological control and biochemistry as metabolic poisons (Jones 2000). The actinomycins are a family of chromopeptide lactone antibiotics that present antitumoral properties, being employed in the treatment of several human neoplasies. Structurally, they have a chromophorous group, identical in all actinomycins, and two pentapeptide chains with a variable composition of amino acids (Kurosawa *et al.,* 2006). Among the actinomycins, actinomycin D has been studied most extensively and is used for treatment of malignant tumors, such as Wilms' tumor (Green 1997), and childhood rhabdomyosarcoma (Womer1997). Actinomycin D is produced by a range of Streptomyces species as part of a mixture of actinomycins, and by some strains of Micromonospora While soil actinomycetes have been extensively studied for their antibiotic production, Sudanese soil samples have been relatively poorly investigated. Due to the large degree of geographical variation, there are a wide variety of soil types found throughout Sudan, many of which are rich in flora and fauna and in microbial diversity. Thus, we have focused on Sudanese soil samples as a potential source of microbial diversity and hence new molecules of better therapiotic effects. This paper describes the isolation of new Streptomyces spp. from Sudanese soil, the identification of these strains and the isolation and identification of bioactive secondary metabolites with anticancer activity a as the major active component is described.

## Materials and Methods

### Isolation, Characterization and Identification of Actinomycetes Strains

*Streptomyces* strains designated as AH 47, AH 11.4 and AH 4.4 were isolated from Sudanese soil samples, collected from different locations in the Sudan. Isolation of the strains was performed by soil dilution plate technique using starch-casein nitrate agar (SCNA) supplemented with 10 µg/ml cyclohexamide (Singh and Agrawal, 2002 and 2003). The pure isolates were maintained as lyophils and as spore suspensions at -80 0C.The isolates were characterized morphologically and physiologically following the directions given by the International Streptomyces Project (ISP), Shirling and Gottlieb (1966) and Bergey's Manual of Systematic Bacteriology (1994).The bioactive isolates were grown in nutrient broth for the preparation of genomic DNA which was extracted according to methods described by Nicodinovic *et al.* (2003). PCR amplification and sequencing of 16S rRNA gene was carried out as described previously (Abdelhalim *et al.*, 2013) using a Peltier thermal cycler (BIO-RAD). Amplified fragments were purified using Qiaquick PCR clean up kit (Qiagen) according to the manufacturer's instructions, and sequenced commercially by MWG. Trees were generated using CLUSTAL X programme (Larkin *et al.*, 2007).

### Extraction, Purification and Isolation of Bioactive Secondary Metabolites

Baffled Erlenmeyer flasks (250 ml), containing 50 ml of TSB medium, were inoculated from a spore suspension, and incubated on a rotary shaker (200 rpm) at 30 °C for 48 h. The cultured broth (1 L) was centrifuged at 6000 rpm for 15 minutes to remove the biomass. Activities against test organisms (*Staphylococcus aureus, Bacillus subtilis, Streptococcus faecalis, Escherichia coli, Pseudomonas aeruginosa, Candida albicans, Aspergillus niger*, and *A. flavus*) were monitored during the isolation, using agar well diffusion assay method as described by Holder and Boyce (1994). Ethyl acetate extracts from both supernatant and mycelium were combined and concentrated under vacuum. The crude organic extract was separated by solid phase extraction (SPE) on a Hypersil C18 column, and eluted with a stepwise gradient of methanol (20-100 per cent). Fractions containing highest antibiotic activity were purified further by HPLC (Varian Prostar system) using an isocratic elution (80 per cent methanol-water) on a ZorbaxStableBond column. Peak purity was assessed by analytical HPLC with a gradient elution of acetonitile using a ThermoHypersil C18 column (4.6 x 150 mm 5 µm). Purified compounds were Spectroscopical analyzed by ESI MS, $^{1}$H and $^{13}$C NMRspectra data the compounds were chemically characterized as actinomycin-Dactinomycin X2actinomycin XαB and Cyclo-(-Pro–Phe) (Figures 17.1 and 17.2).

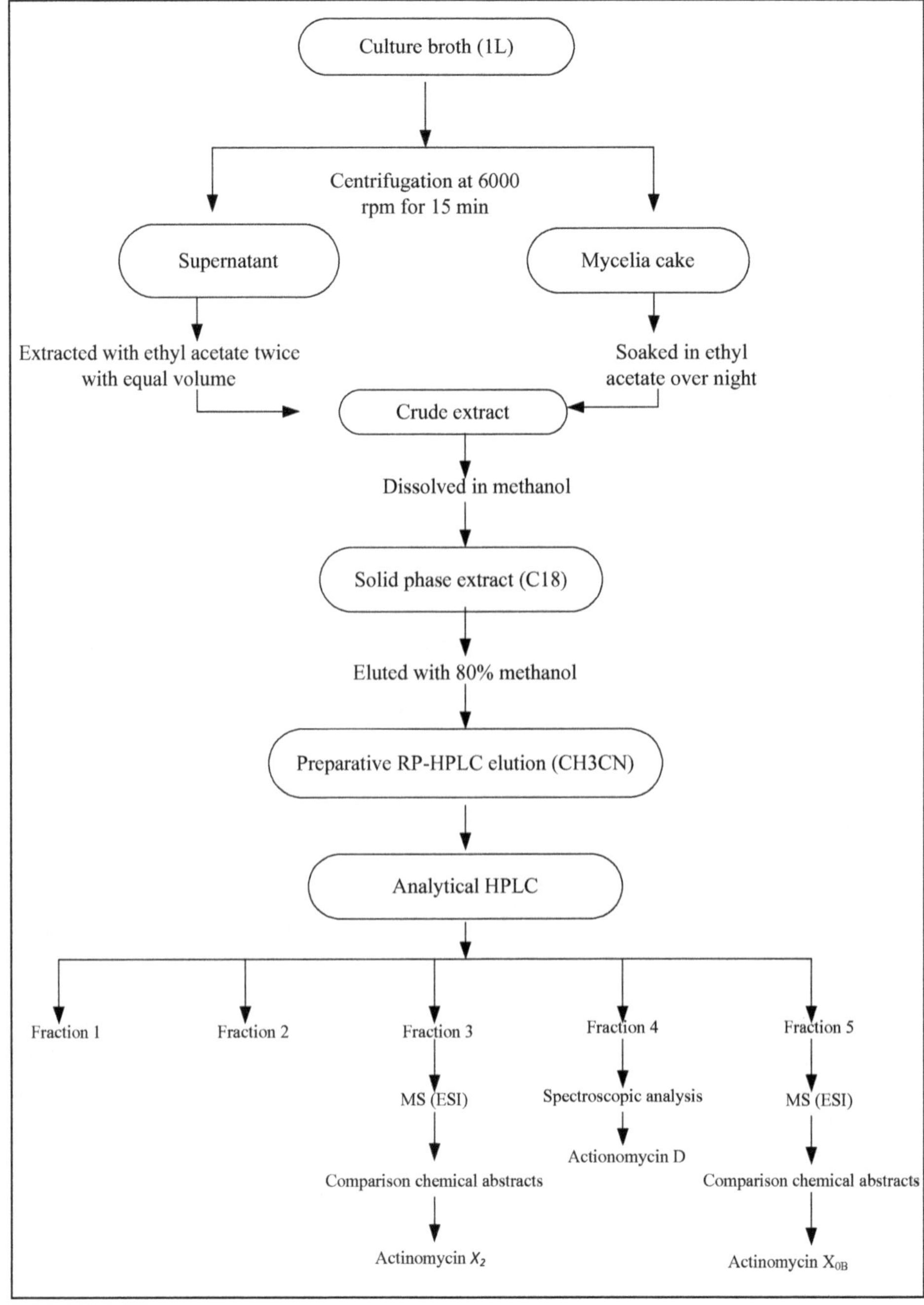


**Figure 17.1: Steps towards Extraction and Identification of Actinomycin D from *Streptomyces* sp. AH47.**

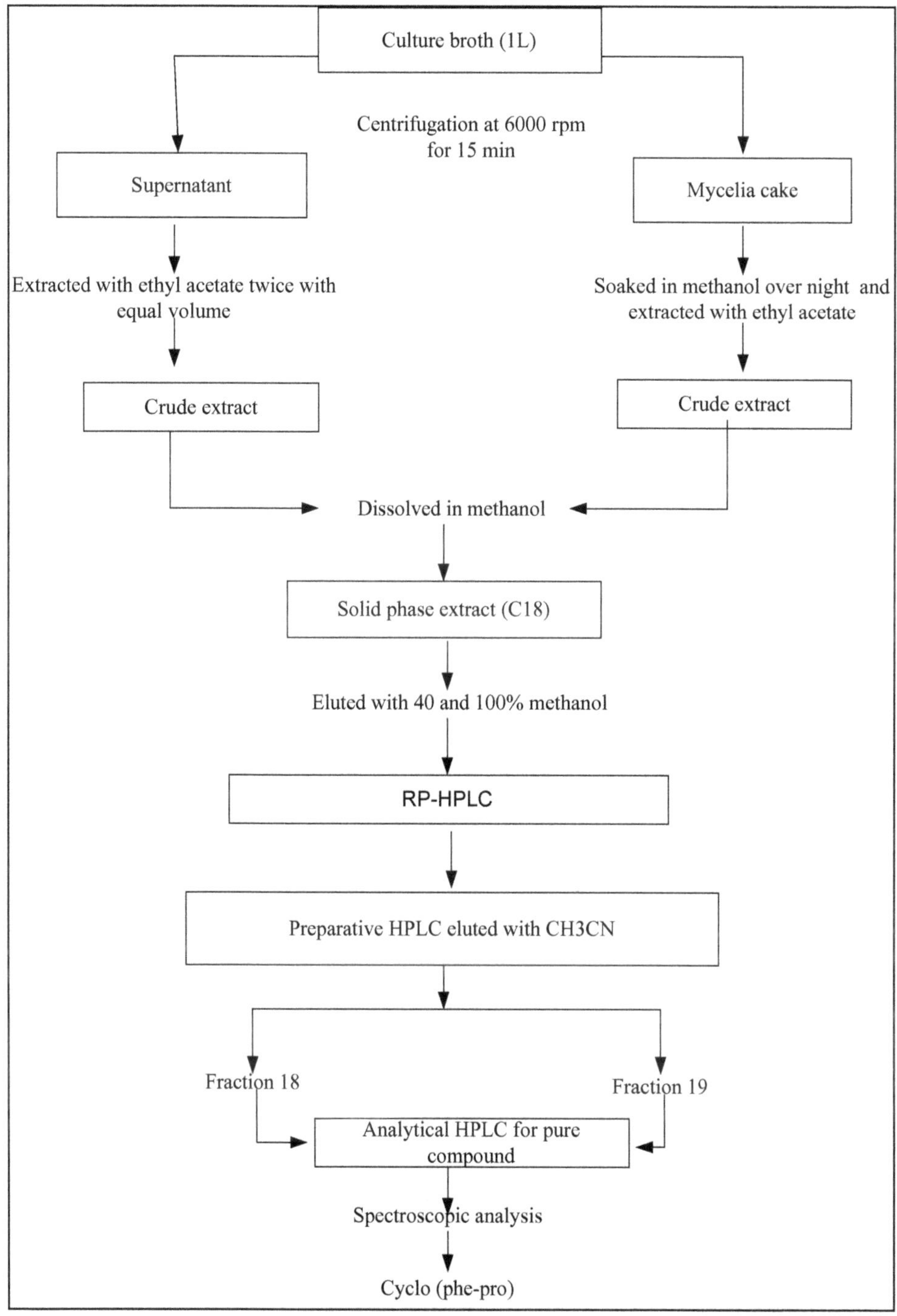


**Figure 17.2: Steps towards Extraction and Identification of Cyclo (L-phenyl, L-prolyl).**

### Production of Actinomycin D by *Streptomyces* sp. AH11.4

It is well established that antibiotic production is affected by carbohydrate (El-Tayeb *et al.*, 2004) and Shanmugaiah, (2008).In order to increase the production of acinomycin-D, ten different carbon sources: (Soluble starch, maltose, sucrose, xylose, raffinose, glycerol, D- galatose, L-arabinose and rhamnose and glucose as a control) were added to the TSB media in the shake flask at a concentration of 1 per cent (w/v), each carbon source was prepared in 50 ml broth that had been seeded to ten baffle flasks with 500 µl spore suspension of *Streptomyces* sp. Strains AH11.1, then incubated in shaker incubator at 30°C with shaking at 220 rpm for 48 hours. Actinomycin D production was tested by agar well diffusion method, against *Bacillus subtilis, S. aureus* and *E. coli.*

### Antitumor Activity of the Actinomycin D and Cyclo (L-phenyl, L-prolyl)

Various cell lines, such as cervical carcinoma cells and Glioma cells UG- 87, were used to evaluate the *in vitro* antitumor effects of the actinomycin-Dand cyclo (L-phenyl, L-prolyl) in the University College Dublin (Ireland) Conway institute of biomolecular and biomedical research. Growth inhibitory effect of glioma cells (UG- 87) and hela (cervical) cells with various treatments was measured by 3-(4,5-dimethylthiazol-2-yl)-2,5- diphenyltetrazolium bromide (MTT, Sigma Chemical Co) assay as described by Qing Chen *et al.* (2003) and by Lu *et al.* (2005). Cells were grown in MEM medium and incubated at 37 °C in a humidified atmosphere containing 5 per cent CO2. Tumor cells (1500 cell per well) in their exponential growth phase were transferred into 96 well plates, Then cells were exposed to different concentrations (1µg $ml^{-1}$, 10µg $ml^{-1}$, 20µg, 30µg $ml^{-1}$ and 40µg $ml^{-1}$) of the compounds for 24 h, and each treatment was tested in triplicate wells. At the end of exposure, 20 µL of MTT (5 g/L) was added to each well and the plates were incubated at 37 °C for 4 h. Incubation was carried out for 48 h in 5 per cent $CO_2$ incubator. the medium was removed, rinsed with phosphate buffer solution and trypsin were added. The trypsinised cells were counted by mixing equal volumes of the cell suspension and trypan blue dye. Morphological changes and death in cells were evaluated by phase-contrast microscopy.

## Results and Discussion

### Cultural Characteristics of Biologically Active *Streptomyces* spp.

During screening of Actinomycetes from Sudanese soils for bioactive natural products, different Streptomyces bacteria were isolated and tested for their antibiotic activity against a range of target organisms. Three isolates designated as strains AH47, AH11.4 and AH 4.4 which appeared to be actinomycetes, displayed a broad antimicrobial spectrum were selected for further analysis.

The results of the cultural and physiological characteristics of these isolates were shown in Table 17.1 and Figure 17.3. The comparison of these observed cultural characteristics with those of the known actinomycete species described in Bergey's manual of Systematic bacteriology, strongly suggested these strains AH

**Table 17.1: Cultural Characteristics of Strains AH 47, AH 11.4 and AH 4.4 on different Media**

| | *Microorganisms* | | | | | | | | | | | |
|---|---|---|---|---|---|---|---|---|---|---|---|---|
| | *AH 47* | | | | *AH 11.4* | | | | *AH 4.4* | | | |
| *Medium* | *Growth* | *Spore Colour* | *Vegetative Mycelia* | *Soluble Pigment* | *Growth* | *Spore Colour* | *Vegetative Mycelia* | *Soluble Pigment* | *Growth* | *Spore Colour* | *Vegetative Mycelia* | *Soluble Pigment* |
| ISP2 | Poor | Grey, white edges | Cream | None | Poor | None | None | None | Abundant | Pink | Brown | None |
| ISP3 | Abundant | Grey | Cream | Green-yellow | Abundant | Grey, white edges | Yellow-green | Orange | Abundant | Rose | Yellow | None |
| ISP4 | Abundant | Dark grey | Yellow | Yellow | Abundant | Dark grey | Orange | Yellow | Abundant | Pink | Yellow | None |
| ISP5 | Poor | None | None | None | Moderate | Cream | None | None | Poor | None | None | None |
| ISP6 | Abundant | None | None | None | Moderate | None | None | None | Moderate | None | None | None |
| ISP7 | Abundant | None | None | None | Moderate | None | None | None | Poor | None | None | None |
| Nutrient agar | Poor | None | None | None | Moderate | None | None | None | Moderate | None | None | None |
| Bennett agar | Poor | None | None | None | Poor | None | None | None | Abundant | Cream | Cream | None |

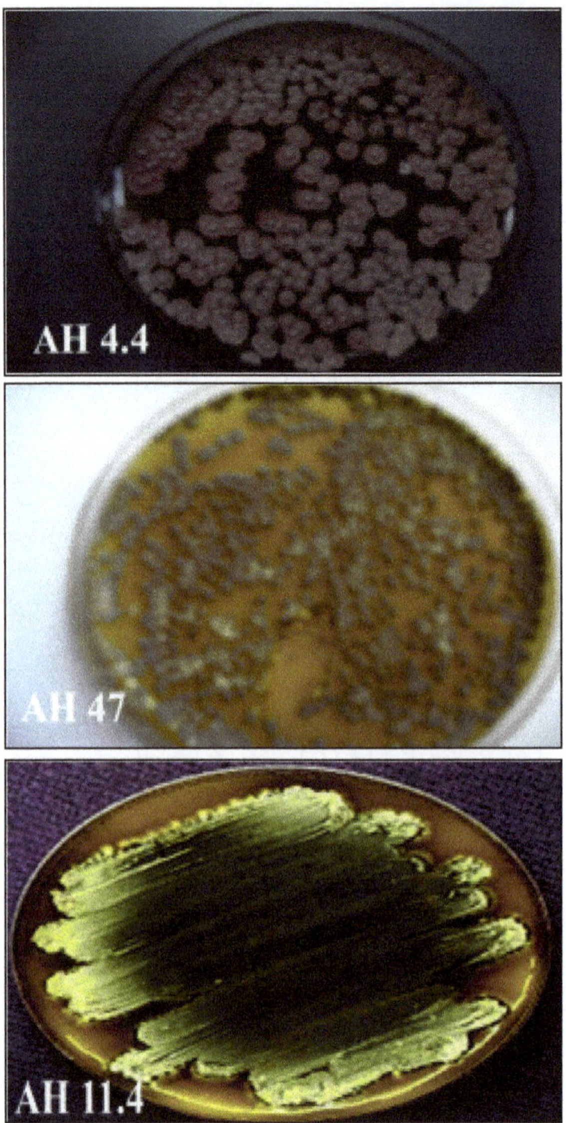


**Figure 17.3: Morphological Types of Colonies of the Selected *Streptomyces* spp.**

47,AH 11.4 and AH 4.4 belong to the genus Streptomyces. Comparison of the 16S rDNA sequences of strains AH47and AH11.4 with sequences in the Gene Bank database demonstrated that the strains was similar to the 16S rRNA sequence *Streptomyces* species. It is clear from phylogenetic analysis that our strains did not cluster with either *N. bachengensis* or any of *Streptomyces* species and represented a distinct phyletic line suggesting a new genomic species.The comparison of the 16S rRNA sequence of the AH 4.4 isolate with those sequences submitted to GenBank demonstrated that the strain was 94 per cent similar to the 16S rRNA sequence to number of isolates all of which were *Streptomyces* species, but phylogenetic analysis demonstrated that the Sudanese strain was on a different node to previously identified strains. Also it was readily distinguished strain AH4.4 from its closet phylogenetic neighbors of these species by using a combination of phenotypic properties; these species are distinct from the known producers of Cyclo (L-phenyl, L-prolyl). On the basis of these results, strain AH4.4 isproposed as the type strain of the novel species, for which the name *Streptomyces sudanensis*. AH4.4 is proposed Figure 17.4.

## Purification, Identification and Structure Elucidation of Antibiotic from *Streptomyces* sp. AH 47, AH 11.4 and AH4.4

The two strains AH 47 and AH 11.4 produced a red/orange-colored active complex. Preliminary HPLC-DAD analysis of ethyl acetate extract identified an absorbance spectrum characteristic of actinomycins. This tentative identification was supported by the observation of strong ions in the ESI (+) MS spectra of the extracts corresponding to the presence of actinomycin D (*m/z* 1255, $[M+H]^+$). Purification of the active compound was carried out using reverse phase SPE and HPLC. NMR analysis (COSY, HSQC, and HMBC) Figure 17.5. Strain AH47 also yielded two minor compounds, which were eluted from the HPLC column at retention times very close to actinomycin D (15.36 and 16.53 min), and had similar UV absorbance maxima to actinomycin D (220, 242 and 443 nm) On the basis of their mass fragmentation data and UV data and after comparison to reported data we suggest to be actinomycin X2 (*m/z* 1269) and actinomycin XαB (m/z 1271) (Kurosawa, *et al.*, 2006). Interestingly, this combination of actinomycins is also produced by *S. padanus* MITKK-103 (Kurosawa, *et al.*, 2006), which is physiologically and phylogenetically distinct from AH47.

The bioactive compound was isolated from the strains AH 4.4 and was revealed to be cyclo (L-phenyl, L-prolyl) by UV, 1H- and $^{13}$C-NMR and MS analyses and by comparison with reference data from literature Table 17.2 and Figure 17.5.

**Table 17.2: Peak No HPLC Data (Rt), Molecular Weight, (m/z), and Assigned Structures of Compounds in the Ethyl Acetate Extract of *Streptomyces* sp. AH 47, AH 11.4 and AH 4.4**

| *Peak No* | *$R_t$(min)* | *M+(m/z)* | *UV nm* | *Metabolites* |
|---|---|---|---|---|
| 1 | 15.36 | 1269 | 220 | Actinomycin $X_2$ |
| 2 | 16.3 | 1255 | 441 | Actinomycin-D |
| 3 | 16.53 | 1271 | 242 | Actinomycin $X_{dinnaB}$ |
| 4 | 23 | 245 | 212 | Cyclo (phenylalanine-proline) |

## Production of Actinomycin-D by *Streptomyces* sp. AH11.4

The antibiotic production by the *Streptomyces* sp. AH 11.4 was strongly influenced by carbon source. The use of starch as a carbon source yielded much higher levels of actinomycin D (306 mg/l) Table 17.3, which compared favorably to other values reported in the literature for shake-flask culture, though much higher

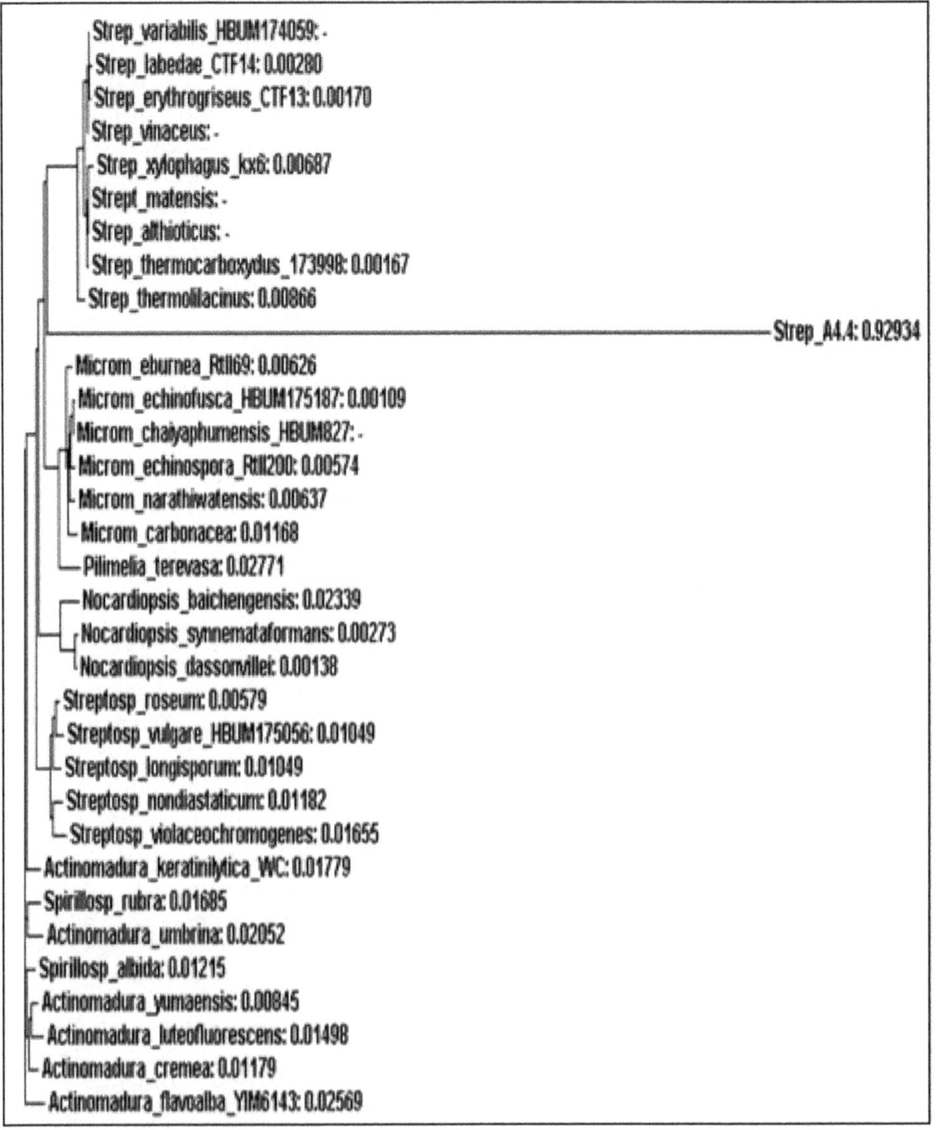


**Figure 17.4: Phylogenetic Tree Showing the Relationship between Strain AH 4.4 and Representative Species of the Genus *Streptomyces* and other Taxa Based on Nearly Complete 16S rRNA Gene Sequences.**

levels have been reported using a bioreactor (Sousa *et al.*, 2002). In comparison to another actinomycin-D producer described in the literature, Streptomyces sindenensis (Vandanaet al., 2008), was shown to produce 80 mg/L actinomycin-D. Sousa *et al.* (2002) reported that *S. parvulus* among three of the species of *Streptomyces* that produce actinomycins has the greatest antibiotic activity (152 mg/L), *S. felleus* 20 mg/L, and *S. regensis*, which did not exceed 12 mg/L. There is continuing interest in the actinomycins and their microbial producers; there are at least more than 20 species of *Streptomyces* capable of producing actinomycins. Examples of such strains include *S. antibioticus* (Waksman and Woodruff, 1940), *S. michiganensis* (Frommer, 1959), *S. parvulus* (Williams and Katz, 1977), *S. nasri* (El-Naggar, 1998), *S. plicatus* (Lam *et al.*, 2002), and *S. sindenensis* (Praveen *et al.*, 2008). These results suggest that *Streptomyces* sp.AH 11.4 is a comparable better producer of actinomycin D, and will be a new source of this important antibiotic. There is continuing interest in the actinomycins and their microbial producers; there are at least more than 20 species of *Streptomyces* capable of producing actinomycins. Examples of such strains include *S. antibioticus, S. michiganensis, S. parvulus, S. nasr, S. plicatus,* and *S. sindenensis.*

## Antitumor Activity of the Actinomycin-D and Cyclo (L-phenyl, L-prolyl)

Activity of actinomycin D against human cervical carcinoma cells and Glioma

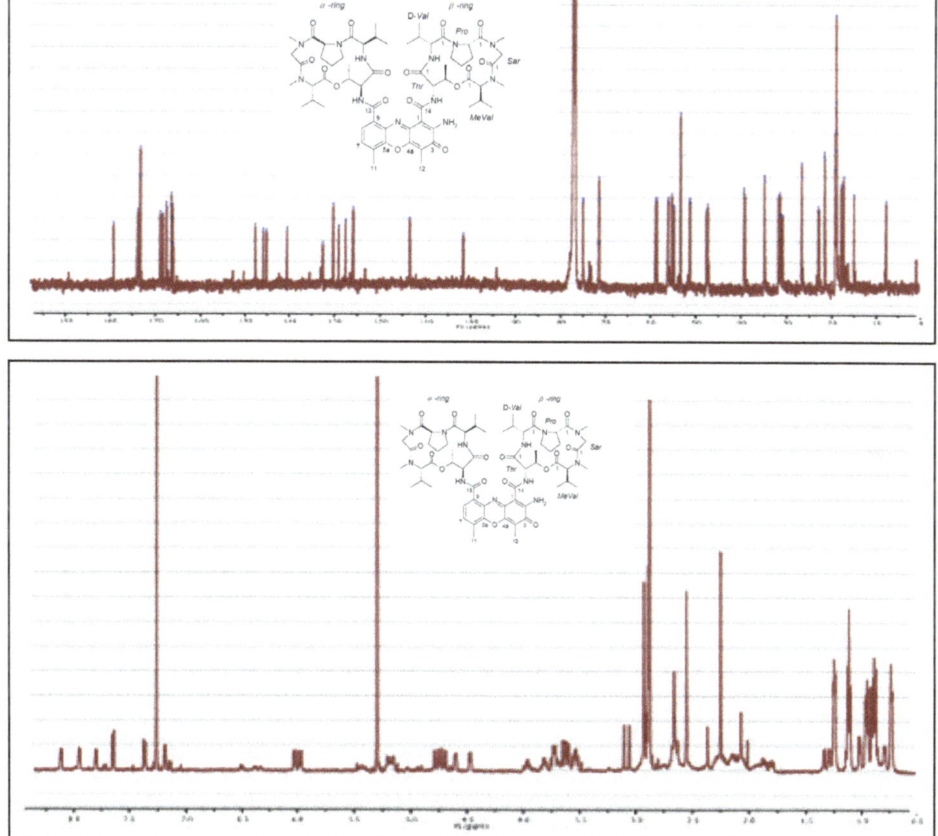


**$^{13}C$ and $^{1}H$ NMR Spectra of Actinomycin D**

**Figure 17.5a: NMR and ESI-MS Spectra and Chemical Structure of Compounds Isolated from *Streptomyces* sp. AH 47, *Streptomyces* sp. AH 11.4 and *Streptomyces* sp. AH 4.4.**

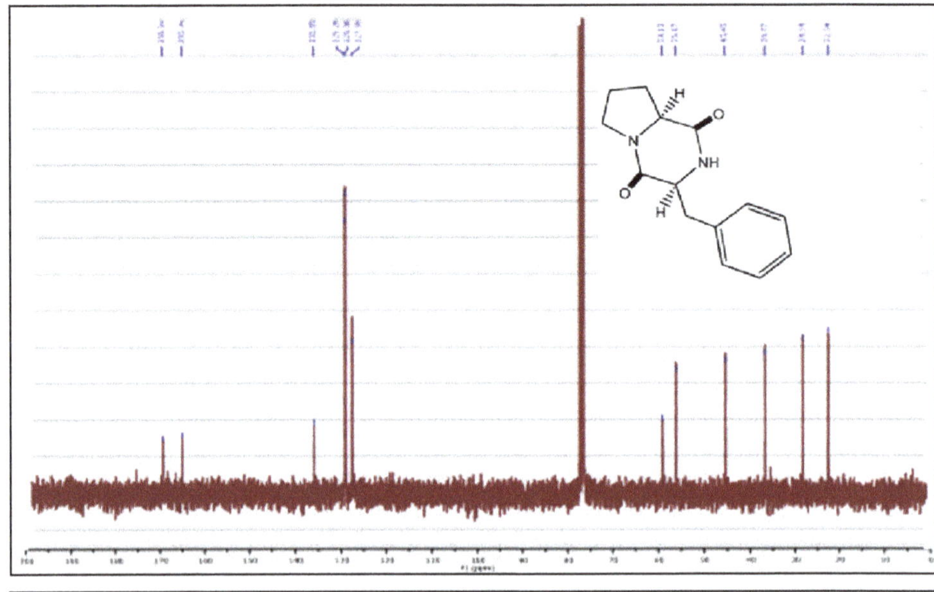


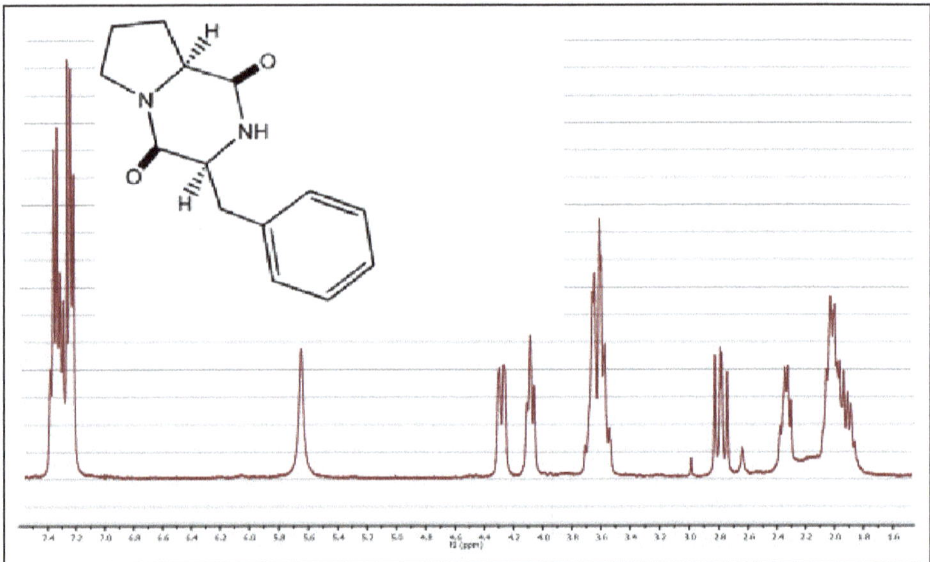


$^{13}C$ and $^{1}H$ NMR Spectra of Cyclo (phenylalanine-proline)

**Figure 17.5b: NMR and ESI-MS Spectra and Chemical Structure of Compounds Isolated from *Streptomyces* sp. AH 47, *Streptomyces* sp. AH 11.4 and *Streptomyces* sp. AH 4.4.**

cells UG as antitumor was assessed in microtiter plate using MTT assay. Figure (6) showed that the actinomycin D and cyclo (L-phenyl, L-prolyl) in concentrations of 1µg ml$^{-1}$, 10µg ml$^{-1}$, 20µg ml$^{-1}$, 30µg ml$^{-1}$ and 40µg ml$^{-1}$ showed significance activity to the human cervical carcinoma cells and Glioma cells UG- 87. Microscopically

**Table 17.3: Actinomycin D Production in Strain AH 11.4 when grown in TSB Containing different Carbohydrates**

| *Carbohydrate Source* | *Acinomycin D Production (mg/L)* |
|---|---|
| Arabinose | 185 |
| Fructose | 192 |
| Glucose | 110 |
| Glycerol | 99 |
| Maltose | 225 |
| Mannitol | 223 |
| Raffinose | 100 |
| Starch | 305 |
| Sucrose | 83 |
| Xylose | 16 |

analysis of the isolated compound suggested antitumor response, because they caused 90 per cent death of the treated cells in compression to the control cells. These results agreed with those of (Takusagawa *et al.*, 2001) who found that the actinomycin D has been shown to have higher activity towards human leukemia cell lines such as HL-60 cells.

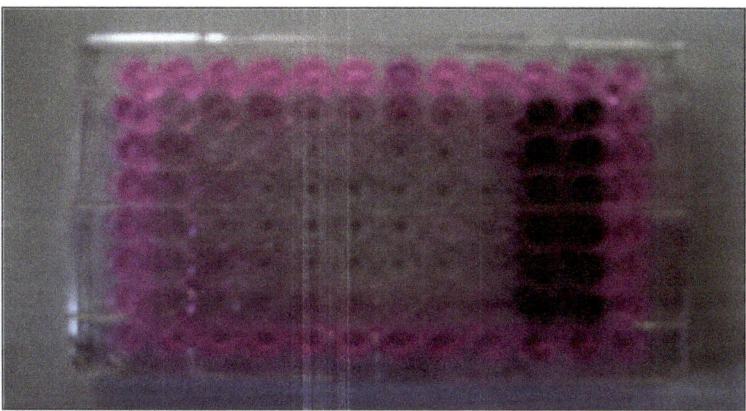

**Figure 17.6: Antitumor Activity of Actinomycin-D with Various Concentrations against Human Cervical Carcinoma Cells.**

## Conclusions

1. A new actinomycin-D producing streptomyces was isolated from Sudanese soil and characterized as *Streptomyces* spp. by 16S rRNA homology.
2. *Streptomyces* sp. AH 47 was the new species of the genus actinomycetes that had the highest level of antibiotic activity and produced mixture of actinomycins.

3. Starch showed to be a better substrate than other carbohydrates for the antibiotic production, by *Streptomyces* sp.AH 11.4 obtaining a maximum actinomycin-D (306 mg/L).
4. TSB medium showed the highest yield of actinomycin-D in shake flask fermentation, with 200 rpm and 30°C, 0.5 ml/50 ml spore suspension and pH 6.
5. The full capacity of AH 11.4 as an actinomycin D producer remains to be exploited as it has the potential for industrial production of this antibiotic.

## Acknowledgments

The author would like to express sincere gratitude to the supervisor Professor. Elshiek.A. Elobied, and he also wish to express his gratitude to Dr. Cormac D. Murphy, and his group University college Dublin (Ireland) UCD. This work was supported by the UNESCO Fellowship Programme (AAH) and the Irish Research Council for Science Engineering and Technology (BC).

## REFERENCES

1. AbdelhalemHamza A, Hiba A. Ali, Benjamin R. Clark, Cormac D. Murphy and Elobaid, A. Elshaik 2013. Isolation and characterisation of actinomycin D producing Streptomyces spp. from Sudanese soil. *African Journal of Biotechnology* 12(9): 2624-2632.
2. Bergey, D. H 1994. Bergey's manual of determinative bacteriology, Baltimore: Williams and Wilkins.
3. El-Naggar MYM 1998. Synergistic effect of actinomycin X-2produced by *Streptomyces nasri* strain YG62 with otherantibiotics. *Biomedical Lett.*, 58: 169-173.
4. El-Tayeb, O. M., Hussein, M. M. M., Salama, A. A. and El-Sedawy, H.F.1 2004. Optimization of industrial production of rifamycin B by Amycolatopsismediterranei. II. The role of gene amplification and physiological factors in productivity in shake flasks. *African Journal of Biotechnology* 3 (5),. 273-280,
5. Frommer, W 1959. ZurSystematik der actinomycinbildendenstreptomyceten. *Arch Mikrobiol.*, 32: 187–206.
6. Gallo, M, and Katz, E 1972. Regulation of secondary metabolite biosynthesis - catabolite repression of phenoxazinone synthase and actinomycin formation by glucose. *Journal of Bacteriology*, 109(2): 659-667.
7. Green, D. M 1997. Paediatric oncology update/Wilms' tumour. *Eur. J. Cancer,* 33: 409–418.
8. Holder, I. A, Boyce, S. T 1994. Agar well diffusion assay testingof bacterial susceptibility to various antimicrobials in concentrations non-toxic for human cells in culture. *Burns*, 20: 426-429
9. Jones, G, H 2000. Actinomycin production persists in a strain of *Streptomyces* antibiotic usphenoxazinone synthase. *Antimicrobial Agents and Chemotherapy,* 44(5): 1322-1327.

10. Kurosawa, K, B., V. P., VanEssendelft, J. L., Willis, L. B., Lessard, P. A., Ghiviriga, I., Sambandan, T. G., Rha, C. K., Sinskey, A. J 2006. Characterization of Streptomyces MITKK-103, a newly isolated actinomycin X2-producer. *Appl. Microbiol. Biotechnol.*, 72: 145–154.
11. Lam K, Gustavson DR, Pirnik DL, Pack E, Bulanhagui C,Mamber SW, Forenza S, Stodieck LS, Klaus DM 2002. Theeffect of space flight on the production of actinomycin D by*Streptomyces plicatus*. *J. Ind. Microbiol. Biotechnol.*, 29: 299-302.
12. Larkin, M. A, Blackshields, G., Brown, N. P, Chenna, R, McGettigan, P. A, McWilliam, H, Valentin, F, Wallace, IM, Wilm, A, Lopez, R, Thompson, JD, Gibson, TJ, Higgin DG 2007. Clustal W and clustal X version 2.0. *Bioinformatics*, 23(21): 2947-2948.
13. Liu, Z., Yanlin, S., Zhang, Y., Zhou, Z., LU, Z., LI, W., and Huang, Y., Rodriguez., C. and Goodfellow, M 2005. Classification of Streptomyces griseus (Krainsky 1914) Waksman and Henrici 1948 and related species and the transfer of 'Microstreptosporacinerea' to the genus *Streptomyces* as *Streptomyces yanii* sp. Nov. *International Journal of Systematic and Evolutionary Microbiology*, 55: 1605-1610.
14. Nikodinovic, J, Barrow, K. D, and Chuck, J. A 2003. High yield preparation of genomic DNA from Streptomyces. *Biotechniques* 35 (5): 932-934.
15. Praveen V, Tripathi CKM, Bihari V, Srivastava SC 2008.Production of Actinomycin-D by the Mutant of a New Isolate of *Streptomyces sindenensis. Brazilian J. Microbiol.*, 39: 689-692.
16. Qing Chen, Miao Ze-Hong, Tong Lin-Jiang, Zhang Jin-Sheng, Ding Jian (2003). Actinomycin D inhibiting K562 cell apoptosis elicited by salvicine but not decreasingits cytotoxicity1. *Acta Pharmacol Sin.*, 24 (5): 415-421
17. Shanmugaiah, V. A., Mathivanan, N., Balasubramanian, N., and Manoharan, P.T 2008. Optimization of cultural conditions for production of chitinase by Bacillus laterosporous MML2270 isolated from rice rhizosphere soil. *African Journal of Biotechnology*, 7(15): 2562-2568.
18. Shirling, E. B. and Gottlieb, D 1966. Methods for characterization of Streptomyces species. *International Journal of Systematic Bacteriology*, 16: 313-340.
19. Singh, D., and Agrawal, V.P 2002. Microbial Biodiversity of Mount Everest Region, a paper presented in International Seminar on Mountains-Kathmandu, March 6-8 (organized by Royal Nepal Academic of Science and Technology).
20. Singh, D., and Agrawal, V.P 2003. Diversity of Actinomycetes of Lobuche in Mount Everest 1 Proceedings of International Seminar on Mountains-Kathmandu, March 6 – 8, 2022 pp. 357-360.
21. Sousa. M. F.V.Q. .Lopes. C. E and Pereira Jr. N 2002. Development of A bioprocess for the production of Actinomycin-D. *Brazilian Journal of Chemical Engineering*, 19(3): 277–285.
22. Takusagawa, F., Carlson, R. G., Weaver, R. F 2001. Anti-leukemia selectivity in actinomycin analogues. *Bioorg. Med. Chem.*, 9: 719– 725.

23. Vandana, C., Praveen, K. M., Tripathi1,A., Vinod, C., Bihari1, S.C. and Srivastava, F 2008. Production of Actinomycin-D by the Mutant of a new isolate of *Streptomyces sindenensis*. *Brazilian Journal of Microbiology*, 39: 689-692.

24. Waksman, S. A. and Woodruff, H. B 1940. Bacteriostatic and bactericidal substances produced by a soil actinomyces. *Proc. Soc. Exptl. Biol. Med.*, 45: 609-614.

25. Williams WK, Katz E 1977. Development of a chemically defined medium for synthesis of actinomycin-D by *Streptomyces parvulus*. *Antimicrob. Agents Chemother.*, 11: 281-290.

26. Womer, R. B 1997. Soft tissue sarcomas. *Eur. J. Cancer*, 33: 2230– 2234; discussion 2234–2236.

# Appendix

## 16S rRNA Gene Sequence of the Isolate 47

TTCGCAGTACGCAGCATGCTGATCTGCGATTACTAGCGACTCCGACT-
TCATGGGGTCGAGTTGCAGACCCCAATCCGAACTGAGACCGGCT-
TTTTGAGATTCGCTCCACCTCGCGGTATCGCAGCTCATTGTACCGGC-
CATTGTAGCACGTGTGCAGCCCAAGACATAAGGGGCATGATGACTT-
GACGTCGTCCCCACCTTCCTCCGAGTTGACCCCGGCGGTCTCCCGT-
GAGTCCCCAGCACCACAAGGGCCTGCTGGCAACACGGGACAAGG-
GTTGCGCTCGTTGCGGGACTTAACCCAACATCTCACGACACGAGCT-
GACGACAGCCATGCACCACCTGTACACCGACCACAAGGGGGGCAC-
CATCTCTGATGCTTTCCGGTGTATGTCAAGCCTTGGTAAGGTTCTTCG-
CGTTGCGTCGAATTAAGCCACATGCTCCGCCGCTTGTGCGGGCCCCCGT-
CAATTCCTTTGAGTTTTAGCCTTGCGGCCGTACTCCCCAGGCGGGG-
CACTTAATGCGTTAGCTGCGGCACGGACGACGTGGAATGTCGCCCA-
CACCTAGTGCCCACCGTTTACGGCGTGGACTACCAGGGTATCTAATCCT-
GTTCGCTCCCCACGCTTTCGCTCCTCAGCGTCAGTATCGGCCCAGAGATC-
CGCCTTCGCCACCGGTGTTCCTCCTGATATCTGCGCATTTCACCGCTA-
CACCAGGAATTCCGATCTCCCCTACCGAACTCTAGCCTGCCCGTATC-
GACTGCAGACCCGGGGTTAAGCCCCGGGCTTTCACAACCGACGCGA-
CAAGCCGCCTACGAGCTCTTTACGCCCAATAATTCCGGACAACGCTCG-
CGCCCTACGTATTACCGCGGCTGCTGGCACGTAGTTAGCCGGCGCTTCT-
TCTGCAGGTACCGTCACTTGCGCTTCTTCCCTGCTGAAAGAGGTTTA-
CAACCCGAAGGCCGTCATCCCTCACGCGGCGTCGCTGCATCAGGCTTG-
CGCCCATTGTGCAATATTCCCCACTGCTGCCTCCCGTAGGAGTCTG-
GGCCGTGTCTCAGTCCCAGTGTGGCCGGTCGCCCTCTCAGGCGGGC-
TACCCGTCGTCGCCTTGGTGAGCCGTTACCTCACCAACAGCTGATAGG-
CGCGGGCTCATCCTGCACCGCCGGAGCTTCGATCACAGGATGCCCAA-
GATGATCAGTATCGTATTAGACCCGATsTTCCCAGCCTGGTCGAGTG-
CAGCAGATGGCCCACGGTTTACTCAACCTCGTTCGCCCAACATTA-
GACTCCCACTCCC

## 16S rRNA Gene Sequence of the Isolate 11.4

agaccggctTTTTGAGATtcgCTCCACCTCGCggtaTCGCagctcatTGtACCGGC-
CATTGTAGCACgtgTGCAGCCCAAGACATAAGGGGCAtgATGacTTGAC-
GTCGTCCCCACCTTCCTCCGagtTGACCCCGGCGGTCTCCCgtgAGTC-
CCCAGCACCACAAGGGCCTGCTGGCAACACGGGACaAGGGTTGCGCTC-
GTTGCGGgACTTAACCCAACATCTCACGACACGAGCTgaCGAcagCCATG-
CACCACCTGTACACCGACCACAAGGGGGGCACCATCTCTGATGCTTTcc-
GGTGTATGTCAAGCCTTGGTAAGGTTCTTCGCGTTGCgtcgaATTAAGC-
CACATGCTCCGCCGCTTGTGCGGGCCCCCgtCAATTCCTTTGAGTTTTAG-
CCTTGCGGCCGTaCTCCCCAGGCGGGGCACTTAATGCGTTAGCTGCGG-

CacgGACGACGTGGAATGTCGCCCACACCTAGTGCCCACCGTTTacGGCGT-
GgaCTACCAGGGTATCTAATCCTGTTCGCTCCCCACGCTTTCGCTCCTCAG-
cgTCAGTAtcggcCCagagaTCcgcCTTCGCCAccgGTGTTCCTcCTGATATCTGC-
GCATTTCACCGCTACAcCaGGaATTCCgaTCTCCCCTACcGAACTCTAGCCT-
GCCCGTATCgacTGCagacCCGGgGTTAAgCCCCGGGCTTTCAcAACCgaCgc-
gaCAAGCCGCCTAcgAgctCTTTACGCCCAATAATTCCGgaCAACGCTCGcg-
cCCtacGTATTAccgCGgcTGCTgGCacGTAGTTAGCCggcgcttctTctgCAGGTAc-
CGTCACTTgcgcTTCtTCCcTgctgAAagAGgtTtacaacccgaAGGCCGtcatcCctCAC-
gcGGc

## 16S rRNA Gene Sequence of the Isolate AH 4.4

GCGTCATTCGCGCATGCTGATCTGCGATTACTAGCGACTCCAACT-
TCATGGGGTCGAGTTGCAAACCCCAATCCGAACTGAGACCGGCT-
TTTTGAGATTCGCTCCACCTCGCGGTATCGCAGCTCTTTGTACCGGC-
CATTGTAGCACGTGTGCAGCCCAAGACATAAGGGGCATGATGACTT-
GACGTCGTCCCCACCTTCCTCCGAGTTGACCCCGGCGGTCTCCCGT-
GAGTCCCCAGCACCACAAGGGCCTGCTGGCAACACGGGACAAGGGTTG-
CGCTCGTTGCGGGACTTAACCCAACATCTCACGACACGAGCTGACGA-
CAGCCATGCACCACCTGTACACCGACCACAAGGGGGCACCCATCTCT-
GGGTGTTTCCGGTGTATGTCAAGCCTTGGTAAGGTTCTTCGCGTTG-
CGTCGAATTAAGCCACATGCTCCGCCGCTTGTGCGGGCCCCCGT-
CAATTCCTTTGAGTTTTAGCCTTGCGGCCGTACTCCCCAGGCGGG-
GAACTTAATGCGTTAGCTGCGGCACGGACGACGTGGAATGTCGCCCA-
CACCTAGTTCCCAACGTTTACGGCGTGGACTACCAGGGTATCTAATCC-
TGTTCGCTCCCCACGCTTTCGCTCCTCAGCGTCAGTATCGGCCCA-
GAGATCCGCCTTCGCCACCGGTGTTCCTCCTGATATCTGCGCATTTCAC-
CGCTACACCAGGAATTCCGATCTCCCCTACCGAACTCTAGCCTGCCCG-
TATCGAATGCAGACCCGAGGGTTAAGCCCCGGGCTTTCACATC-
CGACGCGACAAGCCGCCTACGAGCTCTCTACGCCCAATAATTCCGGA-
CAACGCTTGCGCCCTACGTATTACCGCGGCTGCTGGCACGTAGTTAGC-
CGGCGCTTTCTTCTGCAGGTACCGTCACTTTCGCTTCTTCCCTGCTGAAA-
GACGTTTACAACCCGAAGGCCGTCATCCCTCACGCTCTGTCGCTG-
CATCACGCTTTCGCCCAATGTGCAATACTCCCTCACTGCTGCCTCCCG-
TAGAGTCTGGGCCGTGACTCAGTACCAGTGTTGCCCGTCGCCGTCT-
CAGGTCAGCTACTCGTCGTCGCCATGATGAGTCGTTACGTGACAA-
CATGCTGATACGACGACGGGCTCATCCTGCACCGCAGAGCTTTCAC-
CACGATCGATGCCTGCAGCTGTTCGTTATCCAGTATTAAACCCGATTAC-
CAGGGCCTGTTCCACGGTAGGCCAATTGCCACGGATATCCTCACGCGT-
TATGCCCCACTAATCCCCCCACCGAACTTA.

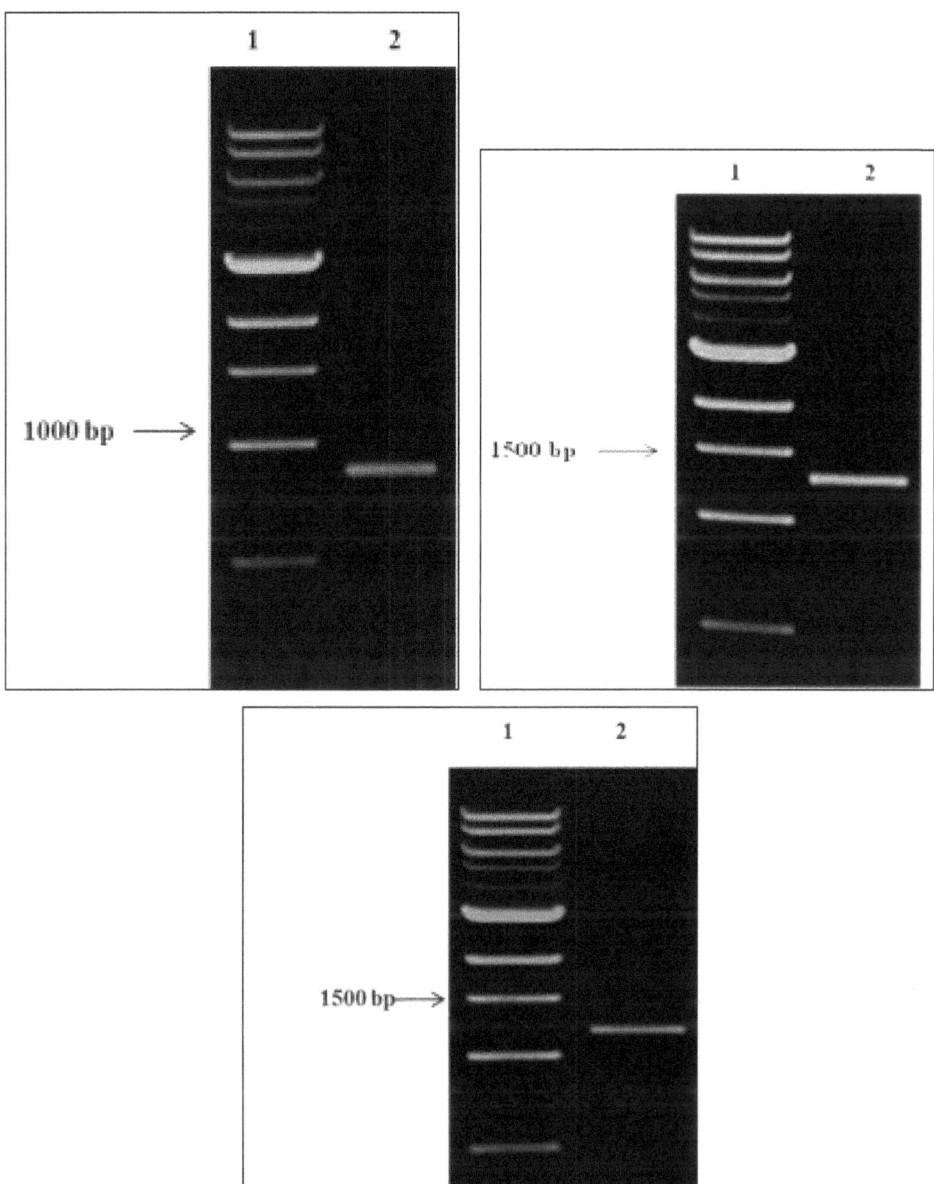


**Amplified 16S rRNA gene fragment total genomic DNA.**
**Lanes 1-2 (1= 1.5 kb DNA ladder).**

**A. Streptomyces sp. AH 47. (1277 bp); B. Streptomyces sp. AH 11.4. (886 bp)**
**C. Streptomyces sp. AH 4.4. (1288 bp).**

# *Chapter 18*

# Isolation and Evaluation of *Streptomyces* Species from Harare Agricultural Soils for Production of Vitamin $B_{12}$

***Tapiwashe Claudious Madeya, Eunita Chidziya and Cephas Mawere***

***Biotechnology Department,***
***Harare Institute of Technology, Harare, Zimbabwe***
***P.O Box BE277 Belvedere, Harare, Zimbabwe***
***E-mail: tipoclaudious@gmail.com, eunitachidziya@gmail.com, cmawere@gmail.com***

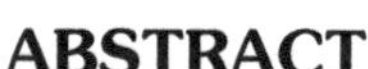

## ABSTRACT

The project sought to isolate and evaluate *Streptomyces* species from Harare agricultural soils for production of vitamin $B_{12}$. The soil samples collected from agricultural farms were cultured in enrichment and selective media. A total of five isolates were isolated from three different soil samples. The biochemical tests performed identified that the isolates obtained were *Streptomyces* species according to the Bergey's Manual of Systematic Bacteriology for Actinomycetes and the International Streptomyces Project. Fermentation growth media was used to access the ability of these isolates in production of vitamin $B_{12}$. The extraction process of vitamin $B_{12}$ was done and determination of vitamin $B_{12}$ production was carried out using the microbial assay method. Lactobacillus species were used as test organisms in the determination of vitamin $B_{12}$ production. Only three isolates were found to produce vitamin $B_{12}$ and these are isolates were *S. lydicus, S. calvus* and *S. oliveceuscleroticus*.The results of this study demonstrate that *Streptomyces* species isolated from local areas in Harare present a significant capacity to produce vitamin $B_{12}$.

***Keywords:*** *Streptomyces, Actinomyces, Species, Isolates, Fermentation, Extraction, Microbiological assay, Lactobacillus.*

# INTRODUCTION

The genus *Streptomyces* are gram-positive bacteria that grow in various environments with filamentous form that is similar to fungi. These ubiquitous soil saprophytes have been studied mainly because they are characterized by a complex secondary metabolism. They produce many secondary metabolites with antibiotic, antifungal and antiviral activity just to mention a few. They produce over two-thirds of the clinically useful antibiotics of natural origin for example neomycin, chloramphenicol just to mention a few. *Streptomyces* is the most well-known genus of *Actinomycetes* family which always has been noted to produce and secrete a large variety of industrial, medical, biotechnological and agricultural secondary metabolites (Locci, 1989).

The project sought to isolate *Streptomyces* species from local (Harare) agricultural soils for possible production of vitamin $B_{12}$. To the best of my knowledge, isolation of *Streptomyces* species has not been done in Zimbabwe. The vitamin $B_{12}$ used in the food and pharmaceutical industry is being imported from other countries and is very expensive.

Vitamins are essential micronutrients that cannot be synthesized by mammals and are required in trace quantities. Microorganisms and plants produce vitamins that are essential for metabolism of all living organisms. Vitamins are now increasingly being introduced as food or feed additives, medical-therapeutic agents, health aids and as technical aids. Nowadays many processed foods, feeds, pharmaceuticals, chemicals and cosmetics contain added vitamins or vitamin related compounds (Martens *et al.*, 2002).

Vitamin $B_{12}$ or cobalamin is a water-soluble vitamin that plays a very fundamental role in neurological function, DNA synthesis and optimal haemopoiesis. It is the only known metabolite that contains cobalt and is an anti-pernicious dietary factor. Natural forms of vitamin $B_{12}$ are methylcobalamin, adenosylcobalamin and hydroxocobalamin. Cyanocobalamin is the industrially produced stable cobalamin form which is not found in nature and it is a cofactor in two enzymes that are fundamental in facilitating growth in humans. When vitamin $B_{12}$ is in the form of adenosylcobalamin, it is the cofactor in methylmalonyl-coenzyme-A-mutase and in the form of methyl cobalamin, it is the direct cofactor of methionine synthetase, an enzyme that recycles homocysteine back to methionine (Berlin *et al.*, 1968).

Vitamin $B_{12}$ is provided as a supplement in many processed foods and is also available in vitamin pill form, liquid, transdermal patch, nasal spray, or injection. It is a common ingredient in energy drinks and energy shots. The production cost of vitamin $B_{12}$ by chemical synthesis are complicated and expensive so there is need to isolate *Streptomyces* species for use in the production of vitamin $B_{12}$.

## Materials and Methdology

### Sampling, Media Preparation and Isolation

Soil samples were collected into sterilized plastic bags from 3 different locations in Harare. These include: Chitungwiza farm, Belvedere farm and Kuwadzana farm.

The soil samples were taken from 15-20 cm depth after removing approximately 3 cm of the earth surface and were then air-dried at room temperature for two days.

Glycerol Yeast Extract Agar (GYEA) media was prepared by dissolving 2g glycerol, 0.8g yeast extract, 0.04g potassium phosphate, 10g peptone, 6g agar into 400ml of distilled water and autoclaved at 121°C for 15 mins at 15psi. The media was then supplemented with nystatin (50µg/ml) and with 1 µg/ml of penicillin after autoclaving.

Tryptone Soy Agar (TSA) was prepared by dissolving 11.25 grams of tryptone soy agar in 250ml of distilled water and autoclaved at 121°C for 15 mins at 15psi. Yeast Extract-Malt Extract Agar (YEMEA) was prepared by dissolving 4g yeast extract, 10g malt extract, 4g glucose, 20g agar in 100ml of distilled water and autoclaved at 121°C for 15mins at 15psi. Nutrient agar (NA) was prepared by dissolving 38g of nutrient agar in 1000ml of distilled water and autoclaved at 121°C for 15min at 15psi (Wacksman and Lechevalier, 1953).

Isolation of *Streptomyces* was performed by the soil dilution plate technique (Waksman, 1961). In this technique, 1g of each soil sample was taken in 9ml of sterilized distilled water in a pre-sterilized test tube. The tubes were then agitated vigorously and heated at 50°C for 30 minutes in a temperature-controlled water bath. Serial aqueous dilution ($10^{-1}$ to $10^{-7}$) were prepared by transferring 1ml of the soil suspension into 9ml of sterilized distilled water in sterilized test tubes. Different aqueous dilutions ($10^{-3}$; $10^{-5}$; $10^{-7}$) of the soil suspensions were applied separately into sterilized Petri-dish and 20ml of warm melted (at around 50°C) Glycerol Yeast Extract Agar (GYEA) medium was added to it. After gentle rotation, the plates were incubated at 27°C for 7-14 days (Wacksman and Lechevalier, 1953).

Another method was used for isolation of the *Streptomyces* when one gram of the soil sample was mixed with nine milliliters of 10 per cent calcium carbonate and incubated at 30°C for 10 days. After that the soil samples were serially diluted from $10^{-1}$ to $10^{-6}$ and the $10^{-6}$ was cultured in GYEA, YEMEA, TSA and NA. The cultures were incubated at 28°C for 7-14 days (Wacksman and Henrichi, 1943).

After growth the isolates were given laboratory reference numbers: 1CX, 1CY, 1AX, 1BX, 1BY, 2AG and 2AS. There were then Mineral Yeast Extract (MYE) broth was prepared as fermentation growth medium for the *Streptomyces* isolates according to Lechevalier and Lechevalier, 1970. The extraction process of vitamin $B_{12}$ was done according to Martens *et al.*, 2002.

## Results and Discussion

### Microscopic, Cultural and Biochemical Characteristics

Five *Streptomyces* isolates were recovered from 3 farming soil samples collected from different areas in Harare. All the tested isolates were Gram-positive, acid-fast negative and filamentous. At maturity the aerial hyphae of all isolates differentiate into long spiral chains of cylindrical immotile spores that are 0.5-2.0µm in diameter as noticed by Anderson and Wellington, 2001.

All of the isolates were considered as *Streptomyces* depending on their mycelial growth nature (Appendix A) and on their ability to grow on Glycerol Yeast Extract Agar (GYEA) supplemented with nystatin (50μg/ml) and with 1 μg/ml of penicillin. This medium is specific and sensitive for *Streptomyces* since it contains glycerol that most Actinomycetes use as a sole carbon source. Nystatin reduce fungal growth (Porter *et al.*, 1960) whereas penicillin reduces the development of non-filamentous bacteria and *Actinomycetes* other than *Streptomyces*.

The results of cultural characterization after 7-14 days of incubation are shown in Table 18.1. All isolates grew on a range of agar media showing morphology typical of *Streptomyces* (Anderson and Wellington, 2001; Locci, 1989; Wendisch and Kutzner, 1991; Williams *et al.*, 1989). The colour of the substrate mycelium and aerial spore mass was varied. The colonies of the tested isolates were all round in shape with opaque and their sizes were different ranging from small, medium and large. The isolates were relatively smooth-surfaced but later developed aerial mycelium that appears granular and powdery. Firstly, all isolates have whitish colonies but later they produced a variety of pigments that colored the vegetative and aerial mycelia. Five isolates produced white colored mycelia, one isolate brown and the other isolate green. Some of the isolates produced spores and others did not produce spores. Colony elevation was flat, raised, umbonate and convex. The edges of the isolated scalloped, wrinkled, smooth and filamentous. All tested isolates grew on Glycerol Yeast Extract Agar.

**Table 18.1: Cultural Characteristics of Isolated Species on different Media**

| *Isolates* | *Media* | | | |
|---|---|---|---|---|
| | *GYEA* | *YEMEA* | *TSA* | *NA* |
| | *Colour, Appearance, Size and Shape* | *Colour, Appearance, Size and Shape* | *Colour, Appearance, Size and Shape* | *Colour, Appearance, Size and Shape* |
| **1CX** | White, granular, large and round | White, powdery, large and round | White, smooth, large and round | Cream, large and round |
| **1CY** | White, scalloped, large and round | White, powdery, large and round | White, wrinkled, large and round | Cream, smooth, large and round |
| **2AS** | White, medium and round | White, medium and round | White, medium and round | White, medium and round |
| **2AG** | Green, wrinkled, medium and round | Green, powdery, medium and round | Green, wrinkled, medium and round | Green, medium and round |
| **1BX** | Brown, powdery, small and round | Brown, granular, small and round | Brown, scalloped, small and round | Light Brown, small and round |
| **1BY** | White, wrinkled, small and round | White, powdery, small and round | White, small and round | White, small and round |
| **1AX** | White, powdery, medium and round | White, granular, medium and round | White, medium and round | White, smooth, medium and round |

All isolates grew on a range of agar media showing morphology typical of *Streptomyces* (Anderson and Wellington, 2001; Locci, 1989; Wendisch and Kutzner, 1991; Williams *et al.*, 1989). These isolates grew on TSA, YEMEA, GYEA, NA, Casein agar Starch agar showing morphological characteristics of *Streptomyces*. As described in the results of cultural characteristics above, these characteristics are the same as obtained by Huang *et al.* (1988). All the tested isolates grew on Glycerol Yeast Extract Agar and these characteristics are the same as characteristics shown by the *Streptomyces* isolates previously isolated by previous researchers (Wendisch and Kutzner, 1991).

**Table 18.2: Biochemical Tests Performed on different Isolates**

| *Test Performed* | *Isolates and their reaction to test* | | | | | | |
|---|---|---|---|---|---|---|---|
| | *1CX Isolate* | *1CY Isolate* | *2AS Isolate* | *2AG Isolate* | *1BX Isolate* | *1BY Isolate* | *1AX Isolate* |
| Methyl red | - | - | - | - | - | - | - |
| Vogues-Proskauer | - | - | - | - | - | - | - |
| Motility | + | + | + | + | + | + | + |
| Indole | + | + | + | - | + | + | - |
| Oxidase | + | + | + | + | + | + | + |
| Catalase | + | + | + | + | + | + | + |
| Urease | + | + | - | - | + | + | + |
| $H_2S$ | + | + | - | + | + | + | + |
| Citrate | + | + | + | + | + | + | + |
| Peptization and coagulation of milk | + | + | + | + | + | + | + |
| Hydrolysis of : | | | | | | | |
| Casein | + | + | + | + | + | + | + |
| Starch | + | + | + | + | + | + | + |
| Gelatin | + | + | + | - | - | - | + |
| Utilization of carbon sources | | | | | | | |
| D-glucose | + | + | + | + | - | + | + |
| Maltose | + | - | + | + | - | + | + |
| Lactose | + | + | + | + | + | + | + |
| Fructose | - | + | + | + | - | + | + |
| Sucrose | + | - | + | + | - | + | + |
| D-xylose | + | + | + | + | + | - | - |
| D-mannitol | + | + | + | + | + | - | - |
| Inositol | + | + | + | + | + | + | + |
| D-raffinose | + | + | + | + | + | + | + |
| D-cellobiose | + | + | + | + | + | + | + |
| Utilization of nitrogen sources | | | | | | | |
| L-lysine | + | + | + | + | + | + | + |
| Cysteine | + | + | - | - | + | + | + |

+: Positive; -: Negative.

The biochemical activities of pure cultures allow genera and species characterization and identification. The selection of a range of biochemical tests to be used depends upon the diversity and nature of the group of bacteria under study. Biochemical characterization of isolates involves diagnostic characters that are recommended in International Streptomyces ISP and are successfully utilized by various investigators in the field (Anderson and Wellington, 2001).

The utilization of carbohydrates and nitrogen sources of growth characteristics are shown in Table 18.2. It is clear that all of the isolates tested were motile, oxidase, catalase, lactose, cellobiose, raffinose, inositol and citrate positive. All of the tested isolates can hydrolyze starch and casein. The results of catalase and urease tests are in accordance with the findings of Anderson and Wellington (2001). All the isolates showed that they are able to produce oxidase enzymes that play an important role in the operation of the electron transport system during aerobic respiration. The production of catalases was shown by all isolates meaning that enzymes catalyze the destruction of hydrogen peroxide to produce water and oxygen. The presence of ureases was shown by all isolates except 2AS and 2AG. The presence of ureases shows that these isolates were able to breakdown urea to produce ammonia, carbon dioxide and water as end products in the media. However, the results of urease test after 24 hours of incubation are not consistent with the results obtained by Oskay *et al.* (2004) who reported negative urease results for 6 of their tested isolates.

All of the tested isolates can hydrolyze starch and casein. This means that all isolates secreted proteolytic enzymes (caseinase) that catalyze the hydrolysis of casein to yield amino acids which are then transported into the cell and catabolized. All isolates produced hydrolases enzymes that catalyze the splitting of organic molecules into smaller molecules in the presence of water. They hydrolyze both amylopectin and amylose using alpha amylases to produce glucose, maltose and dextrins. A wide range of variation was shown by the isolates in their abilities to peptonize and coagulate milk, produce $H_2S$ on triple iron sugar media, liquefy gelatin and produce organic acids from carbohydrate fermentation. All of the tested isolates were able to produce $H_2S$ except for 2AG and 2AS. This shows that these isolates were able to break down of cysteine in the media and take up sodium thiosulfate and reduced by thiosulfate reductase with the release of hydrogen sulfide gas. Isolated species were able to secrete proteolytic enzymes called gelatinase which hydrolyze gelatin (Shirling and Gottlieb, 1968).

The utilization of different carbohydrates as sole carbon source was shown by most of the isolates since they were able to utilize all of the carbohydrates under test except for a few that could not utilize maltose, xylose, sucrose, fructose and mannitol as shown. The ability of microorganisms to ferment carbohydrates and the types of products formed are very useful in identification. All the isolated species that were able to ferment the carbohydrates showed that they produced end products such as alcohols, organic acids, gases or other organic molecules that lower the media's pH and change the medium from its original color to yellow or orange (Williams and Cross, 1971).

These characteristics of *Streptomyces* species is supported by Huang *et al.*, 1998 who reported that *Streptomyces* species possess several metabolic pathways that are supported by large-sized genomes. For example, *S.avermitilis* possesses the largest bacterial genome consisting of 8.7 million base pairs (Pullen *et al.*, 2002). This provides intuitions into the fundamental abilities of *Streptomyces* to utilize different carbohydrate sources. Based on these characteristics all of the isolates were classified in the order *Actinomycetes*; family *Streptomycetaceae* and genus *Streptomyces*. The results of this study demonstrate that *Streptomyces* strains isolated from diverse geographical locations present a significant capacity to produce vitamin $B_{12}$.

Based on the morphology, colour and biochemical analysis the isolates were identified as *Streptomyces* species. As members of genus *Streptomyces* according to Bergey's Manual of Systematic Bacteriology for Actinomycetes four out of five species were presumptively identified as *S. lydicus* (2AS and 2AG), *S. calvus* (1CX), *S.oliveceuscleroticus* (1CY) and *S. rimosus* (1BY and 1AX). Isolate 1BX did not match any of the species in the Bergey's Manual of Systematic Bacteriology for Actinomycetes and may be regarded as a new species.

## Vitamin $B_{12}$ Assay

The growth of *Lactobacillus* species on basal medium around the paper disks soaked with extracted solution from the fermentation media shows that the vitamin $B_{12}$ was successfully produced by the *Streptomyces* species isolated. *Lactobacillus* species are widely used to assay the vitamin $B_{12}$ since they require the vitamin $B_{12}$ for their growth. Without the presence of vitamin $B_{12}$ in the media, they will not be able to grow so their growth confirms that there was presence of vitamin $B_{12}$ on the soaked paper discs with the extracted solution meaning that vitamin B12 was produced in the MYE broth during the fermentation process. These results are the same as those obtained by Martens *et al.* (2002). Only three media plates with soaked paper disks from extracted solution from species *S. lydicus, S. calvus* and *S. oliveceuscleroticus* showed growth. These results conclude that these species were the ones able to produce vitamin $B_{12}$. The other two isolates were not able to produce vitamin $B_{12}$ since *Lactobacillus* could not grow on basal medium with extracts.

## Conclusions

In conclusion, Harare agricultural soils provided a rich source of *Streptomyces* isolates. The results of this study demonstrate that *Streptomyces* species isolated from local areas in Harare present a significant capacity to produce vitamin $B_{12}$. Among the five isolated species only three isolates: *S. lydicus, S. calvus* and *S. oliveceuscleroticus* were able to produce vitamin $B_{12}$.

## Recommendations

There is need for molecular characterization of the isolated *Streptomyces* isolates for further confirmation of the isolated species. Since *Streptomyces* isolates are capable of producing a large number of secondary metabolites there must be a long-term screening programme in order to discover new metabolites. There is also need for evaluation and optimization of the vitamin $B_{12}$ production under different fermentation conditions using locally available substrates in order to minimize costs.

## Acknowledgements

I wish to express my greatest gratitude to my supervisor Mrs. E. Chidziya for her guidance, help and encouragement during the course of this study. My deep thanks to all members of the Biotechnology department for their continuous help and encouragement. My deep thanks also to Mrs. Berejena the chief technologist at UZ Medical Microbiology for her support towards my project. My gratitude and warm thanks are extended to my family for their encouragement and financial support. Many thanks for the help during the preparation of this thesis. I am deeply thankful to all those who have assisted me during this study.

## Abbreviations

TSIA: Triple Sugar Iron Agar
GYEA: Glycerol Yeast Extract Agar
YEMEA: Yeast Extract Malt Agar
TSA: Tryptone Soy Agar
NA: Nutrient Agar
ISP: International Streptomyces Project
MR: Methyl Red
VP: Vogues Proskauer

## REFERENCES

1. Alexander, M 1967. Introduction to Soil Microbiology. John Wiley and Sons, INC. New York, London, Sydney. 472 pp.
2. Anderson, A. S. and Wellington, E. M. H 2001. The taxonomy of Streptomyces and related genera. *Int. J. Syst. Evol. Microbiol.,* 51: 797-814.
3. Atlas, R. M. (1989). Microbiology Fundamentals and Applications.2nd edition, Mac Millan publishing company, New York, 806 pp.
4. Atlas, R. M 1997. Handbook of Microbiological Media, 2nd edition, CRC Press, Boca Raton, New York, London, Tokyo, 1706 pp.
5. Berlin H, Berlin R, Brante G 1968. Oral treatment of pernicious anemia with high doses of vitamin B12 without intrinsic factor. *Acta Med Scand.,* 184: 247-58.
6. Brock, T. D 1970. Biology of Microorganisms. Prentice – Hall, INC. Englewood Cliffs, New Jersey, 737 pp.
7. Cross, T 1989. Growth and Examination of Actinomycetes Some Guidelines. In: Bergey's Manual of Systematic Bacteriology. Williams and Wilkins company, Baltimore, 4. pp. 2340-2343.
8. Embley, T. M. and Stackebrandt, 1994. The molecular phylogeny and systematics of the Actinomycetes. *Annu. Rev. Microbiol.,* 48: 257-289.
9. Goodfellow, M. and Williams, S. T 1983. Ecology of Actinomycetes. *Annu. Rev. Microbiol.,* 37: 189-216.

10. Gottlieb, D. and Shirling, E. B 1967. Co-operative description of type cultures of Streptomyces. I. The International Streptomyces Project. *Int. J. Syst. Bacteriol.*, 17: 315-322.

11. Holding, A. G. J. and Collee, J. G 1971. Routine Biochemical Test. In: *Methods in Microbiology*. Norris, J. R and Ribbons, D. W. (eds). Vol. 6. Academic Press, London. pp 1-32.

12. Huang, C. H., Lin, Y. S., Yang, Y. L., Huang, S. W. and Chen, C. W 1998. The telomeres of *Streptomyces* chromosomes contain conserved palindromic sequences with potential to form complex secondary structures. *Mol. Microbiol.*, 28: 905-916.

13. Koneman, E. W., Allen, S. D., Anda, W. M., Paul, C. S. and Winn, W. C 1992. Introduction to Microbiology, Part 1. In: Color Atlas and Textbook of Diagnostic Microbiology. 4th edition. J. B. Lippincott co., Philadelphia, Ch. 1. pp. 1-60.

14. Lacey, J 1973. Actinomycet ales: Characteristics and practical importance. Edited by G. Sykes and F. Skinner. The Society for Applied Bacteriology Symposium Series, No.2. Academic Press London-New York.

15. Lechevalier H.A 1989. The Actinomycetes III, A Practical Guide to Generic Identification of Actinomycetes. *Bergey's Manual of Systematic Bacteriology*. Williams and Wilkins Company, Baltimore. Vol. 4. pp. 2344-2347.

16. Locci R 1989. Streptomyces and related Genera. Bergey's Manual of Systematic Bacteriology. Williams and Wilkins Company, Baltimore. Vol. 4: pp. 2451-2508.

17. Lechevalier, M. P. and Lechevalier, H 1970. Chemical composition as a criterion in the classification of aerobic Actinomycetes. *Int. J. Syst. Bacteriol.*, 20: 435-443.

18. Martens J.H, Barg H, Warren M.J, Jahn D 2002. Microbial production of vitamin B12. *Appl. Microbiol. Biotechnol.*, 5: 275–285.

19. Marwaha S.S, Sethi, R.P, Kennedy J.F 1983. Role of amino acids, betaine and choline in Vitamin B12 biosynthesis by strains of Propionibacterium. *Enzyme Microb. Technol.*, 5 454–456.

20. McCarthy, A.J. and Williams, S.T 1990. Methods for Studying the Ecology of Actinomycetes.Methods in Microbiology. Ed. by R. Grigorova and J. R. Norris, Academic Press Limited, London, 22: 533-563.

21. Oskay, M., Tamer, A.Ü. and Azeri, C 2004. Antibacterial activity of some Actinomycetes isolated from farming soils of Turkey. *Afr. J. Biotechnol.*, 3: 441-446.

22. Ozaki, H. and Yamada, K 1991. Isolation of *Streptomyces* sp. producing glucose-tolerant-glucosidases and properties of the enzyme. *Agri. Biol. Chem.* 55: 979-987.

23. Porter, J. N., Wilhelm, J. J. and Tresner, H. D 1960. Method for the preferential isolation of *Actinomycetes* from soils. *Appl. Microbiol.*, 8: 174-178.

24. Prescott, L. M., Harley, J. P. and Klein, D. A 1993. Microbiology, 2nd edition. WM. C. Brown publishers.912 pp.

25. Pridham, T. G. and Tresner, H. D 1974. Family VII.Streptomycetaceae In: *Bergey's Manual of Systematic Bacteriology*. 8th edition. Buchanan, R. E. and Gibbons, N. E. (eds). The Williams and Wilkins Company, Baltimore, 1268 pp.

26. Pridham, T. G., Hesseltine, C. W. and Benedict, R. G 1958. A guide for the classification of *Streptomyces* according to selected groups. *Appl. Microbiol.*, 6: 52-79.

27. Pullen, C., Schmitz, P., Meurer, K., Bamberg, D., Lohmann, S., Franca, S., Groth, I., Schlegel, B., Mollmann, U., Gollmick, F., Grafe, U. and Leistner, E 2002. New and bioactive compounds from *Streptomyces* strains residing in the wood of celastraceae. *Planta*, 216: 162-167.

28. Sahin, N., Ugur, A 2003. Investigation of the antimicrobial activity of some *Streptomyces* isolates. *Turk. J. Biol.*, 27: 79-84.

29. Shirling, E. B. and Gottlieb, D 1968.Co-operative description of type culture of *Streptomyces*. II. Species descriptions from first study. *Int. J. Sys. Bacteriol.*, 18: 69-189.

30. Shirling, E. B. and Gottlieb, D 1969. Co-operative description of type cultures of *Streptomyces*. IV. Species description from the second, third and fourth studies. *Int. J. Syst. Bacteriol.*, 19: 391-512.

31. Shirling, E. B. and Gottlieb, D 1972. Co-operative description of type species of *Streptomyces*. V. Additional descriptions. *Int. J. Sys. Bacteriol.*, 22: 265-394.

32. Trejo, W. G 1970. An evaluation of some concepts and criteria used in the speciation of *Streptomyces. Transactions of the New York Academy of Sciences* 32: 989-997.

33. Waksman, S. A 1961. The Actinomycetes.Classification, Identification and Descriptions of Genera and species Vol. 2, Williams and Wilkins Company, 363 pp.

34. Waksman, S. A. and Henrici, A. T 1943. The nomenclature and classification of the *Actinomyces. J. Bacteriol.*, 46: 337-341.

35. Waksman, S. A., Lechevalier, H. A 1953. Guide to the Classification and Identification of the Actinomycetes and their Antibiotics. The Williams and Wilkins Company. Baltimore. 246 pp.

36. Wendisch, F. K. and Kutzner, H. J 1991.The Family Streptomycetaceae in Prokaryotes. A. Ballows (eds), Springer Verlag. Vol. 1, 2nd edition, pp. 922-995.

37. Williams, S. T. and Cross, T 1971. Actinomycetes. In: *Methods in Microbiology*. Booth, C. (ed). Academic Press, London and New York.795 pp.

# APPENDIX

## Appendix A: Cultural Characteristic Results of *Streptomyces* Isolates

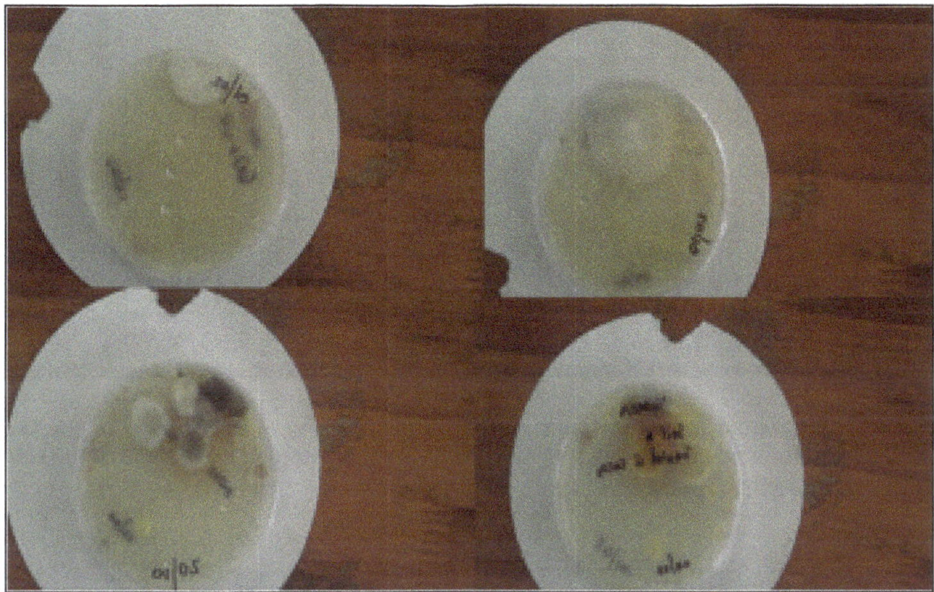

**Figure 18.1: Different *Streptomyces* Isolates on GYEA Isolated *Streptomyces* Species are: *S. lydicus, S. calvus, S. oliveceuscleroticus, S. rimosus.***

## Appendix B

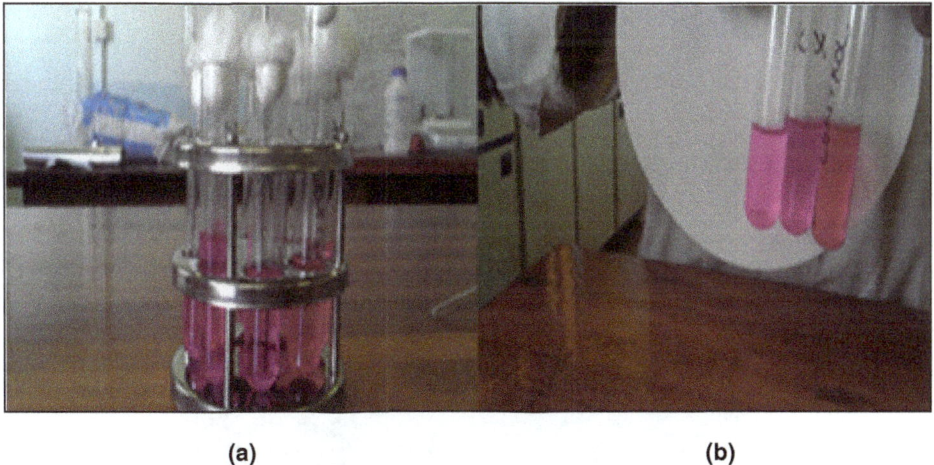

(a) (b)

**Figure 18.2: Urease Test. The urease test results (a) left and (b) right both shows test tubes with urea broth after inoculation and incubation for 72hrs for 37oC. The results of the urea test shows tubes with pink color indicating a positive result.**

## Appendix C

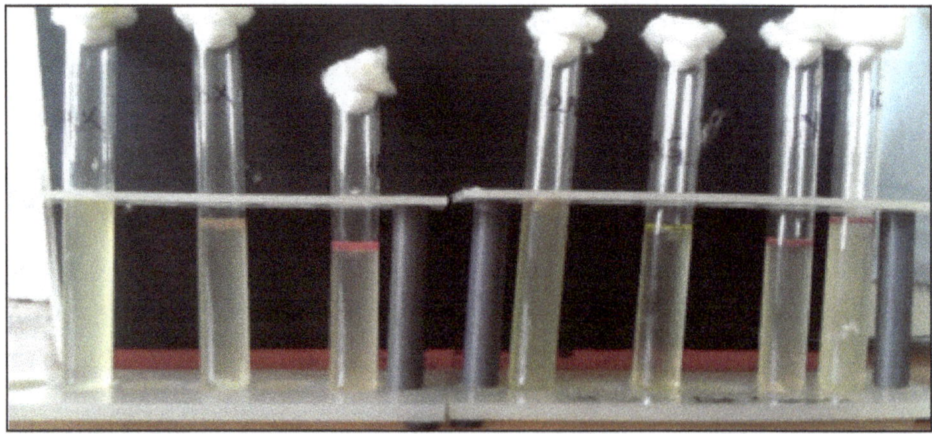

**Figure 18.3: Indole Test. The tubes with a bright red ring at the surface of the test tubes indicate a positive result and tubes with a yellow ring at the surface of the tube indicate a negative result.**

## Appendix D

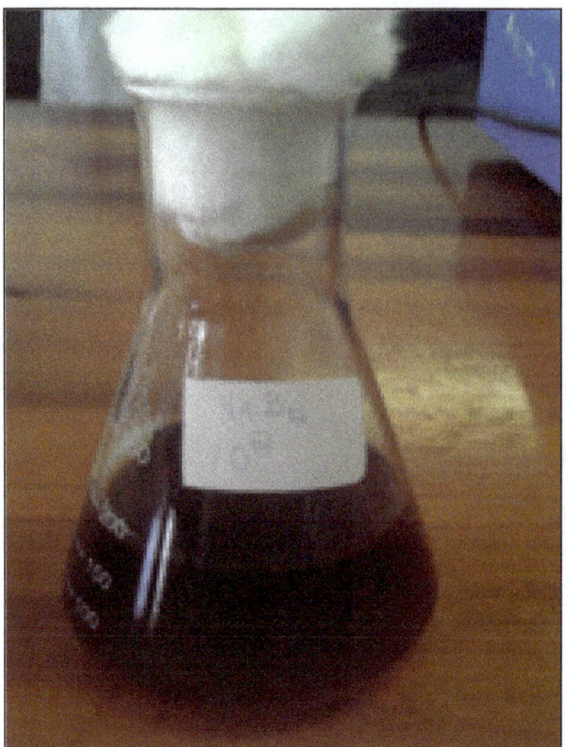

**Figure 18.4: Shows Vitamin $B_{12}$ after Extraction.**

# Chapter 19

# Optimization of Bio-Ethanol Production from Barley Waste Using Response Surface Methodology

*S. Manhokwe and T. Chikuru*

*Midlands State University,*
*Department of Food Science and Nutrition,*
*P Bag 9055, Gweru, ZIMBABWE*
*E-mail: manhokwes@staff.msu.ac.zw*

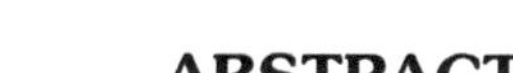

## ABSTRACT

The aim of this study was to optimize bio-ethanol production from barley waste using acid hydrolysis. Currently, barley waste is underutilised and sometimes converted to stock feeds which are then sold at a low cost to farmers at a local malting company. Optimisation was done using the Response Surface Methodology (RSM). A central composite design (CCD) was used in the design of experiments. The independent variables used were the weight of barley waste and sulphuric acid concentration. The weight of barley waste ranged from 10g -30g. It was pre-treated with acid concentrations ranging from 3-10 per cent. Hydrolysis was carried out at 131°C for 30 minutes and pH was adjusted to 4.0-4.5 after hydrolysis prior to fermentation. The dependent variables were sugar concentration and alcohol concentration. Total sugar concentration of the hydrolysate ranged from 4-17 per cent and alcohol from 0.6-1.5 per cent.The optimized conditions were 30g weight of barley waste, 9.9 per cent acid concentration, yielding 14 per cent sugar and 1.2 per cent alcohol. The results indicate that the method is feasible for production of bio-ethanol from barley waste. However, the alcohol yield is low and fermentation conditions need to be optimised.

***Keywords**: Barley waste, Acid hydrolysis, Fermentation, Bio-ethanol.*

# INTRODUCTION

Barley is the major cereal crop employed in the making of malt worldwide. Treatment of barley into malt is an important stage which allows the employment of barley grains in brewing. The received grain is expected to have moisture levels ranging from 10 to 12 per cent (FAO, 2009). The malting process involves three stages: steeping, germination and kilning (Briggs, 1998). In approximately nine days, the processing cycle is completed (FAO, 2009). During malting barley is categorized by kernel size (width) into sizes of more than 2.5 mm, 2.2to 2.5mm, and less than 2.2mm. The fragmented kernels together with grain less than 2.2mm in width are separated by screening and can be collected into silos for final use as animal feed (Guido and Moreira, 2014).

Waste disposal has been a major cost factor as well as a significant feature in the progress of a brewery operation (Fillaudeau *et al.*, 2006). Modification of processes is being done in nearly all industrialized and unindustrialised countries in order to ensure recycling of the residues. Therefore, many big companies have moved to adapting residues not as waste, but as feedstock for further various processes (Mussato *et al.*, 2006). Production of ethanol from any raw material is principally categorised into three processes: attaining fermentable sugars, ethanol release from conversion of the sugars as well as purification done by distillation (Asgher *et al.*, 2013). Non-food based feed stocks used for second generation of bioethanol comprises of cellulosic biomass such as wood, herbaceous crops, farming remains (wheat straw, barley husks), energy plants (switch grass), municipal solid waste.

Lignocellulosic material is increasingly considered a good raw material because it is cheap and easily available. Production of bioethanol from these compounds appears to be potentially viable and economically sustainable (Kumar *et al.*, 2009). Pre-treatment is a critical phase for the biochemical transformation of lignocellulose raw material into bio-ethanol. Approximately 90 per cent of the dry weight in many plants material is stored as celluloses, hemicelluloses, lignin as well as pectin. Hemicellulose is a linear and branched heterogeneous polymer typically made up of five different sugars-L-arabinose, D-galactose, D-glucose, D-mannose, and D-xylose as well as other components like acetic, glucoronic and ferulic acids. The backbone of the chains of hemicellulose can be homopolymer or heteropolymer (Mussatto and Teixeira, 2010).

According to Zheng *et al.* (2009) dilute acid hydrolysis is the most commonly used method of breaking the chain. In this process diluted acids (1-4 per cent) under moderate temperatures of 120 -160°C have proven to be adequate for the hydrolysis. Sulphuric acid is usually used although hydrochloric acid and phosphoric acid are also used. The acid catalyses the breakdown of long hemicellulose chains to form shorter chain oligomers and then to sugar monomers. Since hemicellulose is amorphous, less severe conditions are required to release hemicellulose sugars. Steam explosion is also a method commonly used in hemicellulose hydrolysis (Mussatto and Teixeira, 2010). The biomass is heated using high pressure saturated steam 0, 69-4.83Mpa, 160°C-260°C for a short period. In autohydrolysis the process uses compressed liquid hot water at approximately 200°C and the acids resulting from hydrolysis of acetyl and uronic groups originally present in hemicelluloses catalyse the hydrolysis of links between hemicellulose and lignin as well as between the carbohydrates. Autohydrolysis is a process that can take a few minutes with high yield, low by products formation and no significant lignin solubilisation. Specific microorganisms or a suitable cocktail of enzymes known as hemicellulases can also promote the hemicellulose hydrolysis. Wyman *et al.*(2005) asserts that hemicellulases are produced by many species of bacteria, fungi as well as by several plants.

The process of fermentation is typically done using yeast species *Saccharomyces*. The sugars from the lignocellulosic materials are converted to organic acids that react to form aldehydes, esters and various chemical constituents in addition to alcohol (Isitua and Ibeh, 2010). Distillation is one of the steps of purification of ethanol after fermentation. It is a refining process wherein a subastance is heated to its boiling point, then the vapour formed upon boiling is permitted to move away from the boiling liquid, and the vapour is cooled to condense it back to liquid(Kimbrough, 2000).

Response surface methodology (RSM) is a collection of mathematical and statistical methods useful for the modelling and analysis of problems in which a response of importance is influenced by several variables and the objective is to raise the best conditions for this response. It is a significant subject in the statistical design of experiments (Montgomery, 2005 and Bradley, 2007).

## Materials and Methods

The experimental design and statistical analysis were accomplished with the Response Surface Methodology using Design Expert 6.0.8. The central composite design (CDD) approach with cubic model (Box and Wilson, 1951) was used in this study since it is an effective design which generally displays performance for the process optimization, (Kumar *et al.*, 2015). The combined effects of the independent variables namely weight of barley in gram and acid concentration ($H_2SO_4$) in percent, were investigated using CDD. The dependent variables or responses were the final sugar content after hydrolysis and the alcohol content after fermentation. The experimental design was developed using Design Expert 6.0.8., and resulted in 13 runs as indicated in Table 19.1

**Table 19.1: Design Summary**

| *Study Type* | *Initial Design* | *Design Model* | *Experiments* | *Blocks* |
|---|---|---|---|---|
| Response surface | Central composite | Cubic model | 13 | No blocks |
| *Response* | *Name* | *Units* | *Observations* | |
| Y1 | sugar concentration | per cent | 13 | |
| Y2 | Alcohol Concentration | per cent | 13 | |

| Factor | Name | Units | Type | Low Actual |
|---|---|---|---|---|
| A | Weight | g | Numeric | 10 |
| B | $H_2SO_4$ | per cent | Numeric | 3 |

## Acid Hydrolysis

Acid-based starch hydrolysis was done using Sulphuric acid ($H_2SO_4$). The acid concentration, ranged from 3-10 per cent as shown in Table 19.1. A temperature of 131 °C and 30 minutes was used. Sulphuric acid was added to the barley waste of weight ranging from 10 to 30 g, to hydrolyze hemicellulose and cellulose into fermentable sugars. After hydrolysis, there was a drop in pH of the hydrolysate and it was adjusted to 4.0-4.5 using potassium hydroxide (2N KOH). Brix value was used to estimate the amount sugar present in a solution. The analysis was carried out using handheld refractometer 0-32 per cent (Atago). The cooled hydrolysate was evaluated for sugar concentration using Lane-Enyon method.

### Fermentation

The 13 samples were transferred into separate 500ml fermentation vessels, 3g *S. cerevisiae* was added into each broth and sealed with fermentation corks.Gas collection system was connected to a volumetric gas displacement container with water, connected to a measuring cylinder for measuring water. The fermentation vessels were placed in the shaking water bath at a constant temperature of 30°C for 72hours. Fermentation was set up with the pH ranging from 4.0-4.5. Alcohol determination was done using the Potassium Dichromate method.

### Statistical Analysis

The F-test analysis of variance (ANOVA) was used to analyse the statistical significance of the model equation. The advantage of the model is that it can be tested using different criteria. The Fischer's F-test shows the overall significance of the model, and its probability P (F), correlation coefficient R, Coefficient of determination $R^2$ measure of the goodness of fit of regression model (Pradeep *et al.*, 1996).

## Results and Discussion

Figure 19.1 illustrates the effect of the different combinations of weighed barley waste and sulphuric acid concentration on the resulting sugar concentration after hydrolysis of the samples. Generally, from the results, the amount of sugar concentration increased as the weight of barley waste increased. The highest value of sugars was observed at 34.14 g barley waste and 6.50 per cent acid concentration and the lowest value was observed at 5.86 g barley waste and 6.50 per cent acid concentration.

Contour plots view the response surface in a less complicated manner, indicating contour lines and gives the minimum and maximum ranges which are easy to interpret (Bradley,2007). The regions of sugar concentration are illustrated with colors ranging from light green to the darkest green (Figure 19.2) while

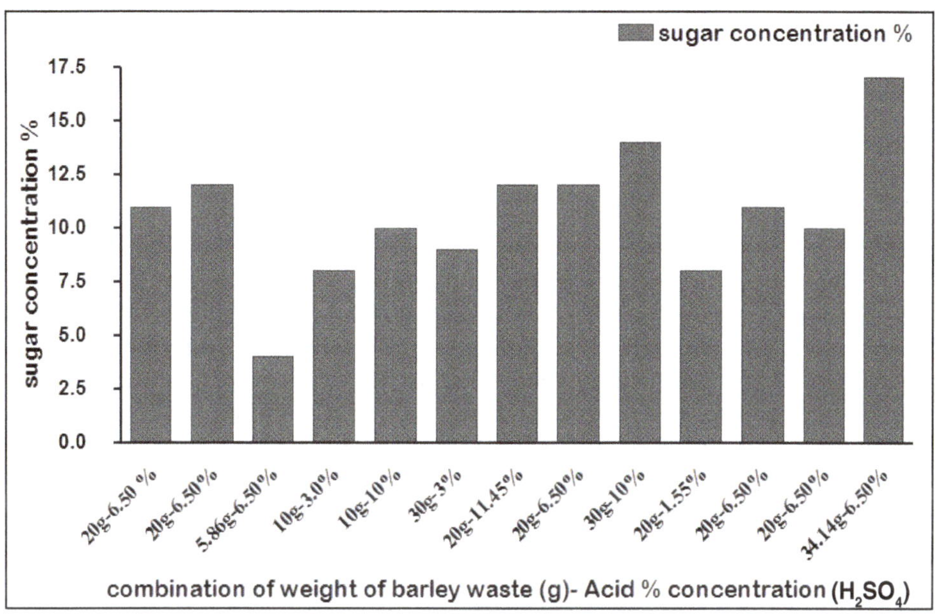


**Figure 19.1: Summary of Sugar Concentration in the Hydrolysate using Lane Eynon Method.**

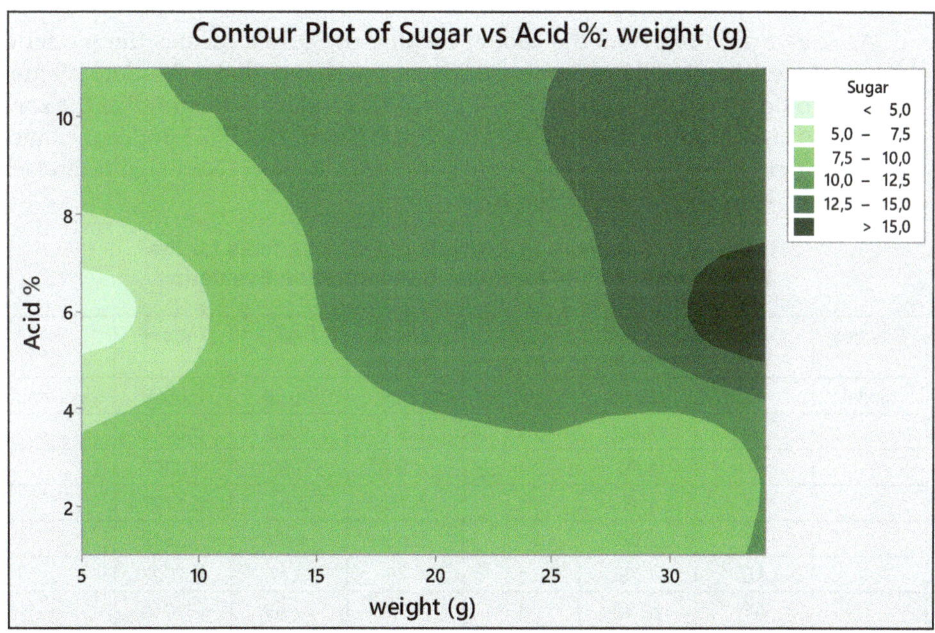


**Figure 19.2: Contour Plot for Total Sugar Concentration at different Weights and Acid Concentrations.**

the plot indicates that as the weight of barley increased the sugar concentration increased. The lowest concentration of sugar was 4 per cent indicated by the first light green spot and the maximum sugar concentration was 17 per cent indicated by the darkest green spot. The highest sugar concentration was obtained at 34.14g of barley waste and 6.50 per cent sulphuric acid concentration, while the lowest was obtained at 5.86g of barley waste and 6.50 per cent sulphuric acid concentration. This generally indicates that the sugar concentration obtained was in the range of 4 per cent to 17 per cent.

However, pre-treatment with dilute sulphuric acid using concentration between 0.5-1.5 per cent is tolerable to hydrolyse for 5 to 60 minutes at 130-200°C. In a study carried out by Carvalho (2009) on dilute acid and enzymatic hydrolysis of sugarcane bagasse for biogas production, optimal hemicellulose recovery conditions were at 2 per cent sulphuric acid concentration at 122°C in 20 minutes, with a recovery of 92 per cent xylan as xylose.But at 100 °C and 128 °C, the highest values of xylose concentration was 19 and 16 g/l, respectively, Wyman *et al.*(1996) reported an increase of the overall sugar yield from 56.8 per cent (when using water pre-treated corn stover) up to 93 per cent by diluted sulphuric acid pre-treatment. Valdes and Planes (1999) also indicated that the maximum overall sugar yield of olive tree (36.3 g sugar/100 g raw material) was obtained at 180°C and 1 per cent sulphuric acid concentration, representing 75 per cent of all sugars in the olive tree biomass (48.7 g/100 g) in their study on pre-treatment of olive tree with sulphuric acid. The dilute range of acid concentrations require more time for pre-treatment, which may take hours for acid action to complete hydrolysis.

As shown in Table 19.2 the Model F-value of 36.59 indicates the model is significant meaning that there is only a 0.05 per cent chance that a "Model F-Value" this large could occur due to noise. The "Lack of Fit F-value" of 0.09 implies the Lack of Fit is not significant relative to the pure error. There is a 77.73 per cent chance that a "Lack of Fit F-value" this large could occur due to noise. Non-significant lack of fit is good, because the model has to fit.

**Table 19.2: Summary of Analysis of Variance Table for the Model Used in RSM for Sugar Concentration Evaluation**

| *Squares* | | *Sum of Squares* | *DF* | *Mean Square* | *Fvalue* | *Prob>F* | |
|---|---|---|---|---|---|---|---|
| Model | | 120.96 | 7 | 17.28 | 36.59 | 0.0005 | Significant |
| | A | 3.53 | 1 | 3.53 | 7.48 | 0.0410 | |
| | B | 4.20 | 1 | 4.20 | 8.89 | 0.0307 | |
| | $A^2$ | 1.15 | 1 | 1.15 | 2.44 | 0.1793 | |
| | $B^2$ | 2.65 | 1 | 2.65 | 5.60 | 0.0642 | |
| | AB | 1.78 | 1 | 1.78 | 3.77 | 0.1097 | |
| | $A^3$ | 22.43 | 1 | 22.43 | 47.49 | 0.0010 | |
| | $B^3$ | 0.25 | 1 | 0.25 | 0.53 | 0.4995 | |
| | $A^2B$ | 0.000 | 0 | | | | |
| | $AB^2$ | 0.000 | 0 | | | | |

| *Squares* | | *Sum of Squares* | *DF* | *Mean Square* | *Fvalue* | *Prob>F* | |
|---|---|---|---|---|---|---|---|
| Residual | | 2.36 | 5 | 0.47 | | | |
| | Lack of fit | 0.053 | 1 | 0.053 | 0.092 | 0.7773 | Not significant |
| | Pure error | 2.31 | 4 | 0.58 | | | |
| Cor Total | | 123.32 | 12 | | | | |

The effects of weight and acid concentration on the total yield of alcohol after fermentation of the hydrolysates are illustrated in Figure 19.3. The resulting sugar concentration of the selected combinations as shown in Figure 19.1 did not show a substantial effect on the alcohol concentration yield. Maximum yield of alcohol was observed at 30 g barley waste and 3.00 per cent sulphuric acid where sugar concentration was 9 per cent and minimum alcohol yield was observed at 5.86 g barley waste and 6.50 per cent sulphuric acid where sugar concentration was 4 per cent. In general, weight of barley waste still played a significant role on the yield after fermentation. It has been reported that Baker's yeast strains cannot break the $C_5$ sugars like xylulose, a situation which gives a tendency of accumulation of unfermented sugars (Kaur and Kocher, 2002). In setups that had higher levels of sulphuric acid from 6.5 to 11.45 per cent, their resultant alcohol content may have been low due to the accumulation of unfermented sugars in the substrate.

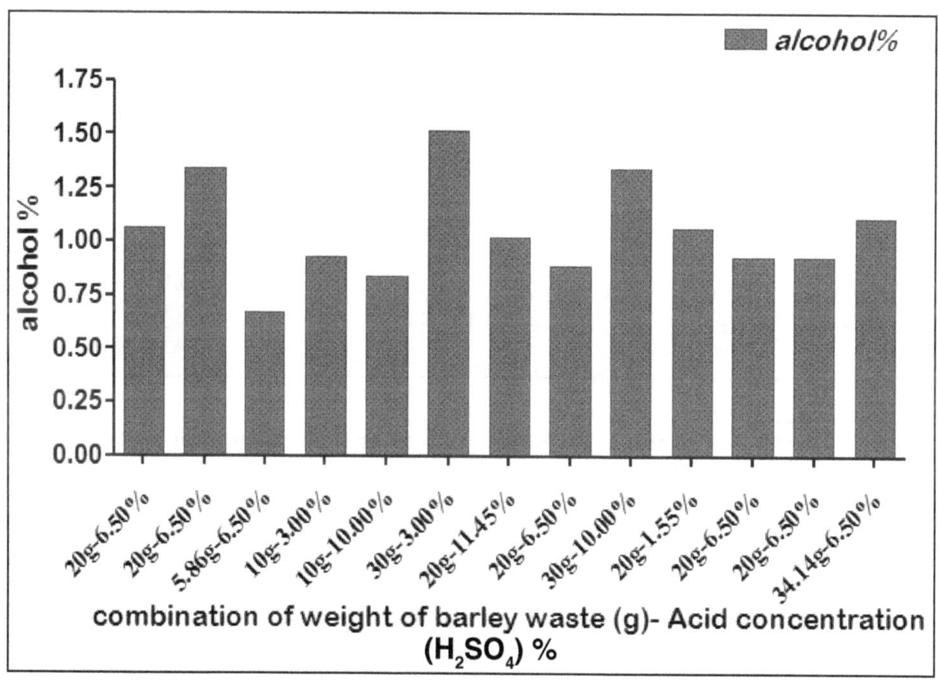


**Figure 19.3: Alcohol Concentration of the Hydrolysates after Fermentation.**

As indicated on the 3D plot in Figure 19.4, alcohol content was increasing constantly with a noticeable increase in weight and a decrease in concentration of sulphuric acid. The peak yield was observed at a range between 27 g and 30g weight. This generally means the optimum alcohol yield could be obtained from the range 27 g to 30g with an acid range of 3 per cent to 6 per cent.

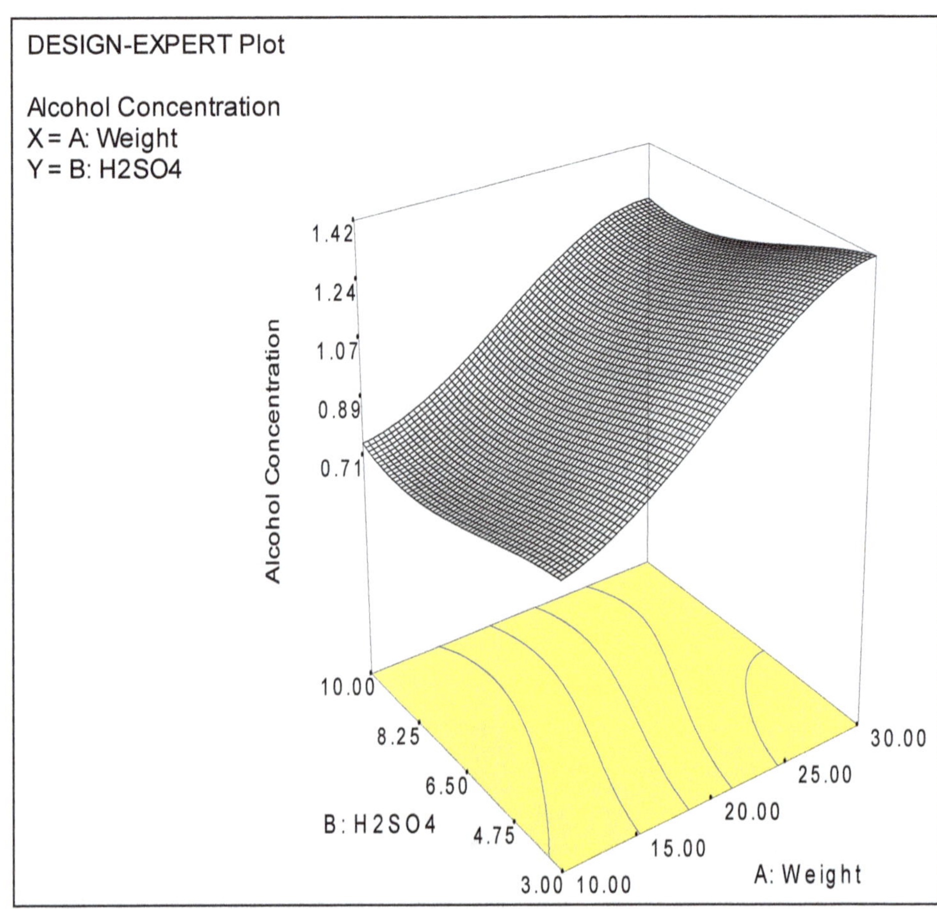


**Figure 19.4: 3D Plot of the effect of weight and acid concentration on the Yield of Alcohol After fermentation of the hydrolysate.**

In Table 19.3, the Model F-value of 7.00 implies the model is significant. There is only a 1.26 per cent chance that a "Model F-Value" this large could occur due to noise. The "Lack of Fit F-value" of 0.66 implies the Lack of Fit is not significant relative to the pure error. There is a 69.28 per cent chance that a "Lack of Fit F-value" this large could occur due to noise. Non-significant lack of fit is good, the model has to fit.

**Table 19.3: Summary of Analysis of Variance Table for the Model Used in RSM for Alcohol Yield Evaluation after Fermentation**

| *Source* | *Sum of Squares* | *DF* | *Mean Square* | *F Value* | *Prob>F* | |
|---|---|---|---|---|---|---|
| Model | 0.38 | 2 | 0.19 | 7.00 | 0.0126 | Significant |
| A | 0.37 | 1 | 0.37 | 13.51 | 0.0043 | |
| B | 0.013 | 1 | 0.013 | 0.49 | 0.4993 | |
| Residual | 0.27 | 10 | 0.027 | | | |
| Lack of Fit | 0.13 | 6 | 0.022 | 0.66 | 0.6928 | Not significant |
| Pure Error | 0.14 | 4 | 0.034 | | | |
| Cor Total | 0.65 | 12 | | | | |

## Process Optimization for Bio-ethanol production

The target goal was to reach a maximum alcohol yield (ethanol), using maximum weight and maximum acid concentration (sulphuric acid) since acid hydrolysis is one of the costly chemical for hydrolysis. The seleceted weight of barley waste ranged from 10-30g, sulphuric acid concentration from 3-10 per cent, resuling in sugar concentrations ranging between values 3.67 -16.69 per cent alcohol content 0.67-1.52 per cent. A solution indicating the best suitable conditions that could yield maximum bio-ethanol from the treatment of the independent variables was selected. The conditions were 30g of barley waste, 9.94 per cent sulphuric acid, yielding 14 per cent sugar and 1.22 per cent alcohol. Its desirability was 0.841 indicating that the estimated regression function may represent that the experimental model and the desired conditions are acceptable.

## Conclusions

The optimum conditions for bio-ethanol production from barley waste were 30 g barley waste and 9.94 per cent sulphuric acid concentration to yield 14 per cent sugars and the 1.22 per cent alcohol. The study demonstrates the technical feasibility of producing bio-ethanol from barley waste at a local malting plant.

## Acknowledgements

The authors would like to thank Kwekwe malting for providing barley waste used in this study. The technical efforts by members of the Food Science and Nutrition department at Midlands State University is gratefully appreciated.

## REFERENCES

1. Asgher, M., Ahmad, Z., Iqbal, H.M.N 2013. Alkali and enzymatic delignification of sugarcane bagasse to expose cellulose polymers for saccharification and bio-ethanol production. *Ind. Crops Prod.*, 44: 488–495.
2. Box P and Wilson K.B 1951. On the experimental attainment of optimum conditions. *J.R. Stat Soc.* 13: 1-45.

3. Bradley N 2007. The Response Surface Methodology. Indiana University of South Bend Briggs D.E. (1998) Malts and malting, Blackie Academic and Professionals, London.
4. Carvalheiro F, Duarte LC, Medeiros R and G´ýrio FM 2004. Optimization of brewery's spent grain dilute-acid hydrolysis for the production of pentose-rich culture media. *Appl. Biochem. Biotechnol.*, 115: 1059–1072.
5. Carvalho R 2009. Dilute acid and enzymatic hydrolysis of sugarcane bagasse for biogas production. *Engenharia Biologica*: France.
6. FAO 2009. Barley Malt Beer. Agribusiness Handbook. Italy.
7. Fillaudeau, Blanpain-Avet, Daufin 2006. Water, Wastewater and Waste Management in Brewing Industries. *Journal of Cleaner Production*, 14: 463-471.
8. Guido L. and Moreira M 2014. Malting. *Contemporary Food Engineering*, pp. 51-70.
9. Kaur, M., and G.S. Kocher 2002. Ethanol production from molasses and sugarcane juice by an adapted strain of *Saccharomyces cerevisiae*. *Indian Journal of Microbiology*, 42(3): 255–257.
10. Kumar P., Barrett D.M., Delwiche M.J., and Stroeve P 2009. Methods for Pretreatment of Lignocellulosic Biomass for Efficient Hydrolysis and Biofuel Production. *Ind. Eng. Chem. Res.*, 48(8): 3713–3729.
11. Kumar, A. Sikder J., P. Sayan and G. Halder 2015. Optimizing the cross flow nanofiltration process for chromium (VI) removal from simulated wastewater through response surface methodology. *Environmental Progress and Sustainable Energy*.
12. Mariam I, Manzoor K., Ali S. and Ikram-Ul-Haq 2009. Enhanced Production of Ethanol from free and immobilized *Saccharomyces cerevisiae* under stationary culture. *Pak. J. Bot.*, 41(2): 821-833.
13. Montgomery D 2005. *Introduction to Statistical Quality Control*, 6$^{th}$Ediiton, John Wiley and Sons, Inc.
14. Mussato *et al.* 2006. Brewer Spent Grain: generation, characteristics and potential. *J. Cereal Sci.*, 43: 1-14.
15. Isitua, C. C. and Ibeh, I. N 2010. Novel method of wine production from banana (*Musa acuminata*) and pineapple (*Ananascomosus*) wastes. *African Journal of Biotechnology*, 9(44): 7521-7524.
16. Onuki S 2015. Bioethanol: Industrial production process and recent studies.
17. Pradeep P., O. Reddy, P. Mohan and Sanghoon K 2012. Process optimization for ethanol production from very high gravity (VHG) finger millet medium using response surface methodology. *Iranian Journal of Biotechnology*, 10.
18. Valdes A. and Planes L.R. 1999. Study of the hydrolysis of rice straw with sulfuric acid under moderate conditions. *Revista de Ciencias Quimicas*, 14: 11-19.

19. Wyman, C. E 1996. Handbook on bioethanol: Production and utilization. Taylor and Francis, Washington DC, USA. opportunies. *Bioresource Technology*,Taylor and Francis.

20. Zheng, Y., Zhongli, P. and Zhang, R. (2009). Overview of biomass pre-treatment of cellulosic ethanol production, *Bioresource Technology*, 2: 51-68.

# Chapter 20

# Synthesis of Hydraulic Brake Fluid from Jatropha Oil

*Damascus Masawi, Soloman Manyere and Shelton Magaiza*

*Department of Bachelor of Technology in Chemical Technology,*
*Harare Polytechnic, Box CY 407, Harare, ZIMBABWE*
*E-mail: damascusmasawi@gmail.com*

## ABSTRACT

This work involved synthesis of hydraulic brake fluid from Jatropha (*Jatrophacurcas*) seed oil obtained from Mtoko, Zimbabwe. The Jatropha oil was transformed into ethyl esters by reacting jatropha oil and ethanol using sulphuric acid as a catalyst at 120°C for 2hs in a stirred reactor. The reaction mixture was cooled down to ambient temperature and the resulting two layers were separated. The upper layer contained a solution of ethyl esters and was characterised for chemical composition by FTIR and GC-MS and for physiochemical properties:boiling point,viscosity, pour point and flash point. GC-MS results gave a conversion of 96-100 per cent of triglyceride into ethyl esters and a yield of 52.36 per cent of ethyl esters. The GC-MS results indicated presence of hexadecanoic acid, octadecanoic acid and 9-12 octadecanoic acid ethyl esters derived from jatropha oil which are biodegradable. Viscosity of 30cSt, at 40°C, 9cSt at 100°C, pour point <-3°C and flash point of 204°C were obtained. FTIR results indicated presence of C-O, C=O and C-H and the combination of these functional groups yielded an ester. The GC-MS results indicated ethyl esters derived from jatropha oil which include hexadecanoic acid, octadecanoic acid and 9-12 octadecanoic acid all of which are biodegradable. The viscocity and flash point test results conform to Dot 3 and Dot 4 hydraulic oil specification requirements. The pour point <-3°C is slightly low, but depressants can be used for modifications. Hence Jatropha oil can be used as an alternative base stock source of hydraulic brake fluid for light motor vehicles.

***Keywords:*** *Jatropha oil, Hydraulic brake fluid, Ethyl esters.*

# INTRODUCTION

Lubricant oils decrease the friction coefficient between two contacting surfaces. Mineral oil and lubricants have saved us over the past decade; they are efficient and cost effective but environmentally unacceptable due to their low biodegradability and toxicity (Krzanet al., 2004). These oils contaminate the air, soil, drinking water and affect human and plant life to a great extent (Lemke *et al.,* 2005). Thus, the demand for environmentally acceptable lubricants is increasing along with the public concerns for a pollution free environment.

Increasing attention has been given to innovative bio-based alternatives for fuel and lubricants mineral products.Vegetable oils have become the subject of interest. Vegetable oils have the attractions of being natural, renewable non- toxic, non- polluting, biodegradable, and cheaper than synthetic. Most vegetable oils are triglycerides which are glycerol molecules with three long chain fatty acids and fatty alcohols of different chemistry. Most vegetable oils have polar and non- polar groups in the same molecule. The presence of polar groups in vegetable oils makes it amphiphilic, thus allowing it to be used as both boundary and hydrodynamic lubricant. In addition vegetable oil have low volatility due to high molecular weight triacylglycerol molecule, good boundary lubrication characteristic due to the polar ester group, high solubilising power from polar contaminants and additive molecules, and lower cost than synthetic oils (Krzan *et al.,* 2004).

The triglyceride structure is also responsible for the inherent disabilities of vegetable oils as lubricant. For many reactions, unsaturated double bonds in the fatty acids act as active sites. There are two major problems associated with vegetable oils as functional lubricants in that they offer low resistance to thermal oxidative stability and poor low temperature properties. Several methods are available to solve the issues regarding the application of plants in lubricants, which include genetic modification, additive treatment and chemical modification (Kucera *et al.,* 2013). Transesterification/esterification of the triglyceride or the esterification of the free fatty acids (FAA) is the most prevalent method for the modification of the carboxyl group of the fatty acid chain.

$$\begin{array}{l} CH_2-O-\overset{O}{\overset{\|}{C}}-R_1 \\ CH-O-\overset{O}{\overset{\|}{C}}-R_2 \\ CH_2-O-\overset{O}{\overset{\|}{C}}-R_3 \end{array} + 3\,R'OH \xrightleftharpoons{\text{Catalyst}} \begin{array}{l} R_1-\overset{O}{\overset{\|}{C}}-OR' \\ R_2-\overset{O}{\overset{\|}{C}}-OR' \\ R_3-\overset{O}{\overset{\|}{C}}-OR' \end{array} + \begin{array}{l} CH_2-OH \\ CH-OH \\ CH_2-OH \end{array}$$

Triglycerides　　Alcohol　　Esters　　Glycerol

*Eqn 1*

**Transesterification of Triglycerides by Alcohol in the Presence of a Catalyst http://www.chemguide.co.uk/physical/catalysis/esterify.html (accessed 8 July, 2016).**

Transesterification leads to the cleavage of esters and the reaction is generally catalysed with acidic or basic catalysts. The features of the substrates directly influence the properties of the ester. The lubricant properties can be changed by the choice of various alcohols and acids. Examples of esterification and transesterification products are; trimethylolpropane (TMP) esters derivatives of TMP, rapeseed oil methyl ester or jatropha methyl ester (JME). They posses cold stability, friction and wear characteristics, and resistivity against oxidation at elevated temperatures. The objective of this research was to synthesise hydraulic brake fluid from Jatropha oil (JO) obtained from jatropha seed oil (JSO) which is abundantly available in Mtoko Zimbabwe, by use of ethanol and sulphuric acid as catalysts.

## Materials and Methods

### Materials

Jatropha seeds were obtained from Mutoko, Zimbabwe and the Jatropha seed oil was mechanically extracted at Harare Polytechnic jatropha biodiesel plant. Ethanol (99.5) per cent and sulphuric acid were purchased from Skylabs, South Africa.

#### JEE Synthesis

The FFA content of the oil was reduced by esterification/transesterification of the JO with ethanol using sulphuric acid as a catalyst. 2000mls of jatropha oil, 200ml ethanol (99.5 per cent) and 0.5mls of sulphuric acid were transferred into a round bottom flask with a reflux condenser on a heating mantle with a magnetic stirrer and temperature controller. The mixture was heated and the temperature was maintained at 120°C for 2hrs. After the reaction was complete, the reaction mixture was cooled for 12hrs to room temperature and transferred into a separation funnel for separation. Two layers were obtained, synthetic hydraulic fluid at the top and glycerol at the bottom.The glycerol was decanted and the synthesised JEE was characterised for its suitability as hydraulic brake fluid

#### GC-MS Qualitative Analysis of JEE

GC-MS Agilant 7890 was used for the determination of conversion, yield and chemical composition of JEE. The following parameters were used, mobile phase pressure25.513KPa (Helium gas), oven temperature 350 °C, and retention time of 24 minutes. 1 ml of hydraulic fluid was pipetted into 100ml volumetric flask and added up to mark using hexane. 1ml of thoroughly mixed solution was pipetted into GC-MS vials. The GC-MS was set on automatic sample injection mode.

#### FT-IR Analysis of JEE

The Fourier transform infrared spectrophotometer (FTIR) was used in order to confirm that the JEE contains esters. FTIR spectra of JEE were collected by taking 32 scan at 2 $cm^{-1}$ resolution. The spectra were scanned from 4000 to 400 $cm^{-1}$ and all samples were taken in potassium bromide (KBr).

#### Physio-chemical Properties Determination of JEE

The following physical properties of the prepared JEE were determined: boiling point, kinematic viscosity, flash point and pour point.

Boiling point was determined by heating the synthetic hydraulic fluid using a burner with a thermometer immersed into the JEE until the solvent reaches a temperature where its vapour pressure equal to that of the atmosphere which is noted by means of a closed capillary

Kinematic viscosities at 40°C and 100°C were measured according to D445 test method. The viscometers were calibrated for 10-50 viscosity range using calibration fluids.

The flash point tester was used to determine the flash point. Sample was placed in a chamber. Temperature was initially set at 150°C and a flame was introduced on thechamber containing the sample. The temperature rose until the chamber flashes indicating the flash point of the sample.

Pour point is defined as temperature where sample still pours. The pour point tells the lowest temperature at which the oil losses its flow characteristic. Pour point determination was carried according to ASTM D97 test method. Sample temperature was measured at 3°C increments until it stopped pouring.

## Results and Discussion

### GC-MS Results of JEE

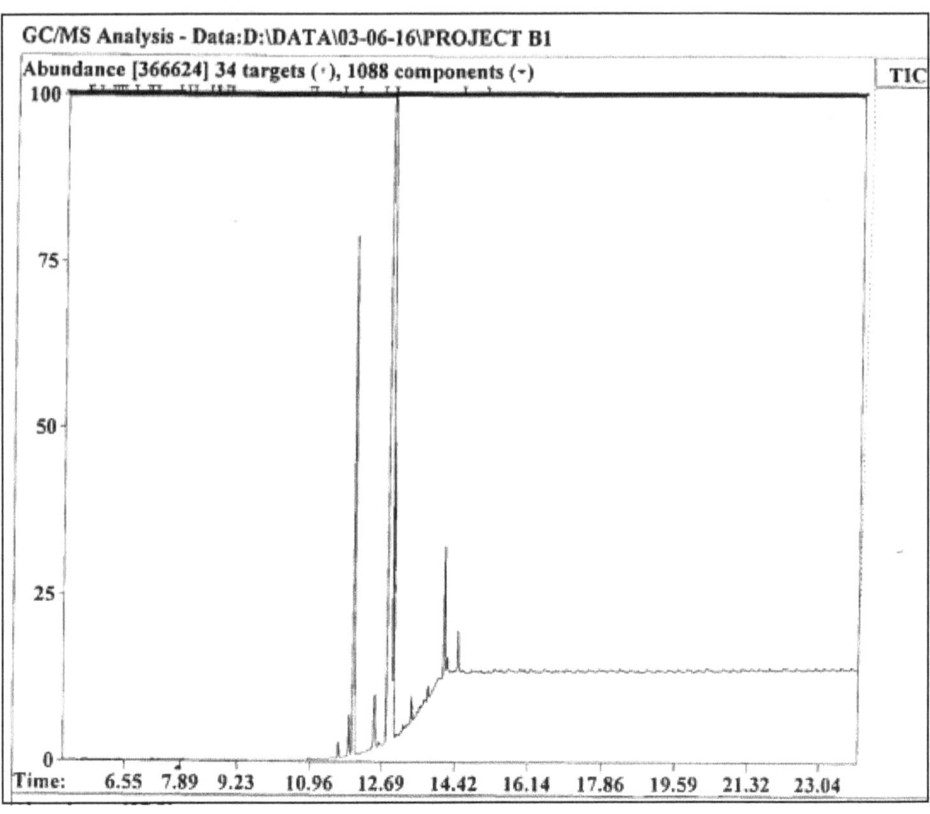


**Figure 20.1: GC-MS of JEE.**

The GC-MS results show that JEE is mainly composed of hexadecanoic acid, octadecanoicacid and 9-12 octadecanoic acid ethyl esters derived from the FFA in jatropha oil.

## Conversion and Yield

Conversion of triglyceride and ethanol reaction into ethyl ester is almost 96- 100 per cent, the reaction almost went to completion because no carboxylic acid was detected by GC-MS.Yield of ethyl ester obtained was 52.36 per cent.

## FTIR Spectra of JEE

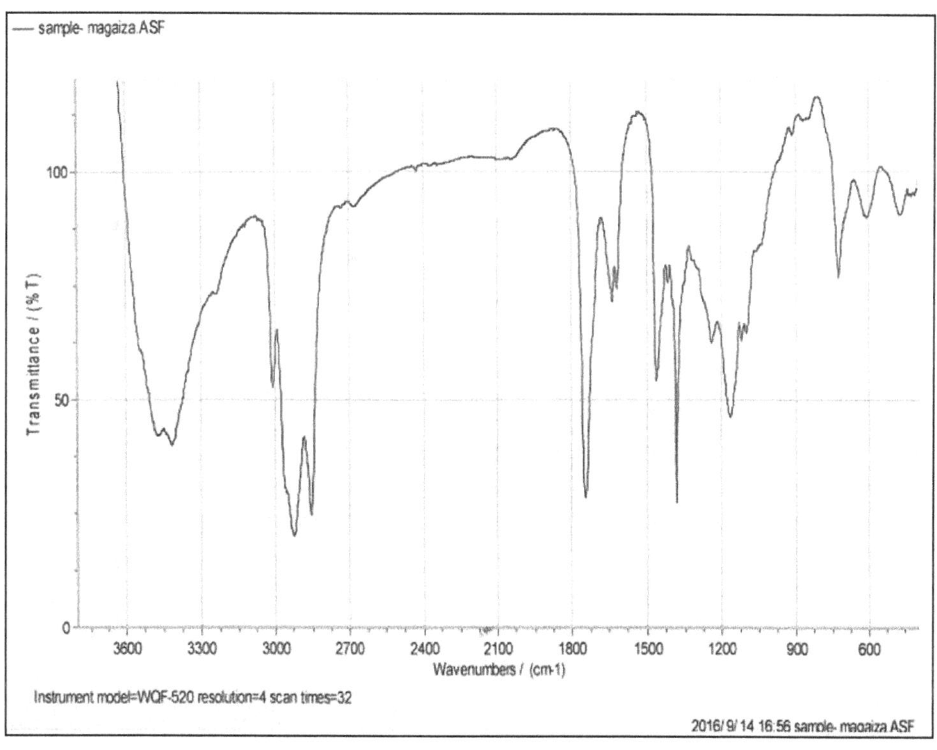


**Figure 20.2: FTIR Spectra of Synthesised JEE.**

The peaks at 1250-1050, 1780-1650, 3300-2700cm$^{-1}$indicate presence of C-O, C=O and C-H bonds. The combination of C-O, C=O and C-H bonds gives an ester.

## Physical Properties of Synthesised JEE

The boiling point of the synthesised JEE was 280°C. The synthesised JEE had a high boiling point indicating that ethyl esters which are the main constituent of the JEE are bonded with intermolecular dipole-udipole bonds which is moderately strong and have morethan 15 carbon atoms as witnessed by the high boiling point. Boiling points of organic solvents increase as the number of carbons is increased.

**Table 20.1: Physical Properties of Synthesised JEE**

| *Physical Characterisation* | *Results* | *Specification DOT 3 and DOT 4 Requirements* |
|---|---|---|
| Boiling point | 280°C | Min155°C |
| Kinematic viscosity@ 40°C | 30 cSt | Max 1500cSt |
| Kinematic viscosity@100°C | 9 cSt | Min 1.5cSt |
| Flash point | 204°C | Min 121°C |
| Pour point | <-3°C | <-2°C |

The kinematic viscosity of the JEE has a kinematic viscosity of 30 cSt and 9cSt at 40°C and 100°C respectively. It implies that kinematic viscosity is inversely proportional to temperature. The viscosity of a liquid decreases as the temperature is raised, while the viscosity of a gas increases as the temperature raised. In a liquid, the increased temperature causes the molecules to move faster, which means that they spend less time pressing against each other and holding each other down. The same heat slows the motion of gas molecules by making them bump into each other more, which makes them move more slow, increasing the viscosity. This is the reason why viscosity of hydraulic fluid at 100°C is much lower than the viscosity at 40°C.

Flash point of JEE was 204°C. Flash point of 204°C is good taking into consideration the fact that hydraulic fluid should have high flash point (>100°C) and those with flush point above 100°C are considered non-flammable liquids. The synthesised JEE has high flash point therefore it can perform better as hydraulic fluid because in hydraulic system heat is released and the presence of volatile substance reduce the efficiency of hydraulic system. If flash point is low the fluid can easily ignite. Flash point of hydraulic fluid should be high.

Pour point was slightly low <-3°C, however depressants can be used to modify it, in order to comply with the specification requirements

## Conclusion

The results obtained from the synthesised JEE complywith DOT 3 and DOT 4 specification requirements of hydraulic brake fluids for light motor vehicles. The synthesised JEE from the JO can be used as an alternative to mineral oil hydraulic brake fluid for light motor vehicles

## REFERENCES

1. Krzan, B. and Vizintin, J. (2004). Ester Based Lubricants Derived from Renewable Resources. *Tribology in Industry,* 26: 1-2.
2. Kucera, M., Ales, Z. Ales, Z., Ivandic Z and Hujo L (2015). Possibility of hydraulic fluids with low environmental impact application in agriculture and transport machinery (http: //www.chemguide.co.uk/organicprops/alcohols/esterification.html) [Accessed on 15 January 2016].

3. Lemke, M., Fernández-Trujillo, R., Löhmannsröbenc, H.-G. (2005). *In situ* LIF analysis of biological and petroleum-based hydraulic oils on soil. *Sensors*, 5: 61-69.

4. United States Department of Transport DOT 3 brake fluid specifications.

6. http: //www.chemguide.co.uk/physical/catalysis/esterify.html (accessed 8 July2016)

# Specific Biotechnology Efforts — *Environment*

*Chapter 21*

# A Comparative Investigation of the Reduction of Coliform Bacteria in Wastewater by *Agaricus bisporus*, *Plerotus sajor-caju* and *Plerotus ostreatus*

*Eunita Chidziya, Marvelous Chikerema and Shumbeyi Muzondo*

*School of Industrial Science and Technology,*
*Biotechnology Department, Harare Institute of Technology,*
*P.O Box BE277 Belvedere, Harare, ZIMBABWE*
*E-mail: eunitachidziya@gmail.com; chikeremamarvelous@gmail.com; shumbeyi@gmail.com*

## ABSTRACT

The ability of *Agaricus bisporus, Pleurotus sajor-caju* and *Pleurotus ostreatus* to reduce the coliform load in partially treated wastewater from a reservoir dam at Firle Sewage Treatment Works in Harare was investigated in this study. Scientists believe that fungi can inhibit and kill bacteria on water agar using the mechanism of competition for nutrients, producing antibiosis, chemo taxis of bacteria to fungi and mycoparasitism. *A. bisporus, P. sajor-caju* and *P.ostreatus* were grown in wastewater using nutrient diffusion method for 20 days at 25°C. The number of coliform bacteria in wastewater was measured using Most Probable Number (MPN) and Standard Plate Count (SPC) tests while the Chemical Oxygen Demand (COD) and pH of the water was also measured at a 5 day interval during the growth period. A decrease in the coliform bacteria of 95 per cent and 90.4 per cent for *P.ostreatus* and *P. sajor-caju* respectively was recorded. COD of the wastewater treated using fungi also decreased. The pH of treated water increased slightly from the initial pH of 8.2 to 8.7 for *P. ostreatus*. *P. sajor-caju* and *P.ostreatus* can reduce the number of coliform bacteria in it wastewater, and lower its COD. *A. bisporus* did not grow well in liquid medium at 25°C. It was concluded that all three fungi can be used for mycoremediation of coliforms in wastewater. *P. ostreatus* was the most effective fungus for mycoremediation of wastewater. An investigation on the ideal growth conditions for *A. bisporus* is recommended.

***Keywords:*** *Mycoremediation, Coliform bacteria, Agaricus bisporus, Pleurotus sajor-caju, Pleurotus ostreatus.*

## INTRODUCTION

Water is the most important inorganic chemical in the world, as well as the most abundant as it forms a quarter of the world. All life forms on earth depend on water in one way or the other. The importance of water to human beings can never be overestimated, as it is used for various purposes like irrigation, fisheries, industrial processes, transport and waste disposal. Water makes up to sixty to seventy percent of the body weight of an adult human and there is need that it is replenished as it is constantly lost.

Zimbabwe's growing population has been faced with lack of clean water. Harare is currently facing acute water shortages as its clean water capacity is able to satisfactorily reach only 40 per cent of the city's population. The demand for clean water has outstripped its supply, as the city uses 450 Million litres (M1) of water per day instead of the 1200 Ml that they require. The major reason for lack of clean water is the inability to effectively treat sewer, so that it can be recycled (ZSA. 2012).

The amount of wastewater that is produced by cities has increased due to the increase in the population; Zimbabwe has a rate of urbanisation that is estimated to be at 3.4 per cent per year. The wastewater infrastructure in most cities of developing countries has deteriorated due to poor maintenance as well as inability to use expensive treatment technologies. This has led to continuously bursting sewer pipes as well as partially treated wastewater being deposited into water bodies. This problem has been faced by many African nations as the 21st century has brought about mass migration from the rural areas to the cities to find better working and living conditions.

The entrance of coliform bacteria into rivers and other static water sources, like lakes and dams, is a major source of concern to the health of human beings and the safety of the environment. There are various diseases that are caused by the presence of microorganisms in water like typhoid fever, cholera, diarrhoea and dysentery.

Crude and inefficient treatment processes result in microorganisms and nutrients being released with treated effluents in the aquatic environment. Bacterial pathogens present in the sewage effluents can result in diseases such as dysentery, typhoid fever, and gastroenteritis upon exposure to the contaminated water. The effluents that enter aquatic ecosystems become a major source nutrient, and this leads to problems of eutrophication and siltation of rivers, lakes and dams.

The major disadvantage of urbanisation is that the cities cannot provide clean water and efficient wastewater treatment methods for the population that already exists (Ekma, 1984). Harare's daily water requirement is estimated at 1200 million litres but the city has capacity to supply an average of 620 million litres daily, a scenario that has left the residents with no option but to find alternative sources. The alternate water sources include urban rivers like Mukuvisi in Harare, shallow wells and boreholes which have since been condemned due to effluent contamination from burst sewer pipes (Muserere *et al.*, 2014).

Mycoremediation is an innovative biotechnology that uses living fungus for in situ and *ex situ* clean up and management of contaminated sites and is therefore a form of bioremediation. The fungal antagonists restrict the growth of bacterial pathogens by the three suggested mechanisms: antibiosis, competition and parasitism (Adebayo *et al.*, 2012).Various species of fungi, particularly the wood-degrading basidiomycetes, are predators of bacteria and nematodes, whereas other species use spores as their specialized food source. For example, *Pleurotus ostreatus*, the oyster mushroom and *Pleurotus sajor-caju* typically preys on fecal coliform bacteria (*e.g.*, *Escherichia coli*) as a source of nitrogen (Srinivas, 2008).In a field demonstration that was done by Thomas *et al.* in 2009 mycoremediation was used in combination with a bioretention cell (*e.g.*, rain garden), incorporating native vegetation, a soil media mix, and natural microbial assemblages to remove and degrade faecal coliforms and nutrients.

Fungi can be used to remediate effluent wastewater by ensuring the removal of pathogenic bacteria from the wastewater before it is deposited into aquatic water bodies. The fungi will also decrease the amount of nutrients that are in the water and this will reduce eutrophication of the rivers and lakes that surrounds the cities. Mycoremediation will provide a cheaper alternative to wastewater treatment and a better more efficient clean up strategy for sewage pipe bursts and increase the quality of effluent before it is disposed (Srinivas, 2008).

The aim of the project was to assess the efficiency of *A. bisporus*, *P. sajor-caju* and *P.ostreatus* in the mycoremediation of coliforms from wastewater effluent.

## Objectives

- ☆ To develop a technique for culturing *A. bisporus*, *P. sajor-caju* and *P. ostreatus* in wastewater.
- ☆ To investigate the ability *of A. bisporus*, *P. sajor-caju* and *P. ostreatus* to reduce the coliform load in wastewater.
- ☆ To compare the coliform reducing capacity of the three fungi.

# Materials and Methods

## Materials

### Wastewater Sample Collection

The sample was collected at a reservoir dam that is downstream of Firle Waterworks in Glenview 1, Harare. The dam is located less than 2 kilometres from residential houses of Glenview 1. The sample was collected in 2 litre capped bottles and refrigerated at 5° C. The collected sample had a greenish colour and a very pungent sewer smell, as well as greenish solid deposits that settled at the bottom of the collection samples.

### Procurement of Spawn

Spawn for *A.bisporus* was bought from Try Mycel located in Ruwa.The spawn was inoculated on wheat grains and weighed 1kg, while the spawn for *P. ostreatus and P. sajor-caju* was bought from the department of Biological Sciences, University of Zimbabwe and it was inoculated on wheat grains and each had a weight of 1kg. All the spawn were kept refrigerated when they were not in use. Before being cultivated, all the spawn were weighed in sterilized glass beakers and then left for 2hrs at room temperature to acclimatize.

The experiments were divided into four sections:

1. Characterisation of wastewater using the MPN, standard plate count, pH and COD tests.
2. Culturing fungi in wastewater.
3. Re-characterization of treated water.
4. Comparison of results.

### Characterization of Wastewater

Four tests were run in order to determine the properties of wastewater before it was treated, and these were the MPN, standard plate count, pH and COD tests.

#### *Standard Plate Count*

The SPC test was done according to the specification in Microbiology: Principles and Applications by Black in 2006. The media used was McConkey agar and the incubation was at 37°C for 24 hrs.

#### *Most Probable Number*

The MPN test was done using the protocol that was proposed by EPA Annex 5 of 2002. The media used was McConkey broth with bile salts that is purple in colour. The test tubes turned yellow in the presence of coliforms and produced visible gas. The incubation was at 37°C for 24 hrs.

#### *Chemical Oxygen Demand*

Five (5) ml of potassium dichromate solution was added to each of the six conical flasks containing10ml of water sample in three 100 ml conical flask labelled as test1, test2 and test3, and also to three (3)100ml conical flasks each with 10ml distilled and labelled as Blank 1, Blank 2 and Blank 3. The flasks were incubated in water bath at 100 ° C (boiling temperature) for 1 hour. The samples were cooled for 10 minutes then 5ml of potassium iodide added into each flask. Ten (10) ml of sulphuric acid was also added in each flask followed by three (3) drops of 1 per cent starch solution.

The contents of each flash were titrated with 0.1N sodium thiosulphate until the blue colour disappeared completely.

### *pH Test*

pH was measured every time before sampling of the experiment. A pH meter was used to measure the pH and it was calibrated every time before being used.

### Culturing Fungi in Wastewater

One of the major drawbacks of mycoremediation was finding a technique of growing the fungi in wastewater. Wastewater is nutrient rich so it is a habitat for many microorganisms, and basidiomycetes will not colonize the culture as it usually rots. Three different techniques for culturing mushrooms in wastewater which are submerged culture, and spawn floatation were improvised in this study as given below:

#### *Submerged Culture*

Trials for submerged culture in fungi was done based on the study of Growth of *Pleurotus ostreatus* on the Wastewater of a Mushroom Farm by Rodriguez *et al.* in 2002. Changes made were that their wastewater was not sterilized before inoculation and there were no nutrient additions to the wastewater to encourage fungi growth.

#### *Spawn Floatation*

This technique is a method that reduces the contact of spawn with the wastewater to avoid rot. This method was simply made up of a filter paper that was placed on top of the wastewater and since filter papers are light the spawn and filter paper float on top of the wastewater.

#### *Nutrient Diffusion*

This method was designed after carrying out submerged culture and spawn floatation which proved to be unsuitable for this project since the mycelia failed to grow in wastewater. The method was more fit for the purpose of this project and it was named nutrient diffusion and it comprised of spawn floatation and submerged culture entities.

#### *Culturing of Mycelia by Nutrient Diffusion*

Fifteen (15) grams of spawn were grown on a filter paper placed on a sterile plastic paper with small holes punched into it (approximate diameter of 4mm) starting from the centre going outwards. The plastic/paper was place on top of the wastewater sample and held in place with a rubber band on the outside of the glass beaker. This design reduced absorption of moisture to the growing mycelia. It was incubated at 25°C for the 20 day period of mycoremediation.

### Re-characterization of Treated Water

This was done by repeating characterisation tests on treated wastewater.

## Analysis of Results

Results were compared by using statistical tools like t-test, standard deviation and also by noting differences in physical characteristics of water

## Results and Discussion

### Developing a Technique for Culturing Fungi in Wastewater

Three methods were assessed for their ability to sustain the growth of fungi in wastewater. These were submerged culturing, spawn floatation and nutrient diffusion. Out of the three (3) methods of Submerged culture Spawn floatation and Nutrient diffusion assessed for their ability to sustain the growth of the fungi, the first two were unsuccessful for all three fungi as the fungal mycelia rotted. The nutrient diffusion method showed vigorous growth with the mycelia reaching confluence within two days. The mycelial growth confluence and into the wastewater through the punched holes is shown in Figure 21.1. These results showed that the fungi can be grown in wastewater using the nutrient diffusion method. The success of this method over submerged culture which equally serves as a habitat for other microbes enables overwhelming of the fungal mycelia before it acclimatised to the that microenvironment thereby resulting into spawn rot.

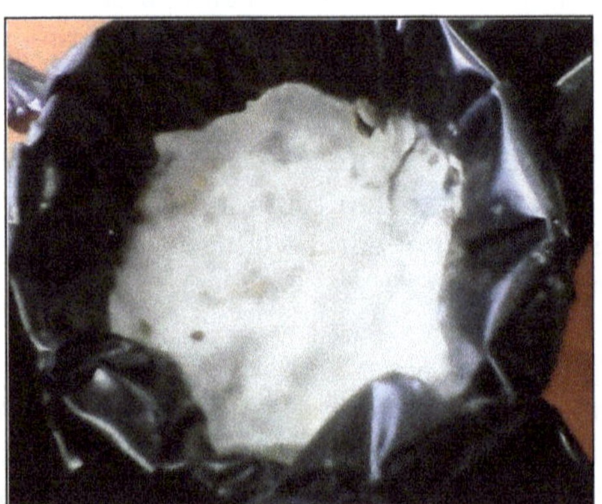

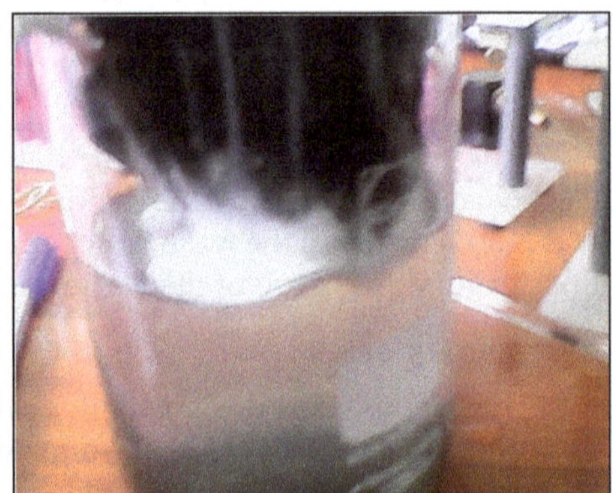

**Figure 21.1: Nutrient Diffusion Set Upshowing 1. Arial view of fungi mycelia growing on top of perforated plastic in contact with wastewater (Left Plate), 2. Side view mycelia of fungi growing on top of wastewater (Right plate).**

### Performance of *A. bisporus*, *P. sajor-caju*, and *P. ostreatus* in Reducing the Coliform Load in Wastewater

*Pleurotus sajor-caju* and *P. ostreatus* managed to grow in the wastewater for the full duration of the mycoremediation period of (20 days) at 25°C. During this period there was a notable significant continual decrease in the number of coliform bacteria as shown by the results (Figures 21.2–21.4)which was confirmed by the t-test in Appendix C, D and E. According to Gregory *et al.*in 2007, the genus *Pleurotus* (oyster fungi) comprises some of the most popular and most cultivated fungi due to their valued organoleptic properties, vigorous growth and undemanding cultivation conditions. Gregory *et al.*(2007) states that *Pleorotus* species grow very well at slightly warm temperatures of 23°C to 33°C. This is very high compared to other edible fungi like *A. bisporus*. *P. ostreatus* grows at an optimum temperature of 23°C to 25°C and *Pleurotus sajor-caju* thrives at marginally higher temperatures than this, usually between 28°C to 30°C (Rodriguez *et al.*, 2002). Consequently the two fungi likely grew and were able to completely colonize both the substrate and wastewater because they were growing at close to their optimum temperatures.

The results that were obtained for most probable number of coliforms and standard plate count of bacteria showed that all the three fungi are capable of mycoremediation of sewer water. According to the results of MPN (not included but with same trend as colony forming units results, Figure 21.2), there was a reduction of the number of bacteria in the sample and the coliform bacteria continued to decrease during the progress of the experiment. At day five coliforms had fallen from 303 to 247, 210 and 157 for *A. bisporus, P. sajor-caju* and *P. Ostreatus* respectively. Figure 21.2 illustrates that there was a decrease in the colony forming units of the wastewater from the first day of treatment using growing fungal mycelia of *A. bisporus, P. ostreatus and P. sajor-caju.* This further proves that all the three species are capable of inhibiting growth and lowering the amount of coliform bacteria thus can be used for mycoremediation of Feacal Coliform Bacteria (FCB)-polluted wastewater. The viable colony forming units of coliform bacteria decreased as the experiment progressed from day 1 to day 20. The growth of mycelia was inversely proportional to the decrease in coliform bacteria, for the three species.

The decrease in coliforms was most probably due to the growth of fungal mycelia since the control (without fungal growth) did not show the same marked reduction. As fungi grow, they secrete extracellular enzymes (ECE) and acids into the environment, in this case wastewater. The ECE like amylases and proteases breakdown polysaccharides and oligosaccharide and polypeptides in the wastewater into simple disaccharides and amino acids that can be absorbed by the growing hyphae (George *et al.*, 2002). Due to the fact that wastewater is a rich carbon source and there is relatively low nitrogen, the mycelia of the fungi can produce toxic metabolites that can kill the coliform bacteria. The coliform bacteria would likely

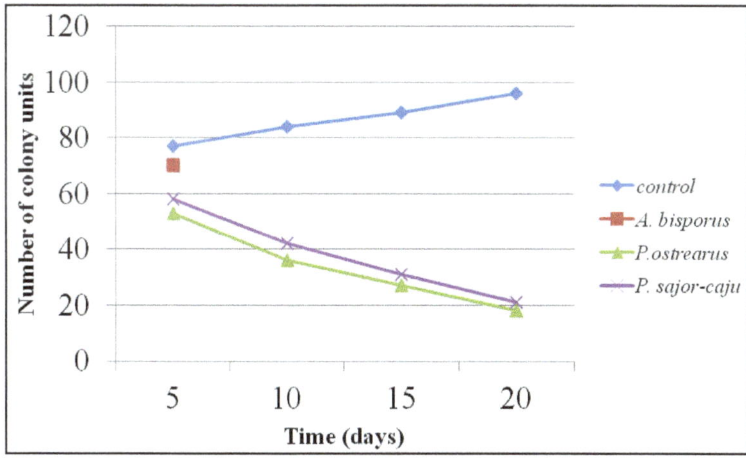


**Figure 21.2: Feacal Coliform Colony Forming Units on McConkey Agar at $10^{-9}$ Dilution Rate for the Control and Wastewater Inoculated with the Test Fungi.**

undergo lysis due to osteolysin produced by the fungi (Rogers, 2012). This causes nutrients to leak from the bacterial cells and fungi can absorb them. During the period of culturing fungi in wastewater there were some mycelial hyphae that were observed inside the wastewater. These were probably directional hyphae which according to Adebayo *et al.*(2002) are used by *P. ostreatus* fungi to attract bacteria in agar as well as excrete toxins that kill them.

*Agaricus bisporus* remediated the wastewater because it reduced the number of coliforms from 77 CFU in the original sample to 70 CFU at $10^{-9}$ dilution rate by the $5^{th}$ day according to Figure 21.2 which shows the number of CFU at different intervals of the experiment. This was also confirmed by the results of MPN, they reveal that upon culturing *A.bisporus* in wastewater, the number of bacteria in it dropped to 247 from 303. *A. bisporus'* spawn grew faster than the others at first, its mycelia had reached confluence and penetrated the wastewater (directional growth) at about 56 hrs. However, the mycoremediation with *A. bisporus* did not continue for the duration of the project because the mycelia stopped growing in some trails while in others it developed yellow and greenish moulds. *A. bisporus* grows at low temperatures (Fermor *et al.*, 1981) and naturally grows at 10-15°C. The incubation temperature for the current study was 25°C which caused it to grow very fast, but made it prone to contaminants as it was not at an optimum temperature.

## Chemical Oxygen Demand

Treating wastewater with *A. bisporus, P. sajor-caju* and *P. ostreatus* also reduced its chemical oxygen demand from an initial 358 mg/L to 322, 304 and 283mg/L respectively at day 5 while at day 20 the COD for water treated with *P. sajor-caju* was 256mg/Land that treated with *P. ostreatus* was 224mg/L as seen in Figure 21.3. The decrease in COD was likely proof that the fungi were utilising the oxidative organic compounds as nutrients through absorption. This is very important because if mycoremediated wastewater is disposed by dilution into aquatic water bodies it will not cause eutrophication and hypoxia (Arceivala, 1998), since there will be

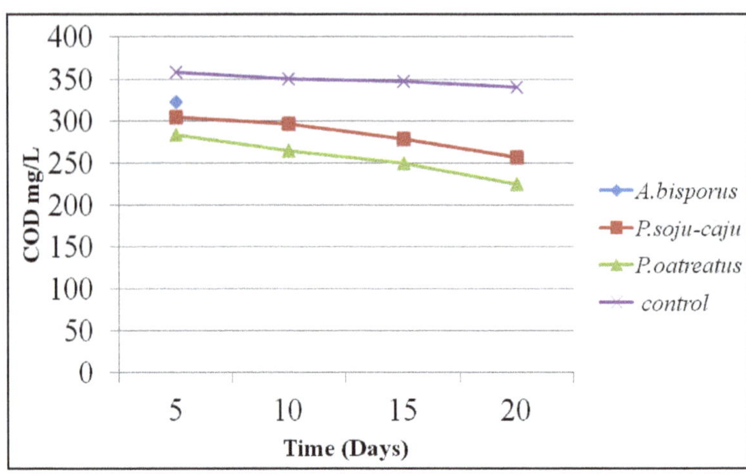


**Figure 21.3: COD for the Wastewater Inoculated with the Test Fungi and Control.**

lower levels of organic compounds than what was initially found in the water. The reduction in COD was significantly greater in *P. ostreatus* than in *A. bisporus* and *P. sajor-caju*, because it grew better than the other two fungi and it is as shown in Figures 21.2 and 21.3. There was a statistically significant difference in the COD levels between the untreated and treated water samples, as shown by the t-test statistical tool and the results are shown in Appendix A.

The percentage decrease in the number of bacteria in the water that was treated with *P. ostreatus* and *P. sajor-caju* was calculated using the formula below. The values were taken from the average number of bacteria in wastewater found from the MPN test.

Per cent reduction =

$$\frac{\text{Initial FCB concentration} - \text{Final FCB concentration}}{\text{Initial FCB concentration}} \times 100 \quad [1]$$

The results were tested for significant difference using a t-test and the results are shown in Appendices A to C.

According to plate counts, COD and per cent reduction results Figures 21.2–21.4, *Plerotus ostreatus* was the best mycoremediator of all the three fungi. Figure 21.4 shows that *Plerotus ostreatus* had reduced by 95 per cent the initial coliform bacteria population that was present in wastewater, while *Plerotus sajor-caju* had reduced by 90.4 per cent after 20 days. *Agaricus bisporus* did not grow past the first five (5) days incubation period. This observation was probably due to suitability of the incubation temperature for culturing (Rodriguez *et al.*, 2002). *Plerotus* species is very tenacious and it can grow even in waste dumps, as it colonizes the substrate completely and so fast that no contaminants can grow in it. This most likely led to its ability to reduce coliforms more than the other two fungi.

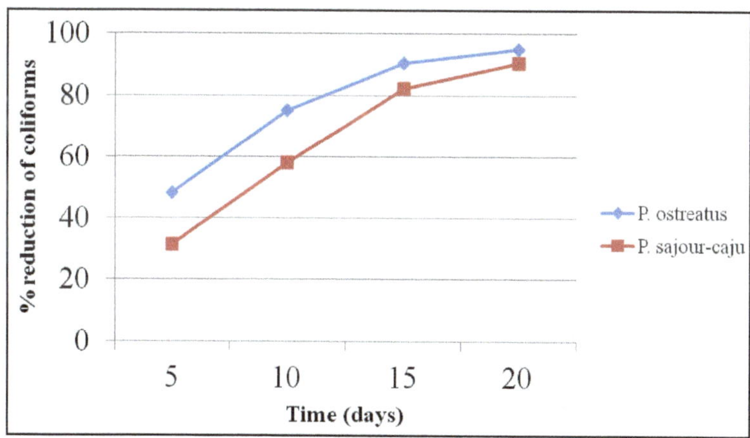


**Figure 21.4: Percentage Reduction of the Number of Bacteria in the Control and Wastewater Inoculated with Test Fungi.**

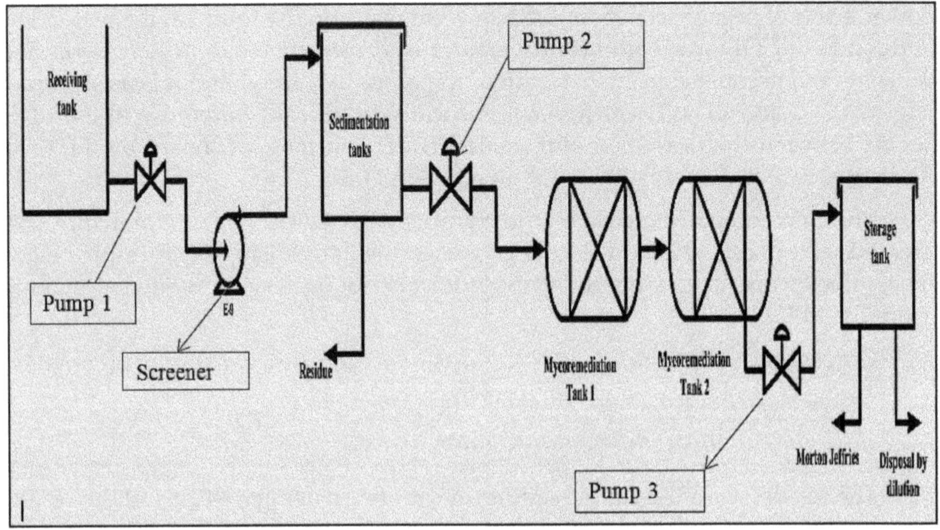


**Figure 21.5: Mycoremediation Process Model Diagram.**

Unrecorded observation on pH measurements showed that there was a slight increase in the pH of the water and it continued until day 20. This was because the coliform bacteria which ferment lactose to lactic acid reduced (Adebayo *et al.*, 2012).

The literature that was gathered during the course of this project along with the experimental data obtained was used to design a process model for mycoremediation of wastewater. This model is proposed to Harare City Council as a secondary stage sewer reticulation process for Firle Sewer works and it can be used as a field run.

This process will be relatively shorter than the sedimentation and separation technique that is currently being used and it will reduce the amounts of chemicals like Chlorine that are used to treat reclaimed water and their effects. The project showed that the fungi that would be most efficient to use in the mycoremediation tanks would be *P. ostreatus* as it was able to significantly lower the number of coliform bacteria, as was shown by t-test at alpha=0.05 shown in Appendices A, B and C.

## Conclusions

*Agaricus bisporus, P. sajor-caju* and *P. ostreatus* can reduce the coliform load of wastewater, and they can lower the amounts of organic matter in wastewater, thus they are all mycoremediators. It was also seen that fungi can be grown in wastewater using nutrient diffusion method. *Plerotus ostreatus* is the most effective fungi for mycoremediation of wastewater.

## Recommendations

- A field run of coliform mycoremediation in wastewater using *P. ostreatus* should be developed.

☆ There is need to develop a protocol and design a lab test that ensures growth of *A. bisporus* in wastewater so its mycoremediation properties can be fully analysed.

☆ Carry out experiments to extract ostelysin from *P. ostreatus* and carry out tests to see if can kill coliform bacteria.

## REFERENCES


1. Adebayo, E.A., Oloke, J. K., Ayandele, A. A., and Adegunlola, C.O., 2012. Phytochemical, antioxidant and antimicrobial assay of mushroom metabolite from *Pleurotus pulmonarius. J. Microbiol. Biotech. Res.*
2. Arceivala, S.J., 1998. Wastewater Treatment for Pollution Control, Tata McGraw-Hill, New Delhi.
3. Ashbolt, N.J. 2004. Microbial contamination of drinking water and disease outcomes in developing regions. *Toxicology* 198: 229-238.
4. Ashbolt, N.J., W.O.K. Grabow, and M. Snozzi. 2001.Water Quality: Guidelines, Standards and Health. Risk assessment and management for water-related infectious disease. L. Fewtrell and J. Bartram (eds). pp. 289-315. IWA Publishing, London.
5. Audic, J., 1990. Evolution des technologies d'élimination des microorganismes IFREMER–Actes de Colloques, 11: 133–148.
6. Berne L.S., Hanscas F.N., 2006. *Mycoremediation: Fungal Bioremediation.* John Wiley and Sons Maryland USA.
7. Black, J., 2006. Microbiology: Principles and Applications 6th edition. Wiley and Sons Maryland USA.
8. Brungs, W. 1973. Effects of Residual Chlorine on Aquatic Life. *Journal of the Water Pollution Control Federation*, 45: 2180.
9. Drechsler, C., 1937. Some Hyphomycetes that prey on freeliving terricolous nematodes. *Mycologia*, 29: 447-552.
10. Droste, R.L., 1997. Theory and Practice of Water and Wastewater Treatment, John Wiley and Sons, New York.
11. Dupray, E., Baleux, B., Bonnefont, J., Guichaoua, C., Pommepuy M., and Derrien, A. 1990. Apport en bactéries par les stations d'épuration IFREMER–Actes de Colloques, 11: 81–88.
12. Ekama, G.A., Marais, G.V.R., 1984. Nature of municipal wastewaters. Theory, design, and operation of nutrient removal activated sludge processes. Water Research Commission, Pretoria.
13. EPA: Wastewater Technology Fact Sheet Chlorine Disinfection. 1999.EPA. Environmental Protection Agency. Office of Water Washington, D.C. EPA 832-F-99-062.
14. EPA: 2002. Guidelines for Drinking Water Quality Annex 5, Environmental Protection Agency. Office of Water Washington, D.C.

15. Fermor, T., and Wood, D. 1981. Degradation of bacteria by *Agaricus bisporus* and other fungi. *Journal of General Microbiology* 126: 377-387.

16. Futscal, T., 2009. Chemical Oxygen Demand Measured, Organic, and Waters - JRank Articles http: //science.jrank.org/pages/1388/Chemical-OxygenDemand.html#ixzz3a2u2yKR

17. Gernaey, K., van Loosdrecht, M., Henze, M., Lind, M., Jorgensen, S. 2004. Activated sludge wastewater treatment plant modelling and simulation: State of the art. *Environmental Modelling and Software*, 19: 763-783.

18. George, I., Crop, P., and Servais, P. 2002. Fecal coliform removal in wastewater treatment plants studied by plate counts and enzymatic methods. *Water Research*, 36(10): 2607-2617.

19. Gregori, A., Kendrick T, Bryce C.A. 2007. Cultivation Techniques and Medicinal Properties of *Pleurotus* spp. *Food Technology and Biotechnology*, 45: 238-249.

20. Jarroll, E., Hoff, J., and Meyer, E., 1984. Resistance of cysts to disinfection agents. In: *Giardia and Giardiasis* (Edited by Erlandsen S. L. and Meyer E. A.). p. 311. Plenum Press, New York.

21. Korich, D., Mead, J., Madore, M., Sinclair, N. and Sterling, C.1990. Effects of ozone, chlorine dioxide, chlorine and monochlor amine on *Cryptosporidium parvum* oocysts viability. *Appl. Environ. Microbiol.* 56(5): 1423-1428.

22. Muserere, S.T., Hoko, Z., and Nhapi, I. 2014 characterisation of raw sewage and performance assessment of primary settling tanks of Firle sewage treatment works in Harare. *Physics and Chemistry of the Earth*, Vol. 67-69.

23. Parr, L. 1936. Sanitary Significance of the Succession of Coli-aerogenes Organisms in Fresh and Stored Feces. *American Journal of Public Health Nations Health*, 26(1): 39-45.

24. Peeters, J., Mazas, E., Masschelein, W., Martinez de Maturana, I., and Debacker, E. 1989. Effect of drinking water with ozone or chlorine dioxide on survival of *Cryptosporidium parvum* oocysts. *Appl. Environ. Microbiol.*, 55(6): 1519-1522.

25. Rodríguez, S. M., Fernández, R. C., Bermúdez, H., Morris and N. García 2002.Growth of *Pleurotus ostreatus* on the Wastewater of a Mushroom Farm. Mushroom Biology and Mushroom Products. Sánchez *et al.*, UAEM. ISBN 968-878-105-3

26. Rogers, T., 2012. Experimental evaluation of mycoremediation of *Escherichia coli* bacteria in solution using *Pleurotus ostreatus*. The Evergreen State College, USA.

27. Rose, J., Dickson, L., Farrah, S., and Carnahan, R. 1996. Removal of pathogenic and indicator microorganisms by a full scale water reclamation facility. *Wat. Res.*, 30(11): 2785-2797.

28. Snow, J., 1855. On the Mode of Communication of Cholera. London, England: J and A Churchill. John Churchill, Princes Street, Soho, London, England

29. Srinivas, T., 2008. *Environmental Biotechnology* New Age International Publishers, New Delhi.

30. Thomas, S.A, Aston L.M., Woodruff D.L, Cullinan V.I., 2009. Field Demonstrations of mycoremediation for removal of fecal coliform bacteria and nutrients in the dungeness watershed, Washington, Battelle: The Business of Innovation, PNWD-4054-1.

31. U.S. EPA, 2010. National Recommended Water Quality Criteria, http: //www.epa.gov/waterscience/criteria/wqctable/index.html#U

32. Vidali, M, 2001. Bioremediation: An overview. *Pure Applied Chemistry*, 73.

33. Water Environment Federation and the American Society of Civil Engineers. 1991. Design of Municipal Wastewater Treatment Plants. 2 vols. WEF Manual of Practice No. 8. Alexandria, VA: Water Environment Federation.

34. Wolverton, B., and McDonald, R. 1979. Upgrading facultative wastewater lagoons with vascular aquatic plants. Water Pollution Control Federation. 51(2): 305-313.

35. Zimbabwe Statistical Agency, 2012. Preliminary Report Census 2012. Harare Zimbabwe, Government of Zimbabwe.

## APPENDIX A: (t-test results for MPN)

| *Days* | *P. ostreatus vs. Control* | | *P. sajor-caju vs. Control* | | *P. ostreatus vs. P. sajor-caju* | |
|---|---|---|---|---|---|---|
| | *T Stat* | *T Crit* | *T Stat* | *T Crit* | *T Stat* | *T Crit* |
| 5 | 29.44 | 4.3 | 3.35 | 4.3 | 1.83 | 4.3 |
| 10 | 13.67 | 4.3 | 13.09 | 4.3 | 5.09 | 4.3 |
| 15 | 11.55 | 4.3 | 13.42 | 4.3 | 4.13 | 4.3 |
| 20 | 13.86 | 4.3 | 13.25 | 4.3 | 9.86 | 4.3 |

## APPENDIX B: (t test results for COD)

| *Days* | *P. ostreatus vs. Control* | | *P. sajor-caju vs. Control* | | *P. ostreatus vs. P. sajor-caju* | |
|---|---|---|---|---|---|---|
| | *T Stat* | *T Crit* | *T Stat* | *T Crit* | *T Stat* | *T Crit* |
| 5 | 28.09 | 4.3 | 18.66 | 4.3 | N/A | N/A |
| 10 | 40.85 | 4.3 | 20.9 | 4.3 | 9.02 | 4.3 |
| 15 | 40.36 | 4.3 | 23.45 | 4.3 | 11.3 | 4.3 |
| 20 | 42.56 | 4.3 | 21.83 | 4.3 | 10.32 | 4.3 |

## APPENDIX C: (t-test results for SPC)

| *Days* | *P. ostreatus vs. Control* | | *P. sajor-caju vs. Control* | | *P. ostreatus vs. P. sajor-caju* | |
|---|---|---|---|---|---|---|
| | *T Stat* | *T Crit* | *T Stat* | *T Crit* | *T Stat* | *T Crit* |
| 5 | 4.89 | N/A | 18.66 | 4.3 | 15.55 | 4.3 |
| 10 | 4.75 | 4.3 | 11.67 | 4.3 | 10.23 | 4.3 |
| 15 | 4.88 | 4.3 | 15.09 | 4.3 | 12.59 | 4.3 |
| 20 | 5.23 | 4.3 | 20.99 | 4.3 | 17.64 | 4.3 |

*Harare Resolution on*

# Industrial Biotechnology: Driving Value Addition and Beneficiation, August 2017

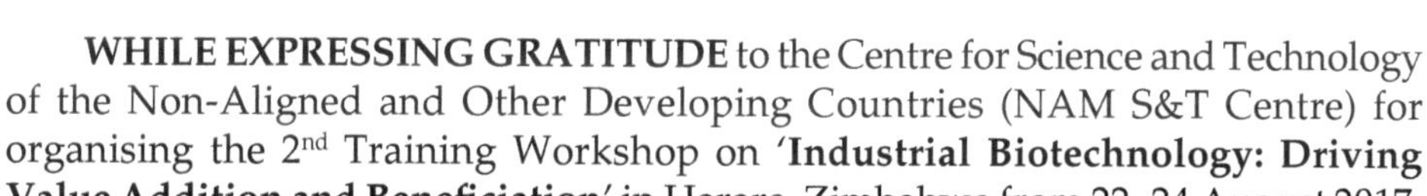

**WHILE EXPRESSING GRATITUDE** to the Centre for Science and Technology of the Non-Aligned and Other Developing Countries (NAM S&T Centre) for organising the 2nd Training Workshop on '**Industrial Biotechnology: Driving Value Addition and Beneficiation**' in Harare, Zimbabwe from 22–24 August 2017;

**EXPRESSING APPRECIATION** to the Government of the Republic of Zimbabwe, the Ministry of Higher and Tertiary Education, Science and Technology Development and the National Biotechnology Authority (NBA) for co-organising and hosting the Training Workshop;

**RECOGNIZING** that Industrial Biotechnology is an enabling tool for NAM and other developing countries to reap multiple socio-economic benefits from natural resources and ensure environmental sustenance;

**HAVING CONSIDERED** the existence of vast opportunities and benefits for value addition and beneficiation in NAM and Other Developing Countries as well as the urgent need for the development, adoption, transfer and promotion of industrial biotechnologies;

**ALSO COGNIZANT** of the major constraints such as inadequate financial resources and R&D infrastructure to promote value addition and beneficiation in NAM and Other Developing Countries;

**HAVING DELIBERATED** on the underlying issues associated with the development, adoption, transfer and promotion of industrial biotechnologies for driving value addition and beneficiation in NAM and Other Developing Countries, consequently concluding that a systematic and holistic multi-stakeholder and multi-national collaborative approach be pursued in driving the value addition and beneficiation agenda in a sustainable manner;

**WHEREAS IT IS RECOGNISED** that environmental issues including, but not limited to climate change and greenhouse gas emissions, need to be taken into account when developing and implementing value addition strategies;

**WE, THE PARTICIPANTS OF THE TRAINING WORKSHOP**, representing the governments, institutions and agencies from Cuba, Egypt, The Gambia, India, Indonesia, Kenya, Malaysia, Mauritius, Myanmar, Nepal, Nigeria, South Africa, Sri Lanka, Sudan, Tanzania, Togo, Zambia and Zimbabwe;

**UNANIMOUSLY RESOLVE AND RECOMMEND THE FOLLOWING:**

1. Research activities should be intensified in the applications of industrial biotechnology in a safe, sustainable and responsible manner, consistent with the provisions of legal frameworks within member states;
2. The governments and concerned agencies of the NAM countries should take appropriate measures to establish research development and innovation funds to support industrial biotechnology within NAM member states;
3. Value addition and beneficiation; intellectual property rights; and biosafety awareness should form an important component of the curriculum in the education system at all levels;
4. Beneficial collaborations and partnerships for generation and exchange of knowledge in the fields of industrial biotechnology among scientists and scientific organizations from NAM member countries should be promoted;
5. Identify industrial biotechnology applications for value addition and beneficiation based on socio-economic potential in NAM member states;
6. Encourage the participation of all stakeholders (government, research institutions, private sector and civil society) in the development, utilization and commercialisation of biotechnologies in industries for sustained development;
7. Efforts should be made to establish a centre each for a short term (4–6 weeks) training course on Industrial Biotechnology in each of the NAM regions (Africa (Zimbabwe, Nigeria, Kenya and Tanzania), Asia (Malaysia, Nepal and Sri Lanka) and Latin America (Cuba)). In this regard, the NAM S&T Centre is requested to facilitate the international travel of the participants from its member countries.
8. Biennial Industrial Biotechnology Conferences under the aegis of the NAM S&T Centre are highly desirable. Nigeria and Kenya have offered to host such a conference subject to internal consultations.

AND FINALLY, given the importance and potential contributions of industrial biotechnology for attainment of sustainable socio-economic development in NAM S&T member states, the Workshop agreed to take urgent measures to establish a committee to work urgently with NAM S&T Centre to craft the roadmap with timelines for the implementation of the above for timely exploitation of the industrial biotechnology. In this regard, Zimbabwe offered to initiate this process, which was highly welcomed by the delegates.

THUS, RESOLVED AT HARARE, ZIMBABWE ON THIS DAY, THE 24TH OF AUGUST 2017.

# Index

## C



## D



## E



## F



## G

## N



## O



## P



## Q



## R



## S

www.ingramcontent.com/pod-product-compliance
Ingram Content Group UK Ltd.
Pitfield, Milton Keynes, MK11 3LW, UK
UKHW021010290726
14059UKWH00001BA/58

9 789389 569087